CH00642633

PRANAYAMA
The Breath of Yoga

By the same author:

Ashtanga Yoga: Practice and Philosophy
Ashtanga Yoga: The Intermediate Series

PRANAYAMA
The Breath of Yoga

Gregor Maehle

Kaivalya Publications

Published by Kaivalya Publications
PO Box 804
Innaloo City, WA 6918, Australia

© Gregor Mahle 2012

This book is copyright. Apart from any fair dealing
for the purposes of private study, research, criticism or
review, as permitted under the Copyright Act, no part
may be reproduced by any process without written
permission of the author.

First published 2012

Illustrations by Roxanne Cox
Copy editing by Allan Watson

National Library of Australia
Cataloguing-in-Publication entry

Author: Maehle, Gregor
Title: Pranayama: the breath of yoga / by Gregor
              Maehle; illustrations by Roxanne Cox
ISBN: 9780977512621 (pbk.)
Notes: Includes bibliographical references
Subjects: Prânayâma
              Hatha yoga
              Breathing exercises
Other authors/contributors: Cox, Roxanne
Dewey no.: 613.192

Every effort was made to contact the holders of
copyright of quoted material, but this did not prove
to be possible in every case.

To the origin and source of this most sacred and ancient teaching, to the Supreme Teacher. To You who projects forth this infinite multitude of universes at the beginning of each world age, sustains them during their entire existence with ease without being affected in the least by this giant effort. Who then without flinching reabsorbs them back into Yourself, annihilating them for the eternally seeming brahmic night, during which this eternal and most precious liberating teaching of yoga is suspended in Your intellect. I bow down to You who then again sends forth this multitude of universes into a new world age and glorious dawn of a new brahmic day. To You who projects forth in each world age this liberating jewel of yoga. To You who has taught our foremost teacher Patanjali and all those others who walked before me. To You who also is the guiding light in this lowliest of your students, this present author.

If there is any truth in my writings on yoga then it is due only to You, who forms the luminous light of my intellect, and to my teachers. If there is any untruth in my writing then it is entirely due to my own defects brought about in my deluded mind through faulty past actions. For there is no fault or ugliness in yoga, which is held in eternal perfection in You, oh foremost and most ancient of all teachers.

DISCLAIMER

This book does not constitute medical advice. Contact a medical practitioner to determine whether you are fit to perform these yogic exercises.

Pranayama cannot be learned from media such as this book, which is not able to give feedback, but must be learned from a qualified teacher. This book can be used only for study and as a supplement to personal instruction. It is also offered as additional education for teachers.

It is aimed at the average student, who exists only in theory. In reality the teacher has to adapt the practice to the individual.

The *pranayama* described here is for spiritual insight for people of average health who are already established in *asana* (posture) practice. Although *pranayama* has manifold therapeutic benefits, the *pranayama* described here is not specifically designed for the alleviation of diseases.

DEFINITIONS

The term Ashtanga Yoga in this text is used to refer to Patanjali's eight-limbed yoga, which includes, apart from posture, also such components as meditation and *samadhi*. The traditional sequential posture yoga of a similar name is called Ashtanga Vinyasa Yoga throughout to disambiguate it from Patanjali's yoga.

The term *yogi* is used to denote masculine and feminine practitioners, the male form of yogi being *yogin* and the female form *yogini*.

The terms God, Supreme Being and Divine are used to denote the masculine, feminine and neuter simultaneously in exactly the sense that the Sanskrit Brahman simultaneously contains all three genders.

Acknowledgements

Many thanks to my wife, Monica Gauci, and to the teachers and students at 8 Limbs in Perth, Australia, who kept sustaining me during a 3-year practice and research retreat. Although during that time they hardly ever got to see me, through their support they have probably contributed more to this book than I have.

I express my gratitude towards the late Yoga Visharada Shri K. Pattabhi Jois. I had the great fortune of receiving 14 months of his instruction and it was this time that firmly grounded me in a daily *asana* practice. Without this bedrock of *asana*, on which all other limbs of yoga rest, however lofty they may be, little can be gained and, even more importantly, little can be retained.

Gratitude also to Yoga Ratnakara Shri B.N.S. Iyengar, from whom I was fortunate enough to receive eight months of often twice-daily one-on-one instruction in *pranayama*, *kriya* and *mudra*. It was his instruction that firmly established me in these aspects of yoga.

Above all, gratitude to the master of both, the late Shri Tirumalai Krishnamacharya, who from our limited view today looks like a towering giant who had mastered all accessories of yoga.

Gratitude to the late Swami Kuvalayananda, founder of Kaivalyadhama, and its current director, O.P. Tiwari. Kaivalyadhama has since the 1920s published an enormous amount of yogic research and scripture, and continues to do so.

Gratitude to the late Dr M.L. Gharote, founder of the Lonavla Yoga Institute and its current director, Dr M.M. Gharote. The Lonavla Yoga Institute specializes in the translation of yoga *shastra*s. Without Kaivalyadhama and the Lonavla Yoga Institute, most modern yogis would have little authentic information available beyond the *Yoga Sutra*, *Hatha Yoga Pradipika*, *Shiva Samhita* and *Gheranda Samhita*.

Gratitude also to Swami Ramdev, who promotes *pranayama* as an important tool in public health, thus taking it and its benefits out of the hands of a select few.

Gratitude then to those ancient sages of India, authors of yoga *shastra*, who in an unceasing stream of teachings compiled and handed down the many ancient yoga scriptures. It was the daily study of their teaching that firmly grounded me in yogic philosophy, meditation and devotion to the Divine.

Contents

INTRODUCTION

This book is the result of almost 20 years of research on *pranayama* and its practice. I received personal instruction on *pranayama* in India from various traditions and sources, most notably 8 months of daily, mainly one-on-one, tuition from Shri B.N.S. Iyengar, student of Shri T. Krishnamacharya. This aroused in me a great interest in researching *pranayama* more deeply. I extensively studied ancient yogic treatises (*shastras*) and more and more integrated their teachings into my *pranayama* practice. Many of the intricate yogic teachings are not handed down in person any more but are concealed in the scriptures waiting to be found by those who are ready to search. With this book

I am not representing any particular lineage or teacher; rather, it contains my attempt to convert into practice the essence of the scriptures.

This book was written in the spirit of passing on what traditional Indian yoga teaches about *pranayama* rather than inventing something new. However, I had to find ways of presenting the original teachings in such a way that a modern audience could digest them without their essence being lost.

I have tried as much as possible to authentically duplicate the atmosphere in which I received *pranayama* in India without watering it down. If in doubt I chose to stick with the original form rather than falling for the temptation to make the book too modern and commercially attractive. Because of that you may find some themes in this book initially somewhat unexpected, but please persist and you will find a treasure within these pages. I am afraid that the more we modernize and commercialize yoga the more we tend to lose its essence. It is my mission to contribute to a renaissance of the original and true yoga, beyond the modern exercise fad and lean, sexy body hype.

1

WHY NEITHER POSTURES NOR MEDITATION
NOR BOTH COMBINED ARE ENOUGH

Although yoga has eight limbs[1] we can discern three main layers of practice of which the others are subdivisions or ancillary techniques. These three layers are posture (*asana*), breath work (*pranayama*) and meditation (*dhyana*). Two of them, posture and meditation, are today very widely practised, but they are usually not linked. Schools that teach yogic postures either do not teach meditation or, if they do, they often teach meditation techniques that are historically not linked to posture practice, such as Buddhist meditation and *Vipassana*. Those schools that do specialize in meditation usually forsake *asana* practice altogether or mistake it for the simplistic keeping in one line of trunk, neck and head. There are currently only a handful of teachers in the world who offer yoga in the way it was designed, which is combining a sophisticated posture practice with technically refined *pranayama* and, additionally, yoga's elaborate and powerful Kundalini-rousing meditation techniques.

Why would we bother to practise three completely independent layers of technique? Does this not place too much strain on teachers and students? Is it not expecting too much of teachers to become competent in three different sets of techniques and students to practise them?

The reason for such a rather complex approach lies in the fact that already the ancient *Upanishads* explained that the human being is made up not of a single layer but of five layers.[2] Succinctly these five layers are:

Sanskrit name	Translation	Area	Technique
annamaya kosha	food sheath	body	postures
pranamaya kosha	pranic sheath	breath	*pranayama*
manomaya kosha	mind sheath	mind	meditation
vijnanamaya kosha	intelligence sheath	intelligence	objective *samadhi*
anandamaya kosha	ecstasy sheath	consciousness	objectless *samadhi*

1. *Yoga Sutra* II.29
2. *Taittiriya Upanishad* II.2–II.5

2

Suffering and mental slavery have come to an end when the nature of the fifth, innermost layer of the human being is revealed. This layer is consciousness, the seat of awareness, and its nature is ecstasy. The method by which this nature is revealed to the yogi is called objectless *samadhi* (*asamprajnata samadhi*). This highest *samadhi* can be entered into once the intelligence of the yogi is fully developed. The development of intelligence is brought about through objective *samadhi* (*samprajnata samadhi*). For the purpose of this text we can look at both *samadhi*s simply as extensions of meditation (*dhyana*) and, since they are advanced yogic techniques that require proficiency in the other more fundamental methods, we need not concern ourselves with them here.

The majority of the work of the yogi takes place in the three lower sheaths, simply because it is where the obstacles are located. Consciousness itself does not contain any obstacles whatsoever, and intelligence will evolve to a certain extent automatically once the three lower sheaths are developed. These three lower sheaths, all of which need development, are body, breath and mind. The yogi usually employs the term *purification* instead of development because development will take place by itself once the so-called impurities are removed.

Impurity in this context is not a moralistic term like sin, but it implies diseases and imbalances of the body, neurotic breathing patterns, subconscious imprints, mental conditioning, *karma*, beliefs and past forms of suffering that we hold on to. Since the layers that contain the obstacles – body, breath and mind – are so different from each other, there is no technique that can remove all obstacles from all three of these sheaths. It is absolutely paramount to understand this. For example, in today's world if your body is sick you go to the medical doctor, if you have mental issues you go to a psychologist and if your car breaks down you go to a workshop. You don't expect one and the same intervention to fix all of your problems.

According to yoga, to remove physical obstacles *asanas* (postures) need to be practised. To remove obstacles from the pranic sheath and the breathing pattern, *pranayama* is advised. To remove obstacles from the mind yogic meditation is engaged in. For swift success, these three methods need to be combined (and accompanied by ancillary techniques such as *kriya, bandha, mudra, mantra, chakra*).

The important information to be understood here is that *asana* alone can prepare only the body and not the mind. Meditation itself can develop only the mind and not the body. You may see an *asana* practitioner with a fully developed body but a mind that lags behind. You may also see a meditator with great mental capacity but a body that is still in the Stone Age. More benefit is obtained if both are practised together, but even then the benefit is not linked, because what links body and mind is the breath, the pranic sheath.

Neither posture practice nor meditation practice can harness the breath, the *prana*, the life force. And it is exactly this that *pranayama* is designed to do. Without *prana* the body is dead and without *prana* the mind is utterly inert. It is *prana* that moves both. For this reason *pranayama* was always considered the axial yogic limb. *Pranayama* is the axis around which the wheel of eight-limbed yoga revolves. *Pranayama* brings success in all other yogic limbs and it is also the axis that connects *asana* and meditation. The purpose of this book is to contribute to a renaissance of *pranayama* and weld together again these three powerful yogic techniques, which are much more potent when practised in sequence and combined.

WHY MODERN POSTURAL YOGA (MAINLY) MISSES THE POINT
In Patanjali yoga[3] the body is transformed into a perfect vehicle on the road to freedom or a perfect vessel to cross the ocean of conditioned existence. Let us have a closer look at the vehicle metaphor.

Suppose the road to freedom was leading through snowy mountains, desert tracks, swamps etc. You would need a vehicle that is robust, in top condition and capable of passing through very diverse terrain. Due to the fact that the trail by itself is already demanding enough, you would need a vehicle that serves you and not one that

3. Patanjali is the ancient sage who wrote the constitution of yoga.

4

needs you to serve it. The last thing you would need is one that constantly lets you know that it needs attention, that it needs to be pampered, spoiled, beautified, upgraded, overhauled, that it wants a photoshoot with itself as the model.

In yoga the body is transformed into such a perfected vehicle. In Patanjali yoga the aim of *asana* (and its ancillary techniques) is to create a body that does not need constant attention because it is sick, or signals pain or discomfort. This is because pain, discomfort and disease force us to deal with the body more and more to the extent that identification with it increases. If you constantly have to go to the doctor, have medical procedures undertaken, swallow daily a multitude of chemicals, all of this will make it more and more likely that you think you are the body. Without giving up this concept, spiritual freedom is not possible. For this reason yoga loosens the identification with the body more and more by not giving you any reason to identify with it. The body is simply there, functioning and supporting you perfectly, without constantly asking you to attend to its needs.

Much different is the notion behind modern postural yoga. It is very much a process of body sculpting and body beautifying, even body building. There are now yoga for abs and yoga for backsides. Glossy magazines sell the body beautiful as a marketing device. Modern postural yoga appears to lead to more identification with the body, not less. But true yoga was always aimed at recognizing us as that which is eternal, infinite and unchangeable. If we practise modern postural yoga, when we are getting old and eventually lying on our deathbeds we are unlikely to fare better than the mainstream population. Afraid, because what we know to be our self, the body, is failing. Concerned, because we do not know where we are going or believe we are going into annihilation.

You will not find yourself, your innermost being that cannot be destroyed by death, merely by practising *asana*. It is only a stepping-stone, a preparation and foundation for venturing into the higher limbs. There is no single yogic *shastra* (scripture) that gives *asana* the role that modern yogis assume it has. Unfortunately – because modern yogis often do not study the classical yogic texts – many have not noticed this fact. It is of utmost importance that modern yogis either study yogic scripture or practise yoga that is actually based on the findings of scripture and not a form of yoga that is watered down to an exercise fad. This brings me to scripture.

USE OF SCRIPTURE AND QUOTATION

You will find ample quotations from scripture in this book, and that may be nauseating to some. I have learned in India that it is very important for yoga teachers to quote from scripture. It is a way of keeping the teacher humble. She is not saying 'I think this and therefore it's right', or 'I am saying this and because of that you do it', but says 'Those great ones who went before me said ...' 'Those giants on whose shoulders I am standing and without whom I wouldn't be here today said ...'

It is very easy to teach a form of yoga where the teacher presents himself as the authority because the students can never challenge or question him. On the other hand to teach according to *shastra* (scripture) is altogether a humiliating affair. The teacher constantly refers to an authority greater than himself and then often has to explain himself when erudite students ask questions like, 'You teach this but here scripture states that ...' Some of these questions the teacher may not be able to answer on the spot, in which case it is good simply to say 'I will get back with the answer'. Sometimes the teacher may have to do additional study and meditation, and the probing of the student may even bring about a change. This is one of the most important aspects of teaching yoga: teaching based on scripture makes the teacher accountable and forces him/her to grow.

The truth is that today we barely know any more what yoga is. If we study the scriptures we have to admit that those ancient ones were greater yogis than we are today. By studying their teachings we will at least know into which direction we need to go. Without scripture we will lose yoga and stop at the 'yoga butt'.

Now to my use of the term *scripture*: I use it to loosely translate the Sanskrit *shastra*. *Shastra* actually means 'path to truth'. According to yoga *shastra*, yoga was originally taught through divine revelation.[4] It was then that it was at its purest and greatest. From that source onwards an almost endless stream of ancient teachers like Patanjali, Vyasa, Yajnavalkya, Shankara and Goraksha Natha described this great teaching in more and more detail. This entire canon of texts comprises a sacred tradition; hence I refer to it as scripture, fully aware that there are details in this canon that are less than sacred, even explicit, but that is probably the same in all sacred traditions on Earth.

Thus my habit of quoting scripture is an attempt to live up to that initial purity and vision of yoga, because it is only too easy to lose one's path in this modern jungle of opinions. If we do not base yoga on what is taught in scripture we will lose it and reduce it to an obsession about posture, health and beauty. But yoga is so much more. Through acquiring skill in *asana*, *pranayama* and meditation as taught in scripture, something can be gained that death cannot take away from us. By practising the complete bandwidth of yogic methods, that which cannot be cut by blades, pierced by thorns, burned by fire or drowned by waves can be experienced.[5] And it is this teaching that the scriptures have preserved for us. We need to be careful not to fall into the reductionist traps of modern fads.

WHY THIS BOOK IS IMPORTANT AND YOU STILL NEED A TEACHER
Just as when learning *asana*, when studying *pranayama* the student encounters the following predicament: A typical yoga class is 90 minutes long and packed full of students. There is so much happening that, apart from correcting your most obvious mistakes, the teacher will not have the time to sit down with you and explain minute details that you need to understand. In a class situation the teacher will repeat the most basic information over and over again

4. *Yoga Sutra* I.26, *Bhagavad Gita* IX.55
5. *Bhagavad Gita* II.23, *Yoga Sutra* III.39

and tailor it to the most inexperienced students. In a class, yoga cannot but be reduced to the lowest common denominator.

In the olden days students entered the household of the teacher and worked as odd-job men while being returned lodging, food and instruction. Such arrangements lasted from several years to a few decades. The teacher had a lot of time to explain the details and correct the practices of the students. This ancient institution, known as *guru shishya parampara* (teacher–student transference), has today fallen by the wayside. There are no more households that you can enter for several years and acquire all this knowledge in return for tending to the fire and herding the cattle. Yet you will need additional information apart from that obtainable in class, because otherwise learning yoga would be as unachievable as learning to fly a large commercial jet plane simply by looking for a few hours over the pilot's shoulder.

You will have to put in a fair amount of formal study apart from your practice in order to succeed. After all, although about 90% of all Sanskrit *shastras* have been lost, there are still more than 100,000 in existence. At the peak of the Indian culture, called *Satya Yuga*, an estimate of 1,000,000 shastras were in circulation. Why do you think all this knowledge was recorded? There was no vanity publishing in those days. In many cases the sages composed under pen names so that today we can't even be sure who exactly the author is. The reason for recording this knowledge was simply that students needed it in order to obtain success in yoga or other sacred disciplines.

You need to have in your mind an inner map of the territory that you are navigating. Imagine driving across a large metropolis or countryside without a map, whether electronic or hard copy. If you don't know where you are going you will end up somewhere else. In the example that I have used here several times, if you don't know that yoga leads to spiritual freedom and how exactly to get there you will instead merely arrive at physical empowerment and a buff body. It is important then that, apart from getting personal instruction, you study your subject so that you get a grasp of it.

Let's now look at the opposite scenario. Even if you have taken to studying ancient yogic treatises or modern books that are based on them, like this one, you will still need a teacher. Recently I read a review of a yoga book in which the reviewer was outraged that, having paid $17 for the book, he found the author additionally recommending the instruction of a teacher.

It's not as simple as paying a few dollars for a book. Here is the rationale: If ever you have taught a yoga class and demonstrated a posture, then watched the class emulate your actions, you will note that there are as many versions of your posture as there are students. What somebody tries to convey through words and actions, and what somebody else believes they have understood and replicated, are two entirely different things. For example if the teacher uses certain words, phrases or metaphors that have no meaning for you, you will simply delete them. You will only understand that part of the teacher's communication when she uses words with exactly the same meaning as you do. But very often we use words that have different meanings for either of us.

For this reason a teacher needs to watch what you do and give you feedback, depending on whether or not your actions can be considered to vaguely resemble what the instruction intended. It would be great if a complex art like *asana* or *pranayama* could be learned from a $17 or even a $150 book. Similarly, I would enjoy obtaining a pilot's licence (and many other things too) from such a small input. The reality, however, is that even after 30 years of practice and 17 years of teaching I have yet to see a student who attained a practice worth mentioning merely from reading books and watching DVDs. Although the sales of my book would increase if I could call it *The Definitive Step-by-Step Guide to Pranayama*, I am afraid I would do neither you nor the subject a service.

SEQUENTIAL AND SIMULTANEOUS NATURE OF YOGIC LIMBS

In the introductions to my previous books, *Ashtanga Yoga: Practice and Philosophy* and *Ashtanga Yoga: The Intermediate Series*, I explained in detail both the sequential and simultaneous nature of the eight limbs of Patanjali's yoga. First a certain base is created in *asana*. Without this base the body will constantly signal discomfort and in this way interfere with any sitting practice. Once you have reached a certain level in *asana* you can start practising *pranayama*. And once you have integrated this stage, you then go on and learn meditation. After you learn the basic method, meditation is then placed within *pranayama*, which itself is situated within *asana*. In this way the yogic limbs are stacked, like Russian dolls, within each other. The initial learning takes place in sequential steps but the application is a simultaneous process.

For this reason it is very important to learn the yogic limbs properly and one after the other. Without *pranayama*, *asana* produces only health. Without *asana*, *pranayama*'s benefits cannot be sustained and integrated into the body. Without *asana* and *pranayama*, meditation is a toothless tiger. Yes, it does give some relief from stress, suffering and excessive attachment, but this is akin to reducing posture to its health benefits.

When all three together are learned through direct practical instruction, along with an understanding of the underlying philosophy that is gained through study, then yoga will succeed. In this spirit I am offering this new presentation of classical yogic *pranayama*. May it support a new appraisal of yoga as a down-to-earth, hands-on and realistic path to spiritual emancipation.

Shastras quoted in the text

Amrita Nada Upanishad
Balakrishna's commentary on the *Hatha Yoga Pradipika* (10 chapters)
Bhagavad Gita
Brahma Sutra
Brahmananda's commentary on the *Hatha Yoga Pradipika*
   (4 chapters)
Brhad Aranyaka Upanishad
Brhadyogi Yajnavalkya Smrti
Chandogya Upanishad
Darshana Upanishad
Dhyana Bindu Upanishad
Gheranda Samhita
Goraksha Shataka
Hatha Ratnavali of Shrinivasayogi
Hatha Tatva Kaumudi of Sundaradeva
Hatha Yoga Manjari of Sahajananda
Hatha Yoga Pradipika (4 chapters)
Hatha Yoga Pradipika (10 chapters)
Jogapradipyaka of Jayatarama
Kumbhaka Paddhati of Raghuvira
Mahabharata
Mandala Brahmana Upanishad
Manu Smrti
Ramayana
Shandilya Upanishad
Shatapatha Brahmana
Shiva Samhita
Shiva Svarodaya
Taittiriya Upanishad
Vasishta Samhita
Vyasa's commentary on *Yoga Sutra*
Yoga Chudamani Upanishad

Yoga Kundalini Upanishad
Yoga Rahasya of Nathamuni
Yoga Sutra of Patanjali
Yoga Taravali of Shankaracharya
Yoga Yajnavalkya
Yuktabhavadeva of Bhavadeva Mishra

The Fundamentals
of Pranayama

DEFINITION AND PURPOSE
OF PRANAYAMA

DEFINITION

Pranayama is a compound noun made up of *prana* and *ayama*. The term *prana* can mean breath, but more often it refers to its subtle equivalent, the life force. *Ayama* means extension. *Pranayama*, then, means extension of life force. Although etymologically 'control of *prana*' cannot be read into the term *pranayama* (because of the central long *a*), many later traditional authors have interpreted it exactly in this way. Ramana Maharishi went as far as using the term *prana rodha*, which clearly means control of *prana*, to make the point. For this reason 'control of *prana*' or 'direction of *prana*' must also be accepted as a meaning of the term, as it is this that you will eventually do in *kumbhaka*.

Yoga has become very popular around the world, but unfortunately this popularity extends only to *asana* (posture). It has gone so far that students now use the term yoga to refer to *asana* only, and *pranayama* is thought of as something exotic or strange. However, in yogic tradition *pranayama* has always taken centre stage and *asana* was looked at only as a preparation or groundwork for *pranayama*. I will endeavour to show the pre-eminence of *pranayama* through quotations from the history of yoga and modern authorities as well. I do so in the hope that this will generate renewed interest in this most potent technique of yoga.

PATANJALI ON PRANAYAMA

The author of the *Yoga Sutra* offers several definitions of *pranayama*. Firstly he describes it as the removing of agitation and turbulence from inhalation and exhalation.[6] Lack of agitation and turbulence of the breathing pattern equates to a smooth flow of mind, making meditation achievable. After this is achieved, various *kumbhakas*

6. *Yoga Sutra* II.49

14

(breath retentions), such as internal, external and midway suspension, are practised with consideration of mental focus, time span and count until the breath is long and subtle.[7] This second definition makes clear that Patanjali saw *pranayama* not only as an extension of *prana* using *Ujjayi* breathing, but also as formal *kumbhaka*, with its length measured by count, while sitting in a meditation posture such as *Padmasana*.

Wilful manipulation of the breath is transcended once the fourth, spontaneous *kumbhaka* is experienced, which other texts call *Kevala Kumbhaka*.[8] With this final *kumbhaka*, *tamas* (torpidity) and *rajas* (frenzy) are removed from the mind and the original *sattva* (intelligence) shines through (Patanjali's term for *sattva* is *prakasha*).[9] With these impediments removed and the original state of mind restored, the yogi is now fit to perform the inner limbs, i.e. the higher yoga of meditation.[10]

Patanjali has described in only five sparse *sutras* how mental impediments intercept higher yoga, that the impediments can be removed through *pranayama*, that the removal is complete once spontaneous transcendence from the breathing pattern occurs (various schools differ in their interpretation of this *sutra*) and that this transcendence must be preceded by astute practice of the various *kumbhaka*s taking into account the modification of technical parameters, which is linked to creating a breath rhythm that is long and smooth, leading to a corresponding flow of life force and mind.

Just as he did with *asana*, which he described in only three *sutras*, Patanjali describes the effect of correct *pranayama* practice but not how to practise the actual techniques. This was to be done by a real-life teacher and more than one method was accepted.

MANU AND VAJNAVALKYA ON PRANAYAMA

That *pranayama* is the most important part of yoga has already been confirmed by many of the foremost sages of India such as Manu,

7. *Yoga Sutra* II.50
8. *Yoga Sutra* II.51
9. *Yoga Sutra* II.52
10. *Yoga Sutra* II.53

Yajnavalkya, Vyasa and Shankaracharya. Manu, the ancient Indian lawgiver, stated in his *Manu Smrti* that any accumulated demerit (i.e. bad *karma*) had to be deleted and erased by means of *pranayama*.[11] This is due to the fact that even ancient Indian law was constructed around this most important goal of human life – to reach spiritual emancipation, i.e. *mukti*. The sages noticed that any word, thought or act left a subconscious imprint. The imprint was particularly detrimental to spiritual freedom when the act that produced it was vicious rather than virtuous. Manu also says that *pranayama* is the greatest *tapas*, the greatest spiritually purifying practice of all.[12] Generations of sages confirmed that the most effective means of deleting unwanted subconscious imprint was and is *pranayama*. *Pranayama* is thus the ideal tool for deleting negative conditioning and reconditioning the subconscious in such a way that it supports spiritual freedom.

This same view is corroborated in the ancient text *Brhadyogi Yajnavalkya Smrti*, where sage Yajnvalkya proclaims that practising 100 rounds of *pranayama* will delete all karmic demerit.[13]

The tendency of *pranayama* to destroy demerit is affirmed in both Vedic and tantric scriptures. The *Yoga Chudamani Upanishad* says that karmic demerit is destroyed by *pranayama*,[14] and the *siddha* Goraksha Natha made the same assertion, in identical words, in his text *Goraksha Shataka*.[15]

PRANAYAMA IN THE BHAGAVAD GITA

The *Bhagavad Gita* is the most influential of the Indian scriptures. Containing the teachings of Lord Krishna, it defines *pranayama* in two ways.[16] Firstly it says that some practice *pranayama* by offering *apana* (vital down-current) into *prana* (vital up-current) and *prana*

11. *Manu Smrti* VI.71–72
12. *Manu Smrti* II.83
13. *Brhadyogi Yajnavalkya Smrti* VIII.36
14. *Yoga Chudamani Upanishad* stanza 108
15. *Goraksha Shataka* stanza 54
16. *Bhagavad Gita* IV.29

16

into *apana*, and thus arrest the breath. The *Gita* uses the term *prana apana gati*. *Prana gati* is the inner down movement, which is contained in the rising inhalation. *Apana gati* is the inner rising, which is contained in the descending exhalation. This implies the profound teaching that each force in the universe contains its own counterforce. The pranic movement here is stopped by focusing on the *gati*, which is the inner opposite of the apparent outer force. *Apana gati*, the inner upward movement contained in the exhalation, is one of the main motors to drive Kundalini (the coiled life force propelling spiritual liberation) upwards.

The second definition of *pranayama* mentioned in the *Gita* is the sacrifice of the senses into *prana*. During the movement of *prana*, i.e. inhalation and exhalation, the senses reach out and attach themselves to various objects of desire or aversion. During *kumbhaka* the senses are naturally drawn inwards and the yogi supports this by focusing on the Divine at the time of *kumbhaka*. The yogi forsakes and surrenders the normal outgoing activity of the senses and thus 'offers' it to the *prana* suspended and arrested through *kumbhaka*. Hence, like the *Yoga Sutra*, the *Gita* sees *pranayama* both as perfecting the process of inhalation and exhalation and as mental operations performed during the time of *kumbhaka* (breath retention).

MEDIEVAL TEXTS ON PRANAYAMA AND KARMA

Next we find the idea that *pranayama* deletes bad *karma*s taken up in the medieval Hatha Yoga texts. According to the *Hatha Yoga Pradipika*, all *karma*s are destroyed when *pranayama* is mastered.[17] The *Hatha Tatva Kaumudi of Sundaradeva* agrees that *pranayama* dissolves mountains of karmic demerit[18] while Jayatarama's *Jogapradipyaka* (a text written in Hindi rather than Sanskrit) extends this to mean that *pranayama* destroys all types of karmic demerit.[19] When texts talk of all types of *karma* they are referring to:

17. *Hatha Yoga Pradipika* (10 chapters) VII.18
18. *Hatha Tatva Kaumudi of Sundaradeva* XXXVIII.57
19. *Jogapradipyaka of Jayatarama* stanzas 505–510

• *karma* we have created in the past that has not yet fructified, i.e. is waiting in the karmic storehouse (*sanchita karma*)
• *karma* created in the past that already is fructifying or activated and has formed our present bodies (*prarabdha karma*)
• *karma*s that we are creating now and will lead to future embodiments (*kriyamana karma*).

These are all destroyed together by *pranayama*.

Without wanting to go into too much detail on *karma* in a book essentially on *pranayama*, I would observe that, as you might have noticed, whenever one makes a new start in life, or develops in a new direction, after the initial enthusiasm has worn off old tendencies tend to assert themselves. This can take the form of trying more and more techniques but never managing to overcome a certain level of obstacles. The reason for this is that there are certain *karma*s (*prarabdha karma*s) associated with the creation of your present body and mind. These *karma*s are difficult to overcome and will automatically reassert themselves given the chance. They are so ingrained that some Indian schools suggest looking at them as ordained and accept them.

Similarly there are *karma*s we have accumulated in the past but which have not yet fructified. The problem with these *sanchita karma*s, which wait in the karmic storehouse for the appropriate trigger, is that we cannot know what they will produce for us. Even if our present situation is fortunate, these *karma*s could be negative. There is a common belief that, just because one is in a fortunate position now, one is forever entitled to that. But according to the *karma* teaching you could in fact exhaust your last bit of merit right now. The moral therefore is never rest on one's laurels and strive always for spiritual growth. The yogi aims at intercepting these *karma*s before they bear fruit.

The third type of *karma*s, *kriyamana karma*s, are those we are producing now and that will bear fruit in the future. *Kriyamana* means that we are creating our destiny today. What we will be in the future is determined by our thoughts, expressions and actions today.

We are assured by the *rishis* and *siddhas* of yore that these three types of *karma* can be burnt in the fire of *pranayama*, leading to complete freedom from our past. Sundaradeva makes this particularly clear in his text *Hatha Tatva Kaumudi*.

He explains first that the yogi perceives the three types of *karma* through arousal of Kundalini.[20] Through *pranayama* he then annihilates them. Later in the same text he affirms that intense practice eliminates all subconscious imprints (*samskaras*) and the *karma* that has already started to fructify (*prarabdha karma*).[21] This clear statement is particularly valuable, since this type of *karma* is the most difficult to delete as it has already led to the forming of our present body and is strongly associated with it. To use a modern expression, we could say this *karma* is in our DNA or has formed the DNA of our present body.

MODERN TESTIMONIES

The miraculous properties of *pranayama* have been confirmed not only by authorities long gone but also by recent ones. Swami Niranjananananda, successor of Swami Satyananda, says that *pranayama* destroys *karmas*[22] and Yogeshwaranand Paramahamsa, founder of Yoga Niketan, confirms that focusing on the heart lotus in *kumbhaka* destroys *karma* from previous lives.[23]

The great yogi Nathamuni foresaw the current development, according to which yoga is reduced to the performance of *asana*. In his *Yoga Rahasya*, handed down through T. Krishnamacharya, he differentiates between those who practise only *asana* and those who follow the entire path of Ashtanga Yoga.[24] The sage wanted to assert that limiting one's yoga to practising postures was not

20. *Hatha Tatva Kaumudi of Sundaradeva* XLVI.30
21. *Hatha Tatva Kaumudi of Sundaradeva* LI.20
22. Swami Niranjanananda, *Prana and Pranayama*, Yoga Publications Trust, Munger, 2009, pp. 46 and 136
23. Yogeshwaranand Paramahamsa, *First Steps to Higher Yoga*, Yoga Niketan Trust, New Delhi, 2001, p. 355
24. *Yoga Rahasya of Nathamuni* III.36

Patanjali's traditional eightfold yoga (Ashtanga Yoga). Nathamuni goes on to put great emphasis on *pranayama*.

T. Krishnamacharya, being the fountainhead of modern yoga, needs little introduction. He was the teacher of B.K.S. Iyengar, K. Pattabhi Jois, B.N.S. Iyengar, Srivatsa Ramaswami, T.K.V. Desikachar and A.G. Mohan. He said that *pranayama* was the most important of the eight limbs and the prime means for extending one's lifespan.[25] It did this by counteracting diseases, which in turn it achieved by balancing the three *doshas* (humours) of the body.[26] Krishnamacharya also stated that *pranayama* would lead to the higher limbs of *dharana* and *dhyana*, and he went even further in saying that *dharana* was impossible to attain without the practice of *pranayama*.[27] In his first book, *Yoga Makaranda* of 1934, the great teacher also explained that in eight-limbed yoga one gets benefits only related to the particular limb that one practises.[28]

If the practice is restricted to *asana* only, the benefit is simply a strengthened body and improved blood circulation. If one wants to harvest benefits like health and longevity, intellectual strength, clarity and strength of expression, *pranayama* needs to be added. In the same text Krishnamacharya also explains that *pranayama* enables the yogi to focus on and visualize the *chakras*, resulting in almost endless health benefits.[29] He also proclaims that *dhyana* and *samadhi* are attained through *pranayama*.[30]

Sundaradeva, who authored the monumental 1000-page *Hatha Tatva Kaumudi*, supports this view by saying that *pranayama* is the most

25. A.G. Mohan, *Krishnamacharya: His Life and Teachings*, Shambala, Boston & London, 2010, p. 57
26. A.G. Mohan, *Krishnamacharya: His Life and Teachings*, Shambala, Boston & London, 2010, p. 70
27. A.G. Mohan, *Krishnamacharya: His Life and Teachings*, Shambala, Boston & London, 2010, p. 113
28. T. Krishnamacharya, *Yoga Makaranda*, rev. English edn, Media Garuda, Chennai, 2011, pp. 48–49
29. T. Krishnamacharya, *Yoga Makaranda*, rev. English edn, Media Garuda, Chennai, 2011, pp. 50–54
30. T. Krishnamacharya, *Yoga Makaranda*, rev. English edn, Media Garuda, Chennai, 2011, p. 64

important practice of Hatha Yoga,[31] this being not a separate form of yoga but the lower limbs of Patanjali's eight-limbed Ashtanga Yoga.

A similar view is entertained by Swami Ramdev, the originator of a powerful *pranayama* renaissance in India, who criticises those who teach Ashtanga Yoga as *asana* only. He claims that postures alone are not enough to cure serious and chronic disorders[32] and recommends *pranayama* and traditional ayurvedic medicine to reduce India's dependence on imported Western chemicals. To those who deflect students from practising *pranayama* by making it sound difficult and unattainable, Swami Ramdev says that *pranayama* is so harmless that even children and the elderly can do it.[33]

Swami Ramdev also declares that Hatha Yoga (i.e. the *asana* and *pranayama* parts of the eight-limbed yoga) and Kundalini Yoga (the concentration dimension of Patanjali's Ashtanga Yoga) today are more important than ever because nowadays there are no more teachers who can give *shaktipat*.[34] *Shaktipat* means the revelation of mystical states to others through the power of one's own attainment. Swami Ramdev holds that this power nowadays has become extinct, as there are no more sages of that calibre.

PRANAYAMA AND HEALTH

Let us return to T. Krishnamacharya's statement that the most important yogic limb to power both spiritual development and health is *pranayama* and not *asana*. This view is supported by Jayatarama, who says in his *Jogapradipyaka* that any worldly and spiritual goal whatsoever can be accomplished by means of *pranayama*.[35] We will hear more about this claim when analysing the flow (*svara*) of breath through the left and right nostrils.

The ancient Vedic text *Brhadyogi Yajnavalkya Smrti* confirms that *pranayama* produces the state of perfect health by removing all

31. *Hatha Tatva Kaumudi of Sundaradeva* IV.17
32. Swami Ramdev, *Pranayama*, Divya Yog Mandir Trust, Hardwar, 2007, p. 3
33. Swami Ramdev, *Pranayama*, Divya Yog Mandir Trust, Hardwar, 2007, p. 3
34. Swami Ramdev, *Pranayama*, Divya Yog Mandir Trust, Hardwar, 2007, p. 49
35. *Jogapradipyaka of Jayatarama* stanzas 505–510

disorders of the three humours (*doshas*) *vata, pitta* and *kapha*.[36] This is supported by the co-founder of the *siddha* movement, Goraksha Natha, who says that when *prana* is arrested one becomes free from disease.[37] A similar view is aired in the *Yoga Chudamani Upanishad*, which states that *pranayama* destroys all diseases, and diseases appear only in those who are not able to do it.[38] Sundaradeva, author of the *Hatha Tatva Kaumudi*, attests that by practising *pranayama* continuously, with full devotion, a long life is obtained[39] and that all ailments caused by *vata, pitta* and *kapha* are cured.[40]

This message, confirmed by great yogis of all ages, reverberates also in modern times. The Kaivalyadhama Institute in Lonavla, India, is possibly the most important *pranayama* research laboratory of the last 100 years. Its current director, O.P. Tiwari, agrees that *pranayama* both maintains health and raises Kundalini to empower meditation.[41] Swami Ramdev says about *pranayama* that it is used to keep the *Pranamaya kosha* clean, healthy and disease free.[42] The *Pranamaya kosha* is the pranic sheath that connects the gross body (*Annamaya kosha*) with the mind (*Manomaya kosha*). He elaborates by saying that *pranayama* balances the digestive system, cures pulmonary, cardiac and cerebral diseases, boosts immunity and helps with diabetes, cancer, hormonal problems, allergies, renal problems, degenerative problems such as greying of the hair, failing eyesight and the onset of ageing.[43]

Pranayama is often lauded as a panacea for all possible ailments. This concept, however, applies mainly in its capacity to prevent imbalance of the humours, *vata, pitta* and *kapha*. When suffering from

---

36. *Brhadyogi Yajnavalkya Smrti* VIII.32
37. *Goraksha Shataka* stanza 92
38. *Yoga Chudamani Upanishad* stanza 116
39. *Hatha Tatva Kaumudi of Sundaradeva* XLV.58
40. *Hatha Tatva Kaumudi of Sundaradeva* XLVIII.24
41. O.P. Tiwari, *Kriyas and Pranayama*, DVD, Kaivalyadhama, Lonavla.
42. Swami Ramdev, *Pranayama Rahasya*, Divya Yog Mandir Trust, Hardwar, 2009, p. 2
43. Swami Ramdev, *Pranayama Rahasya*, Divya Yog Mandir Trust, Hardwar, 2009, p. 88

a potentially fatal disease, a responsible use of *pranayama* would be to practise it in conjunction with medical treatment. This is also implied in the title *Yoga in Synergy with Medical Sciences* by Swami Ramdev's aide Acharya Balkrishna.

PHYSIOLOGICAL CHANGES DURING PRANAYAMA AND THERAPEUTIC APPLICATION

As stated in many ancient texts, but also by modern authorities such as Swami Sivananda,[44] *pranayama* can cure and prevent diseases by restoring the balance of the three humours, *vata, pitta* and *kapha*. According to Ayurveda, disease is generally caused by an imbalance of the *dosha*s. So *Surya Bhedana pranayama* is used to reduce the *vata* and *kapha dosha*s, *Ujjayi pranayama* diminishes *kapha*, while *Shitali, Sitkari* and *Chandra Bhedana pranayama*s minimise the *pitta dosha*, while *Bhastrika* curtails all three *dosha*s simultaneously. The *Hatha Tatva Kaumudi* states that diseases due to aggravated *pitta* are healed in three months by practising *Chandra Bhedana* (inhaling through left and exhaling through right nostril), while diseases resulting from aggravated *vata* or *kapha* are removed in the same time by practising *Surya Bhedana* (inhaling through the right and exhaling through the left nostril).[45]

Pranayama can also be used to harmonise the brainwaves, as Swami Niranjanananda says.[46] Yoga also says that *pranayama* increases the lifespan. According to yoga, every being has a set number of breaths. By slowing down the breath they are spaced over a longer time span; hence the overall life expectation increases. Swami Niranjanananda asserts that reducing the normal respiratory rate from 15 or 16 breaths per minute down to 10 will extend the lifespan to 100 years.[47]

44. Swami Sivananda, *The Science of Pranayama*, BN Publishing, 2008, p. 99
45. *Hatha Tatva Kaumudi of Sundaradeva* X.33
46. Swami Niranjanananda, *Prana and Pranayama*, Yoga Publications Trust, Munger, 2009, p. 110
47. Swami Niranjanananda, *Prana and Pranayama*, Yoga Publications Trust, Munger, 2009, p. 155

Pranayama can alleviate chronic diseases by fixating *prana* in the troubled areas. For this purpose the breath is retained so that *prana* can be absorbed. The medieval Hatha text *Yuktabhavadeva* states that for the alleviation of diseases *prana* needs to be concentrated at the location of the disease.[48] Practically speaking, during *kumbhaka* the yogi mentally concentrates on a particular area and *prana* follows the mind to the required location. To increase the efficiency of the method, *kumbhaka* length is extended as the absorption rate of *prana* increases accordingly.

On the other hand the length of *kumbhaka* is limited by the oxygen needs of the heart. For this reason the heart is slowed down by experienced yogis to such an extent that its oxygen use is minimized. This can lead to the impression that the heart has stopped and the yogi is dead. For example T. Krishnamacharya's ability to stop his heartbeat was monitored and confirmed by a team of medical doctors.[49] Others envied Krishnamacharya for this ability but nobody wanted to put in the required three extensive practice sessions of *Nadi Shodhana pranayama* per day over decades, combined with an exclusively milk diet.

MENTAL AND SPIRITUAL BENEFITS THROUGH PRANAYAMA

In the *Shandilya Upanishad* we find the injunction that the fluctuations of *prana* are to be stilled through the practice of *pranayama*.[50] Why should we be interested in stilling these fluctuations? The great *siddha* Goraksha Natha explained in his *Goraksha Shataka* that, as long as *prana* moves, mind moves, and when *prana* is stilled the mind is stilled as well.[51] A still mind can be used like a still lake to see one's own reflection. If the surface of the lake is ruffled, only distorted images are discernible. If the surface of the lake of the mind is still, however, the mind can reflect like a clear crystal whatever it

48. *Yuktabhavadeva of Bhavadeva Mishra* lxvii
49. T.K.V. Desikachar, *Health, Healing & Beyond*, Aperture, New York, 1998, p. 28
50. *Shandilya Upanishad* stanza 46
51. *Goraksha Shataka* stanza 94

is turned towards, in this case the self.[52] Thus self-knowledge is possible. For this reason ways of stilling the mind were explored by the yogis. From this exploration *pranayama* surfaced as the most straightforward method to power meditation, based on the observation that thought is powered by *prana*. When *prana* is stilled thought is stilled, too.

Jagatguru (world teacher) Shankaracharya explores in his *Yoga Taravali* the connection between the higher limbs and *pranayama*. He states that, when *pranayama* is perfected, Kundalini enters what yogis call the central energy channel (*sushumna*) and it is then that *dharana* (concentration, the sixth limb of yoga) and *dhyana* (meditation, the seventh limb) are effortlessly taking place.[53] Shankara states here clearly that *pranayama* causes Kundalini to rise and Kundalini itself powers *dharana* and *dhyana*. Without this motor of Kundalini, *dharana* and *dhyana* take a lot of effort to reach. In fact you can spend hours every day for decades of your life watching your breath without getting far. This is simply due to the fact that if your *prana* is centred in one of the lower *chakra*s your mind will naturally gravitate to themes of survival and fear (*Muladhara Chakra*), procreation and emotion (*Svadhishthana Chakra*) and assimilation and wealth (*Manipuraka Chakra*). If you lift Kundalini to the third eye (*Ajna Chakra*) you will automatically and spontaneously enter deep meditation, as Shankara explains, and his tool of choice is *pranayama*.

In a similar vein, the *Brhadyogi Yajnavalkya Smrti* declares those as ignorant who think that through knowledge alone liberation is possible, a reference to the Advaita Vedantins.[54] Rather than that, through the combined application of knowledge and the eight limbs, particularly *pranayama*, *dharana* and *dhyana*, liberation is possible. This particular philosophy is called *Karma-jnana-samuccaya*, meaning through action and knowledge freedom is possible. This

52. *Yoga Sutra* I.41
53. *Yoga Taravali of Shankaracharya* stanzas 12, 14
54. *Brhadyogi Yajnavalkya Smrti* IX.34

philosophy was also espoused by T. Krishnamacharya, who was critical of Advaita Vedanta.

The tantric text *Hatha Yoga Pradipika* informs us that the *prana*, once it enters the middle channel (*sushumna*), will arrest the mind (*manonmani*) and make it calm.[55] To achieve this aim it recommends various *kumbhakas*, i.e. forms of breath retention. The same is stated by Shrinivasayogi in his text *Hatha Ratnavali*.[56] The *Hatha Yoga Pradipika* gives us some insights into how exactly meditation and its goal, liberation, on the one hand and *pranayama* on the other are connected. The *Pradipika* declares that 12 *pranayama*s make one *pratyahara* (the fifth limb), 12 *pratyahara*s make 1 *dharana* (the sixth limb), 12 *dharana*s make one *dhyana* (the seventh limb) and 12 *dhyana*s make 1 *samadhi* (the eighth limb and culmination of yoga).[57] It also proclaims that those who talk of *Jnana* (knowledge) without having made *prana* steady by means of *pranayama* are hypocrites[58] and that one is considered liberated only when the *prana* does not move during inhalation and exhalation.[59] Again here, achievements in *pranayama* are used to determine or measure one's mystical achievements to distinguish the yogi who has *siddhi* (proof of attainment) from the Advaita Vedantins, who are always prattling on about their knowledge but are often just blowing hot air (pun intended).

Sundaradeva, in his *Hatha Tatva Kaumudi*, confirms the *Hatha Yoga Pradipika*'s jab at the Advaita Vedantins: that without mastery of *pranayama* it is hypocrisy to talk of self-knowledge,[60] but he goes further still. He says that in this *Kali Yuga* (the current age of darkness) success in yoga cannot be gained without *mudra*, *asana* and *pranayama*. He adds that *pranayama* gives rise to *pratyahara* (the fifth limb),[61] which is the prerequisite to *Shakti Chalana* (Kundalini-rousing), called

---

55. *Hatha Yoga Pradipika* II.41–2
56. *Hatha Ratnavali of Shrinivasayogi* II.3–4
57. *Hatha Yoga Pradipika* (10 chapters) I.36–37
58. *Hatha Yoga Pradipika* (10 chapters) VII.15
59. *Hatha Yoga Pradipika* (10 chapters) X.36
60. *Hatha Tatva Kaumudi of Sundaradeva* II.2
61. *Hatha Tatva Kaumudi Kaumudi of Sundaradeva* XLI.44

dharana (the sixth limb) in the *Yoga Sutra*. He encourages us by saying that practice of *asana*, *pranayama*, *mudra* (pranic or energetic seal) and *bandha* (pranic or energetic lock) makes rousing of Kundalini straightforward[62] and that wealth, mastery, liberation, nay everything, is achievable through *pranayama*.[63] The current author does not intend this book to be a guide to riches and power, but nevertheless Sundaradeva's statement that *pranayama* is helpful in other than spiritual matters will be confirmed and explained in the chapter on *nadi* and *svara* balance.

Sahajananda, author of the *Hatha Yoga Manjari* and disciple of the *siddha* Goraksha Natha, assures us that all *pranayama* practitioners will experience bliss.[64] He also confirms that *pranayama* brings about liberation[65] and that it achieves *pratyahara* (the sixth limb of yoga).[66] For the devotionally minded among us, he argues that *pranayama*'s greatness is beyond all doubt because Maheshvara (Lord Shiva) Himself practised it.[67] In numerous other texts we find the reference that Lord Brahma and other celestials (*devas*) practised *pranayama* because they were afraid of death. This carries an implication of the potency of *pranayama* to overcome or at least delay the onset of death.

Swami Niranjanananda explains that *pranayama* can reduce some of the common dangers of meditation. He says that *dhyana yoga*, i.e. the yoga of meditation, may induce hypnosis if mind is not kept sattvic.[68, 69] This is a common occurrence that I have warned of in my previous books. Yoga does not recommend meditation without prior preparation and training. Niranjanananda recommends that the mind be made sattvic and kept that way through the practice of

62. *Hatha Tatva Kaumudi Kaumudi of Sundaradeva* XLIV.51
63. *Hatha Tatva Kaumudi Kaumudi of Sundaradeva* XLVIII.37
64. *Hatha Yoga Manjari of Sahajananda* II.78
65. *Hatha Yoga Manjari of Sahajananda* II.65
66. *Hatha Yoga Manjari of Sahajananda* II.67
67. *Hatha Yoga Manjari of Sahajananda* II.65
68. Swami Niranjanananda, *Prana and Pranayama*, Yoga Publications Trust, Munger, 2009, p. 133
69. *Sattva* means intelligence, wisdom or light.

pranayama. The swami thus echoes what yogic tradition has said about meditation since time immemorial. Of course in these modern days only few heed such qualified advice, and thus head for the abyss of intellectual torpidity and stagnation. Famously, the *Ramayana* shows the dangers of meditation when not done with a sattvic mind. Of the three demon brothers, the demon king Ravana practised meditation with a rajasic mind and wrath became his undoing. His brother Kumbhakarna meditated with a tamasic mind and fell into a deep slumber from which he only rarely woke up. Only the third brother, Vibhishana, meditated with a sattvic mind, and it was only his intellect that gravitated towards the Divine.

The *Ramayana*, although written down after the *Mahabharata*, contains one of the most ancient orally-handed-down epics of humanity. It delivers many subtle teachings on meditation, which, although mastered by sages of a bygone era, are not understood any more by modern practitioners. Hence more and more are heading down the road taken already by Ravana and Kumbhakarna. It is not a general lack of meditation that gnaws at the foundation of this world, for this whole world meditates with profound expertise on Mammon, the mighty dollar. It is what you meditate on that will determine your destiny, for what you meditate on you will attract and become. Before embarking on the voyage of meditation, the intellect has to be made sattvic through *pranayama.*

Andre Van Lysebeth, author of several good books on yoga and the first westerner to visit Krishnamacharya's student K. Pattabhi Jois in Mysore, issues a similar caution but goes into more detail. He says it is essential that *asana* and *pranayama* be mastered before one dares to activate the *chakras*, otherwise pranic short circuits may occur.[70] These are, however, likely to occur only in those who do not prepare themselves properly through *asana* and *pranayama*, and one is inclined to add to this list *kriya*, the purification processes.

To finish off our venture into testimonies on *pranayama* from authorities of the ages, I quote Sir John Woodroffe, the author of *The*

70. Andre van Lysebeth, *Die Grosse Kraft des Atems*, O.W. Barth, Bern, 1972, p. 260

Serpent Power and many other perennial classics on *Tantra*. He states that Shakti, i.e. Kundalini, can be roused by two means, either through *mantra* or through *pranayama*.[71] However, Shyam Sundar Goswami, author of the seminal *Laya Yoga: The Definitive Guide to the Chakras and Kundalini*, makes it clear that *mantra* is enlivened through purification of the *nadis*.[72] The prime means of doing so is *pranayama*. It needs to be practised before venturing into any deeper aspects of yoga, as it powers all upstream methods (meaning all those that belong to higher limbs) of rousing Kundalini.

I hope to have achieved my aim of showing that *pranayama* is the method that is central to yoga, not *asana*. But *pranayama* cannot be undertaken without a proper grounding in *asana* practice, as will be shown in the chapter on *asana*. But to practise *asana* without going on to *pranayama* is like continuing to plough a field without ever sowing the seed, or like washing a garment over and over again without ever wearing it. It is obviously absurd to refuse to take the step that brings the reward for one's efforts, but this is exactly what the modern yoga movement is doing.

In contrast with those who practise *asana* and refuse to move on to *pranayama*, we have those who jump ahead and enter into meditation practices without having any grounding in *asana* and *pranayama*. Meditation is a vehicle that can drive us across the ocean of conditioned existence. The engine of this vehicle is Kundalini (roused life force). This engine is powered by the fuel of *kumbhaka* (breath retention), the essence of *pranayama*. However, this fuel can be ignited only in a body that is forged in the fire of *asana*. In the wake of the visit of certain rock band members to Indian gurus and the subsequent New Age movement, dozens and possibly hundreds of millions of people have started to meditate. Some gurus promised that a daily meditation practice would surely lead to success within 2 years or less. Now, some 40 years later, we can declare that such successes, if any, remain the exception.

71. Sir John Woodroffe, *The Serpent Power*, Ganesh & Co., Madras, 1995, p. 247
72. Shyam Sunder Goswami, *Laya Yoga*, Inner Traditions, Rochester, 1999, p. 115

Like an *asana* practice that does not develop into a *pranayama* practice, a meditation practice that is not powered by *pranayama* is unlikely to produce more than temporary results. It is also the reason why so many spiritual seekers are still relying on their gurus to produce results in them rather than being able to permanently put legs under their own spiritual discipline. Most meditation techniques when taught by the ancient sages were either done during *kumbhaka* (breath retention) or powered by other methods of Kundalini-rousing, which then often included one element of *pranayama* or another. Hence the importance of *pranayama* as the vital link that connects *asana* and *meditation. Asana* prepares the ground on which *pranayama* can be practised. *Pranayama* prepares the ground on which meditation will become successful. Meditation, when done properly, can lead to realization of the Divine.

PRANA

MEANINGS OF THE TERM PRANA AND ITS FUNCTION

Having established the importance and scope of *pranayama*, let us turn to *prana* itself. As is the case with many other terms, *prana* can have several meanings depending on context. For example some yogic scriptures instruct you to draw the *prana* in through the left nostril and expel it through the right and vice versa. Here, *prana* simply means breath.

More often we come across passages that advise us not to let the *prana* enter the head, or consciously push it into the arms to gain strength or direct it into areas of the body that harbour disease. Very common is also the scriptural advice to move *prana* into the central energy channel (*sushumna*), which, once achieved, produces the mystical state. In all of these instances *prana* obviously does not mean breath but 'life force'. Breath is the gross expression of the subtle life force.

In its cosmic form *prana* is also the manifestation of the Great Goddess and is then frequently described in a personalised form – it may be called Shakti when thought of as descending, or Kundalini when thought of as ascending. Again these two terms are often interchangeable depending on context.

The *Brhad Aranyaka Upanishad* identifies *prana* with the Brahman (infinite consciousness / deep reality).[73] The same is said in the *Brahma Sutra*.[74] How can the Brahman, which is pure, infinite consciousness, be the same as the subtle life force, which, although permeating and moving this entire universe, is still a far cry from pure consciousness? The answer we find in the *shanti mantra* 'Sham no mitra' of the *Taittiriya Upanishad*.

In this invocation we find the important passage 'Namo brahmane namaste vayo tvameva pratyaksham bhrahmasi tvameva pratyaksham brahma vadishyami', which means 'I salute you oh Brahman, I

73. *Brhad Aranyaka Upanishad* III.9.9
74. *Brahma Sutra* I.5

salute you, oh Prana. For you, Prana, are indeed the directly perceptible Brahman. You alone I shall call the directly perceptible Brahman.'

The understanding of this passage is very important. The Brahman
is the transcendent aspect of God. Transcendent aspect means it is
not directly perceptible (other than through an act of grace). But it
can be recognised by its immanent aspect, in our case the *prana*. In
this *shanti mantra* the *prana* is called the immanent aspect of Brahman.
The philosophy according to which God is at the same time both
immanent and transcendent is called *panentheism*. Panentheistic
thought is present in all major religions. In Christianity, for example,
the Father is God transcendent and both Jesus and the Holy Spirit
are God immanent. Interestingly enough, *spirit* is the translation of
the original *pneuma* in the Greek New Testament. The term *pneuma*
derives from the Sanskrit *prana* and, even in the English *inspiration*,
the connotation of inhalation and thus breath is still present.

T. Krishnamacharya also linked *prana* to consciousness. He explained that in the waking state *prana* is projected out to both body
and mind.[75] In the dream state it is withdrawn from the body and
extends only out to the mind. In the deep-sleep state, however, *prana*
is withdrawn from both body and mind and abides in consciousness. That is why dreaming is not truly restful and not really
conducive to health.

It also explains the existence of proverbs in some languages that
say in sleep one goes home to God or in sleep one does not sin. It is
reflective of the fact that *prana* is absorbed into our spiritual nature
and absolutely no activity is present.

Some scriptural passages identify *prana* as the *prakrti* (nature,
material cause) of the Samkhya philosophy, and in this case we simply
look at the cosmic impersonal manifestation of what expresses itself
in the individual as breath and life force. The *Shatapatha Brahmana*
describes *prana* as the elixir of immortality (*amrita*).[76] *Amrita* more

75. T. Krishnamacharya, *Yoga Makaranda*, Media Garuda, Chennai, rev. English edn,
2011, p. 44
76. *Shatapatha Brahmana* X.2.6.18

often than not denotes a drug derived from a creeper, but in yoga the *amrita* is the reservoir of *prana* in the centre of the brain, the area of the third ventricle. When the *prana* is arrested there, immortality is gained. This immortality, however, does not necessarily refer to physical immortality, some schools interpreting it as the realization of divine consciousness.

Other textual passages say that *prana* and *apana* need to be united in the navel *chakra* (*Manipura*). In such contexts, *prana* refers to only one of the ten vital airs (*vayus*) that in themselves are subdivisions of the broader life force, *prana*. *Prana* has two storehouses in the body, a lunar, mental storehouse in the centre of the brain (*Ajna Chakra*) and a solar/physical storehouse in the area of the navel (*Manipura Chakra*). *Manipura Chakra* is also the seat of fire (*agni*), and this is why some texts suggest raising Kundalini with fire and air (*prana*), but more about that later.

Some older texts also use the term *vayu* instead of *prana* (as the *Taittiriya Upanishad* above). In this book, if *prana* is used with the meaning of life force it will stand by itself. If it is used to denote the vital up-breath *prana vayu*, a subdivision of the life-force *prana*, then the compound *prana vayu* is used instead of the simple *prana*.

The term *prana Shakti* is also frequently used to denote the efferent (outgoing) function of the *nadi* system, i.e. the ability of individuals to actively express themselves through the body, such as moving it in space and making it perform actions. *Prana Shakti* is thought of as working through the right nostril, and breathing methods that primarily utilise the right nostril therefore make one extraverted and active.

Opposed to that is *manas Shakti*, the collective term for afferent (incoming) *nadi* signals, which are activated through the left nostril. Breathing through the left nostril makes one more inactive, introverted and reflective, this being a function of *manas Shakti* rather than *prana Shakti*.

This is covered in more detail in the chapter on *nadi* balance. To those who reduce the term *prana* to merely mean 'breath'

Swami Ramdev declares that it is not only breath but also invisible divine energy.[77]

Summarizing, *prana* is thus the body and actions of the Great Goddess, with which she causes, produces, maintains and destroys not only the entire world of manifestation but also each and every individual by means of breath. The downward-moving process of manifestation of individuals (Shakti) and the upward-surging process of their spiritual emancipation (Kundalini) are the two directional manifestations of *prana*. *Prana* is the God immanent that permeates and sustains this entire universe and all beings. Additionally the term *prana* is used to denote the vital upward current on the one hand and the efferent (outgoing) currents of the *nadi* system on the other. When trying to understand the significance of the term *prana* one therefore needs to cast one's net as widely as possible to include all of these possible meanings; otherwise certain textual passages will remain opaque.

EFFECTS OF PRANAYAMA

The practice of *pranayama* has several important effects on *prana*, and through it body and mind. *Pranayama* draws *prana* back into the body, it increases and stores *prana*, it equalises the flow (*svara*) of *prana* in the *nadi* system, and directs *prana* into the central energy channel (*sushumna*). Below is a detailed breakdown of these effects. Further, *pranayama* has a profound effect on the humours (*doshas*) of the body and the qualities (*gunas*) of the mind. These effects are such that *pranayama* can be designed to combat any of the obstacles that sage Patanjali listed in *Yoga Sutra* I.30. As an explanation of these effects requires an understanding of the individual *pranayama* techniques, they are described after the practice section in the chapter '*Pranayama* as remover of obstacles' in the back of this text. The main effects of *pranayama* practice are:

77. Swami Ramdev, *Pranayama Rahasya*, Divya Yog Mandir Trust, Hardwar, 2009, p. 15

34

Drawing scattered prana back into the body
The *Vasishta Samhita*, containing sage Vasishta's teachings on yoga, argues that *prana* is larger than the body by 12 *angulas* (finger widths).[78] This means that the pranic body extends by 12 finger widths over the surface of the gross body. Sage Yajnavalkya agrees that *pranayama* draws *prana* into the body,[79] which was previously scattered 12 *angulas* beyond the surface of the gross body. The same information is represented in the Vedic literature. In the *Shandilya Upanishad*, sage Atharvan describes our body as being 96 finger widths in length, with *prana* extending 12 *angulas* beyond the body.[80] He who through the practice of yoga reduces his *prana* so that it does not scatter beyond the body becomes the greatest of yogis, Sage Atharvan adds.

The medieval *siddhas* came to the same conclusion. The *Goraksha Shataka* states that *prana* goes out from the surface of the body 12 *angulas*,[81] but during strenuous activities such as sexual intercourse 36 or more *angulas*; hence it is then depleted. Sage Gheranda cites the same figures.[82] This, according to the sages, scatters one's *prana* and shortens one's life. Decrease the scattering of *prana* and you will live longer. The *Hatha Tatva Kaumudi* supports this view in saying that whoever reduces the outflow of *prana* below 12 digits is an expert in yoga.[83] Scattering of *prana* manifests in our lives through a scattered mind: being talkative and being involved in manifold activities that do not get us anywhere. It leads to restlessness, to 'being out there' instead of resting in one's centre, to 'being all over the place' instead of resting in one's heart, to sustaining relationships even if they are degrading and to developing desires that are unwholesome for oneself. *Pranayama* is used to concentrate *prana* in the body,

78. *Vasishta Samhita* II.7
79. *Yoga Yajnavalkya* IV.8–9
80. *Shandilya Upanishad* stanza 15
81. *Goraksha Shataka* stanza 94
82. *Gheranda Samhita* V.79–82
83. *Hatha Tatva Kaumudi of Sundaradeva* XXXVII.2

to withdraw the projection of *prana* out into the surroundings, and this effect makes us a whole and integrated human being.

Storing and increasing prana

In his book *Pranayama, Kundalini and Hatha Yoga*, Acharya Bhagwan Dev states that only a small amount of the *prana* that could be absorbed from the air through deep and controlled yogic breathing is realistically extracted through normal, shallow breathing.[84] The actual storage of *prana* in the body is effectively improved through *kumbhaka* (breath retention). *Kumbhaka* is used for fixation of *prana* in the body. This statement also makes clear that *pranayama* is only completed through breath retention, i.e. mere *Ujjayi* breathing is *pranayama* only in a preliminary sense.

The *Hatha Tatva Kaumudi* informs us of the effects that holding or fixating of *prana* in various areas of the body has.[85] Fixating is simply done by focusing the mind on the required area during *kumbhaka*. As *prana* will go where mind goes, conscious concentration will automatically divert *prana* to that area. According to Sundaradeva, by holding the *prana* at the navel one overcomes all diseases, by holding it at the tip of the nose, control over *prana* is gained, and by holding it at the big toes one attains lightness. Distribution of *prana* to various areas of the body predominantly takes place during the exhalation phase. While the retention phase is used to absorb the *prana* in the navel area (*Manipura Chakra*), it is actually the exhalation that is used to transport *prana* from the navel to areas where it is needed more urgently.

Drawing prana into the central channel

As previously quoted, the *Hatha Yoga Pradipika* states that in yogic circles (other than those of the Advaita Vedantins) any talk of self-knowledge (*jnana*) is just boastful prattle if it is not accompanied by

84. Acharya Bhagwan Dev, *Pranayama, Kundalini & Hatha Yoga*, Diamond Books, New Delhi, 2008, p. 9
85. *Hatha Tatva Kaumudi of Sundaradeva* XII.13ff.

36

prana being inducted into the central *nadi* (*sushumna*). This *nadi* suspends the mind, which is powered by the two outer *nadis*, Ida and Pingala. These two solar and lunar *nadis* contain the *prana* at times when the mind is activated. When the yogi attains the mystical state, the mind is suspended and *prana* is in *sushumna*. Jayatarama, in his *Jogapradipyaka*, tells us that the induction of *prana* into *sushumna* depends on the practice of *kumbhaka* and nothing else.[86] We have to remember that in contrast to Western culture, which focused for two millennia mainly on technology and how to conquer the outer world, Indians became veritable astronauts of the inner spaces. This meant that somebody who could truly access mystical states in India was as highly esteemed as, for example, a Columbus, Leibniz, Newton or Einstein was in the West.

In between those true inner astronauts, who were authentic yoga practitioners and enjoyed such states, there were, however, many who were not true artisans of *prana*, just blowers of hot air who engaged in the above-mentioned boastful prattle. Jayatarama's definition was used to separate the wheat from the chaff. Within the school of yoga, only those who had mastered *pranayama* and thus *kumbhaka* were invited to make statements about the higher limbs and their related mystical states.

Even distribution of prana

The *Hatha Tatva Kaumudi* then describes the final effect of *pranayama*.[87] It declares that in *Kevala Kumbhaka* the *prana* is evenly spread all over the body. *Kevala Kumbhaka* is the pinnacle of *pranayama*. It is thought to occur spontaneously once the other forms of *pranayama* are mastered, and its non-occurrence should be taken as a hint that the other wilful and structured *pranayama* techniques, collectively referred to as *sahita kumbhaka*s, are still in need of continued attention. Patanjali, in his *Yoga Sutra*, calls *Kevala Kumbhaka*

86. *Jogapradipyaka of Jayatarama*, ed. Swami Mahesananda et al., Kaivalyadhama, Lonavla, 2006, p. 108
87. *Hatha Tatva Kaumudi of Sundaradeva* LIV.67

the fourth *pranayama* (*chaturtha*),[88] which automatically leads to *samadhi*. According to the *Hatha Tatva Kaumudi*, in the samadhic state *prana* will not accumulate in some areas of the body and be depleted in others, but will spread evenly. This is due to the lack of mental activity. It is the mind and the conditioning that cause an uneven distribution of *prana* throughout the body. Compare this with the fact that the Ayurvedic texts describe the mind (*adhi*) as the root cause of all diseases (*vyadhi*).[89] The mind in its normal state not only prevents *samadhi* but also causes diseases in the body and ultimately brings about its destruction.

VAYUS

In some older texts such as the already quoted *Taittiriya Upanishad* the term *vayu* is used instead of *prana* as meaning life force. However in the last few thousand years the term *vayu* in yogic literature implies a subdivision of the life force, *prana*, into 10 vital airs, which we could call sub-*pranas*. Unfortunately one of these sub-*pranas* is called *prana*, which leads to some confusion. In this text the life force is therefore called *prana* throughout, whereas when the vital air *prana* is talked about it is dubbed *prana vayu*.

Of the ten so-called *vayus* (vital airs) five are considered primary (*prana vayu, apana, samana, udana, vyana*) and the other five secondary (*naga, krkara, kurma, devadatta, dhananjaya*). Of these we need to concern ourselves mainly with *prana, apana* and *samana*. These *vayus* are important to us in regard to three areas: meditation, health / life extension and Kundalini-raising. I will cover them in sequence:

Vayus and meditation

Prana vayu is associated with inhalation and intake whereas *apana vayu* is related to exhalation and elimination. *Apana* also powers urination, defecation, menstruation, ejaculation and delivery of the foetus during childbirth. It is thus a downward movement whereas *prana*

88. *Yoga Sutra* II.51
89. Vedic branch of medicine

is an upward movement. Compare for example the rising of the chest during inhalation (*prana*) and the dropping of the thorax during exhalation (*apana*). However, keen meditators will have noticed that the inhalation, although raising the chest, starts at the nostrils and terminates at the perineum. Correspondingly, following the exhalation with your awareness will lead you from the pelvic floor up to the nostrils, where the air leaves the body. Hence during inhalation and exhalation there is both an upward and a downward movement present.

This is confirmed by the *pranayama* researcher Shrikrishna, member of Kaivalyadhama, who says that the subtle movement of *prana* is the reverse of the gross breath.[90] He explains that during inhalation there is a downward flow (called *apana gati*). Correspondingly, during the gross exhalation there is an energetic upward flow (called *prana gati*). To make matters trickier, he points out that in some yogic texts the words *prana* and *apana* are simply equated with breath and in others with the subtle energy flow (*gati*). This is why in some texts *prana* is described as a downward movement and in others as an upward movement. To feel and harness them both simultaneously, as they cross over, is one of the most powerful secrets of meditation. To do so, as you inhale feel how your gross breath fills your torso from the perineum to the throat while at the same time the subtle energy reaches from the nostrils down to the pelvic floor. This means that your awareness has to reach simultaneously up and down. Then feel how, upon exhaling, first the upper lobes of your lungs empty, then the chest drops and finally the abdomen contracts, whereas the subtle energy flow at the same time reaches from the perineum upwards towards the head. To keep feeling this dual movement is one of the most effective ways of quietening the mind.

Vayus and life extension

To study and ultimately master the movements of *apana* and *prana* has other important implications. The *Hatha Yoga Pradipika*, for

90. Shrikrishna, *Essence of Pranayama*, 2nd edn, Kaivalyadhama, Lonavla, 1996, p. 75

example, says that by pulling the *apana vayu* up and forcing the *prana vayu* down, the body of the yogi becomes as that of a 16-year-old.[91] Both *vayus* eventually lead to a depletion of life force as *prana vayu* is projected out of the body in an upward trajectory and *apana vayu* downwards. *Apana vayu* can be turned upwards through use of *Mula Bandha* and *Uddiyana Bandha* (see chapter on *bandhas*) and *prana vayu* can be directed downwards by application of *Jalandhara Bandha* and *Jihva Bandha*. By turning them around, the *vayus*, according to the scriptures, meet at the *Manipura Chakra*, where they are converted into *samana vayu* and absorbed into the solar pranic storehouse of the body. Such absorption of *prana* into the *Manipura Chakra* is thought to be responsible for yogic feats such as being interred for days or weeks and still being alive when dug out. Pilot Baba, for example, has shown that yogis can stay alive for a very long time even when cut off from an oxygen supply. This is not a new teaching: it is already contained in the most ancient *Upanishad*, the *Brhad Aranyaka*, which says that whoever increases *samana vayu* is beyond death. Note here the consistency of yogic tradition over many thousands of years.

Apart from absorbing *prana*, *apana* and *samana vayus* into the solar pranic storehouse, the slowing down of breath and heartbeat to such an extent that both become almost non-discernible is helpful. This capability has been shown by T. Krishnamacharya and others. Slowing down the heartbeat reduces oxygen consumption of the heart and increases time spent in *kumbhaka*. Slowing down the breath also increases the general life expectancy.

Vayus and Kundalini-raising

The third important area where the *vayus* are touched upon, after meditation and health / life extension, is the role of the *apana vayu* as motor for Kundalini-rousing. Apart from *apana*, the primary *vayus* either move upwards (*prana vayu*, *udana vayu*) or are direction neutral (*samana* and *vyana vayus*). It is the *apana vayu*, through its strong

91. *Hatha Yoga Pradipika* II.47

downward flow, that is mainly responsible for depletion of life force and for keeping us chained to our animal nature. *Apana* often also has a strong influence on language, leading to excessive use of faecal and sexual expressions. According to yoga, if *apana* is turned up we can leave our animalistic side behind and embrace the Divine.

This driving up of Kundalini is caused by the mingling of *prana* and *apana* in *kumbhaka* at the *Manipura Chakra*. This is a popular theme in ancient texts. Sage Yajnavalkya explained to his wife, Gargi, that *apana* has to be sent on an upward trajectory by means of applying *Mula Bandha* in *Siddhasana*.[92] Once it arrives at the *Manipura Chakra* (the fire *chakra*), the fire needs to be stoked by drawing *prana vayu* down. The fire will then burn the tail of the serpent Kundalini and, moved by the dual force of *apana vayu* and fire, the serpent will rise through the *chakras*. Sage Vasishta also says that Kundalini is awakened through *apana* with fire and that it moves up like a cobra.[93]

Raghuvira goes into more detail in his *Kumbhaka Paddhati*,[94] a scripture entirely devoted to *pranayama*. He states that mastery over *apana* (*apana jaya*) will produce mastery over *mula bandha* (root lock), *mudras* (energy seals), *dharana* (concentration), *agni* (fire), the raising of Kundalini and an increase in *sattva guna* (intelligence).

A few explanations here: Mastery of *apana* (vital down current) and *mula bandha* (root lock) is close to synonymous. One will lead to mastery over the other. Mastery over *apana* will lead to the stoking of *agni* (fire). A strong *agni* will burn toxins and thus increase health. A strong *agni* combined with an upturned *apana* will rouse Kundalini. When a disciplined practitioner makes Kundalini rise it will make the yogi capable of practising *dharana* (concentration) and after that the other higher limbs.

It needs to be understood that the term Kundalini in the more modern scriptures (i.e. those of the *Kali Yuga*) stands for what Patanjali meant by *dharana*. During Patanjali's age (*Dvapara Yuga*) humanity

92. *Yoga Yajnavalkya* XII.1ff
93. *Vasishta Samhita* II.17–18
94. *Kumbhaka Paddhati of Raghuvira* stanzas 57–59

was more intellectually and philosophically inclined. In that age Patanjali's definition of *dharana* as the ability to bind the mind to one place for three hours was universally accepted.[95] In our current age, *Kali Yuga*, people are much more physically inclined; hence yogis looked for an interpretation of the term *dharana* that involved physical phenomena.

Yogis observed that *dharana*, i.e. binding the mind to a sattvic (sacred) meditation object for three hours, was possible only when the *prana* was raised to the higher *chakras*. If *prana* is limited to the lower *chakras* then one will express oneself in terms of survival (*Muladhara Chakra*), sexual identity (*Svadhishthana Chakra*) or assimilation of wealth, food and objects (*Manipura Chakra*). *Prana*, when rising, is named Kundalini. The physically oriented yogis of the *Kali Yuga* now looked for ways to raise Kundalini in order to empower *dharana*.

Among the chief ways of raising Kundalini are the path of air and the path of fire or the use of both simultaneously. 'Path of fire' means purifying and stoking *agni* (fire), and we will concern ourselves with that later. 'Path of air' means turning the *apana vayu* up and using it as a motor to force Kundalini up. Remember that *apana* is the only *vayu* current that points down, albeit strongly so. If it is turned upwards, all the *vayus* together will suck up Kundalini like a giant vacuum cleaner, and it is this that is referred to as the path of air. The *Yoga Kundalini Upanishad* says that *apana*, which normally flows downward, must be raised up by means of *Mula bandha*.[96] The *Upanishad* continues to say that *apana* rising up will mix with *agni* and together they will rise to the *Manipura Chakra*.[97] Here they will unite with *prana vayu* (vital up current) and Kundalini, being sucked up by the *vayus* and ignited by *agni* (note that the English word *ignite* is derived from the Sanskrit *agni* = fire), will rise up through the *sushumna*.[98] This, in a nutshell, is the method to achieve *dharana* as

95. *Yoga Sutra* III.1
96. *Yoga Kundalini Upanishad* I.64
97. *Yoga Kundalini Upanishad* I.65
98. *Yoga Kundalini Upanishad* I.66–67

described in the more modern yoga *shastras* (scriptures). However, it only clothes the ancient concepts in a more modern language. For example the term *sushumna*, the central energy channel – the path for the ascent of Kundalini – was already used in the *Chandogya Upanishad*,[99] which predates the *Yoga Sutras* by centuries.

I have explained this in some detail to show that there is not, as some Western scholars argue, a yoga of the Vedic seers, then a different yoga of the ancient *Upanishads*, then a classical yoga of Patanjali and then a more modern yoga of the *Hatha Yoga* texts. This is not the case. Over thousands of years there is a continuous, congruent tradition of sages and *siddhas* who had the same mystical experience. What changed was the audience and its capacity to understand the teachings. Hence the one teaching of yoga was clothed in different languages and adapted using different methods to bring the same mystical experience to an audience whose make-up had changed as the millennia went by.

99. *Chandogya Upanishad* XIII.6.6

SVARA AND NADI BALANCE

I consider this the most important chapter in the book, because somebody who really understands it would be insane not to go on and practise *pranayama*. The reason for writing this book is, after all, to get you to go beyond *asana* and practise *pranayama* too.

Imagine how great it would be to have a switch that, when operated, would enable you to consciously choose between your right and left brain hemispheres, intuitive and analytical intelligence, sympathetic and parasympathetic nervous systems, fight/flight reflex and rest/relaxation, and between the male and female, solar and lunar, aspects of your psyche. How great it would be if, when required, you could switch from being compassionate to doggedly determined. Or from charged with energy to completely relaxed within a few minutes. Or from extrovert (physically present, expressive and outgoing) to introvert (reflective and absorbing) within a short time. This switch does in fact exist and it is not at all hidden. It is the prominently protruding olfactory orifice right in the middle of your face: your nose.

How can that be? you may ask. Let's start right at the very beginning. Before the Big Bang and before the appearance of time and space, heaven and earth, mind and matter, only infinite consciousness existed. In yoga we call infinite consciousness Brahman, deep reality. Because it forms the deepest layer of reality, it cannot be reduced any further to elementary particles. It is reality itself. In the *Purusha Sukta* of the *Rig Veda* it is said, 'In the beginning there was darkness only. In this darkness the One silently breathed.' This means that the first sign that there was a God was in fact God's breath. God, then, in order to be able to create the universe, became polar. The infinite consciousness (Brahman) crystallized into a male and a female pole, in many yogic schools called Shiva and Shakti.

And right here is the fundamental truth of *pranayama*. The two poles of creation, the male and female poles of the cosmos, are represented

44

in the hemispheres of the body and brain of the individual, and are associated with the right and left nostrils respectively.[100] In yoga they are called the solar nostril or Pingala (the right one) and the lunar nostril or Ida (the left one).

RIGHT AND LEFT BRAIN HEMISPHERES
The right brain hemisphere, which is more intuitive and holistic, is powered by the left nostril. The left brain hemisphere, which is more analytical and dissecting, is powered by breathing through the right nostril. Try it out: Study an academically difficult subject such as law, medicine or physics and see how far you get when breathing through the left nostril. You are far better at memorizing and dissecting difficult subjects when breathing through the right nostril.[101] Obviously, when studying too much you will become unbalanced, as you keep using the same part of your brain and *nadi* system over and over again.

Then undertake another experiment and try to be empathic and compassionate to the woes and suffering of another being when breathing through the male, analytical right nostril. It won't work. You will, like a computer, analyse what they are doing wrong and suggest improvements to their current strategy. That is not what is needed in this situation. Instead, they need your listening, understanding and empathy to heal and feel the nurturing, human traits that are powered by the left nostril.

Or try to understand complex poetry, music or paintings. You need to holographically feel all the many dimensions that the author felt to really appreciate a great artwork. Feel how all of this becomes suddenly possible when you do use the left nostril, which enables you to sit back, relax, zoom out of a narrow view and receive complex connections, which are far greater than you.

A complete, integrated human being is not just 100% male or female but, depending on circumstance, is capable of activating either male

100. *Shiva Svarodaya* stanza 52
101. *Shiva Svarodaya* stanza 114

or female circuits of their psyche and thus their capabilities. This is reflected in the Indian image of Ardhanarishvara. It is an androgynous form of Lord Shiva and his female aspect, Devi Parvati (Shakti), the god that is half woman and half man.

SYMPATHETIC AND PARASYMPATHETIC NERVOUS SYSTEMS
The next dualistic pair we will look at is the sympathetic and parasympathetic branches of the nervous system. The sympathetic nervous system governs the fight-or-flight reflex. It is activated through stress and, by emitting adrenalin, it mobilises your energy resources. It is activated through the right, solar, male nostril. When breathing through the right nostril you will be able to perform strenuous physical tasks like fighting for your life against foes, running from danger as fast as you can or lifting heavy stones to erect pyramids.[102]

If it is that effective, why don't we always breathe through the right nostril? Because overemphasizing the sympathetic nervous system will cause us to burn out. It is good for short bursts of energy but, if we overemphasise it, we will become irate, suffer insomnia and tend to develop a type-A personality. Not to mention that we will have only 50% of the capabilities of a complete, integrated human being.

The parasympathetic nervous system enables us to recharge, rest and sleep, and experience pleasure. It is activated by breathing through the left nostril. Your work breaks will become more effective when breathing through this nostril. You will find more enjoyment in spending time with friends and loved ones, going to the beach or walking in nature when breathing through this nostril. Nursing and caring for a child will come more naturally when breathing through the left nostril. Try it out.

Whatever subject you speak about, if you need to address a large audience you need to do so while breathing through the right nostril. The right nostril governs efferent (outgoing) nerve impulses such as the ones used when speaking, working with your hands,

102. *Shiva Svarodaya* stanza 115

running, defecating, urinating or when being the active partner during sexual intercourse. However, breathing too much through the right nostril can give people the impression that you like the sound of your own voice, or that you are too physical or cannot surrender when that becomes appropriate. It is hard to see your own mistakes or shortcomings when breathing through the right nostril.

AFFERENT AND EFFERENT NERVE CURRENTS

The left nostril governs the afferent (incoming) nerve impulses. When you need to listen, see, feel, smell or taste, use the left nostril. Use this nostril also when reflecting on yourself or wanting to be self-critical. Afferent also means being receptive. During the moment of conception it is essential that at least the female breathe through the left nostril because she is receiving the spirit of the child into her womb. Some cultures went even further. In the case of some Australian Aboriginal and African tribes the male left the village to receive the child through dreaming. This is a typical lunar, left-nostril function, and it shows maturity of a culture if a fully initiated and integrated male can enter what normally would be considered the female domain to receive and embrace new life.

The afferent (incoming) nerve current, however, can also be too dominant and this will express itself by one being overly introverted, meek, not expressive enough, possibly even depressive, and not being able to stand up for oneself. This can be effectively counteracted through activating the efferent (outgoing) current by inhaling through the solar, right nostril.

CATABOLIC AND ANABOLIC FUNCTION

Catabolism is the metabolic breakdown of complex molecules into simple ones. It happens during digestion of food. When eating and breaking down food in the stomach, breathe through the right nostril. Similarly to powering an analytical, dissecting solar mind, use of the right nostril also powers the breakdown of food in the digestive tract. Anabolism is the metabolic synthesis of simple molecules into complex ones. It is what we colloquially call recovery, rest and nurturing. It takes place mainly during sleep and relaxation, and it is powered by the left, lunar nostril. Assimilating the broken-down elements of food is done more effectively when breathing through the left nostril. That is why around 90 minutes after food intake the *svara* (flow) should ideally switch to the left nostril.

It is because of the anabolic/nurturing character of the lunar nostril and the breaking down / catabolic character of the solar nostril that Raghuvira says in his *Kumbhaka Paddhati* that movement of *prana* in Ida (left nostril) is called nectar, while that in Pingala (right nostril) is called poison.[103] With the tools given so far you will understand this otherwise surprising statement. You will also understand Sundaradeva's claim that the right nostril burns morbidities through heat (a catabolic breakdown).[104]

Note that the metabolic/physical function of each nostril is also related to its mental function. We could call the lunar mind anabolic in that it is nurturing, absorbing and synthesizing. The solar mind is catabolic in that it breaks down by means of dissecting arguments and analyses structures by breaking them down into their constituents. Whereas the solar mind is able to zoom in and dissect / break down a picture into minute details, the lunar mind can synthesise missing contexts and zoom out until the whole is seen. Choose your nostril according to which function is required at any given time.

BODY OR MIND

You may also activate the respective *svara* (nostril flow) according to whether you need to activate your body or your mind. Sundaradeva states in his *Hatha Tatva Kaumudi* that *prana*, the life force (i.e. the body), resides in the right nostril, while *manas* (the mind) dwells in the left nostril. He calls this revelation the great secret.[105] However, it is not a secret any more if we take into consideration the previous

103. *Kumbhaka Paddhati of Raghuvira* stanza 14
104. *Hatha Tatva Kaumudi of Sundaradeva* XXXVI.27
105. *Hatha Tatva Kaumudi of Sundaradeva* XXIII.38

paragraph on afferent and efferent nerve currents. When the left nostril is predominant, afferent currents rule, which are those that carry sensual impressions back to the mind to be analysed. In other words the left nostril activates the mind. When the right nostril flows, efferent (outgoing) nerve currents are predominant. This presupposes that the mind has come to a conclusion and the nerves now carry the mind's signals outwards to activate a physical response. This means that the right nostril activates the body. For this reason the *shastras* (scriptures) state that during strenuous physical activity the right nostril should be activated.

HEALTH THROUGH SVARA

You will also be able to vastly improve your health by mastering the *svara* (flow). Sundaradeva says in his *Hatha Tatva Kaumudi* that disorders caused by aggravated *pitta* are to be treated by breathing through the left nostril, whereas diseases caused through aggravated *vata* and *kapha* subside when breathing through Surya, the right nostril.[106] Additionally there are *pranayama* techniques dedicated to altering your *dosha* constitution. *Shitali pranayama* reduces *pitta*, while *Surya Bhedana pranayama* increases it when required. *Chandra Bhedana*, *Shitali* and *Sitkari* increase *kapha* and reduce *pitta*, while *Ujjayi* reduces *kapha* and increases *pitta*. According to yoga *shastra*, *Bhastrika* reduces and expels all three *dosha*s and thus creates a balance between them. All of these techniques will be explained in detail in their respective chapters.

ACTIVITIES RELATED TO NOSTRIL PREPONDERANCE

Breathing through the appropriate nostril when performing particular activities is said to lead to success. The *Vasishta Samhita* says one should breathe through the right nostril during sexual intercourse (in the case of the male), eating, amassing wealth and participating in martial activity.[107] Notice the penetrating, devouring and aggressive

106. *Hatha Tatva Kaumudi of Sundaradeva* X.33
107. *Vasishta Samhita* V.46

49

nature of all of these activities. The authoritative text on this particular matter is considered to be the *Shiva Svarodaya*, and it would be
worthwhile for everybody interested in *pranayama* to study it deeply.
This text says that obtaining nourishment,[108] giving birth and
dying,[109] and keeping wealth in security need to be done when breathing through the left nostril. Notice the nurturing and surrendering
character of these activities. Other right-nostril activities, according
to the *Shiva Svarodaya*, include researching things that are difficult to
understand (such as science, which is a male, dissecting activity),[110]
studying the scriptures (again analytical, dissecting intelligence),[111]
performing the *shatkarmas* (destroying impurities), teaching or influ-
encing others (a penetrating activity) and mercantile activities like
trading (again analytical).

Yoga should generally be practised during the left *svara* (flow
through Ida) according to the *Shiva Svarodaya*. Yoga is about nurturing
the relationship with the Divine and your true self. It is successful
during left *svara* and inauspicious during right *svara*. This view is supported by Sundaradeva, who says that all *pranayamas* need to start
with the left nostril, while they are useless when initiated through the
toxin- and heat-producing right nostril.[112] He also says that he is a yogi
who always practises through the lunar (left) nostril, which controls
amrita, thus attaining the elusive nectar of immortality.[113]

Summarizing, when studying scripture and analysing yogic technique, such as by reading this book, you need to breathe through
the right nostril because your mind needs to activate its dissecting,
catabolic function. However, once you have digested the rather abstract
content of this book, switch to the left nostril and activate your female
psyche. You will then be able to zoom out, put all of the various
pieces of the puzzle together and assimilate them as a whole. When

108. *Shiva Svarodaya* stanza 104
109. *Shiva Svarodaya* stanza 106
110. *Shiva Svarodaya* stanza 81
111. *Shiva Svarodaya* stanza 116
112. *Hatha Tatva Kaumudi of Sundaradeva* XXXVII.4
113. *Hatha Tatva Kaumudi of Sundaradeva* XLI V.47

practising yogic technique your mind needs to synthesize, put together and function anabolically, so breathe through the left nostril.

We will turn now to the third *svara*, the middle one. This *svara* powers yogic and mystical experience, and while in this state you should do nothing but practise yoga and meditation.[114]

THE BALANCED SVARA OR MIDDLE BREATH

A Tibetan lama with whom I used to study told me that plain meditation without any additional aid would take on average 300 lifetimes to lead to success. I have no way of verifying this statement, but a *pranayama* master might well have uttered it. The core idea of *pranayama* is that meditation is almost a waste of time if it does not take place when the middle *svara* is predominant, that is when *sushumna*, the central *nadi* flows. When *sushumna* flows, however, you can cover ground in meditation that would otherwise take years.

In a state of average health, unstressed and not exposed to any extreme climate, extreme emotions or any other extreme influences, each nostril will be open for approximately 60 to 90 minutes, which corresponds to the fact that brain hemisphere activity generally switches with the same rhythm.[115] But if one switches from one side to the other after approximately 1 to 4 minutes, a balance between both nostrils occurs. This is referred to as the middle *svara* or *sushumna*. The middle *svara* acts as a junction (*sandhi*) between Ida and Pingala. Like the junctions between inhalation and exhalation, waking and sleeping, night and day, dream and deep sleep, life and death, day and night, this junction also suspends for a moment the mind, which casts its fabric of appearance over reality. During this moment of suspension we might be able to look through the coarse texture of the fabric and see the underlying deep reality (Brahman). While the brief junction offers the most auspicious moments for meditation, the penultimate aim of *pranayama* is to extend the middle *svara* for many hours and eventually days to enable the

114. *Shiva Svarodaya* stanza 130
115. Swami Muktibodhananda, *Swara Yoga*, Yoga Publication Trust, Munger, 1984, p. 91

mind to settle profoundly within deep reality, a state that yoga calls objectless *samadhi*.

The balance and finally suspension of both Ida and Pingala leads to the drawing of *prana* into the central energy channel, *sushumna*. According to many yogic schools and scriptures, balance between Ida and Pingala, anabolic and catabolic functions, right and left brain hemisphere, parasympathetic and sympathetic nervous systems, afferent and efferent currents, *manas Shakti* and *prana Shakti*, is of paramount importance to the mystical experience.

A disclaimer here: As great as *sushumna* flow (middle *svara*) is for spiritual exultation, it can provide little for worldly aspirations. The reader must not be duped into believing that mystical insight automatically comes with or leads to material wealth. The *Shiva Svarodaya* says that during times of the middle *svara* no worldly profit can be obtained.[116] In fact if you do perform any commercial activity during that *svara* you are likely to lose everything, as proper judgment is suspended.

You won't become charismatic through middle *svara* either: according to Swami Muktibodhananda one is in fact less likely to captivate people during *sushumna* flow.[117] Conversely, we can deduce that whenever somebody appears charismatic it is definitely not *sushumna* that is flowing but Pingala (the right nostril). Being charismatic means that you get access to somebody else's mental software. It's a code-breaking activity, which requires the flow of the male, penetrating Pingala. A mystic with the middle *svara* flowing couldn't care less about captivating people.

Muktibodhananda also informs us that during *sushumna* flow both spiritual and criminal tendencies may emerge.[118] The important lesson here is that middle *svara* is helpful only during spiritual practice. Certainly do not make any business decisions or any other decisions that require reasoning during *sushumna* flow: all of these

116. *Shiva Svarodaya* stanza 124
117. Swami Muktibodhananda, *Swara Yoga*, Yoga Publication Trust, Munger, 1984, p. 97
118. Swami Muktibodhananda, *Swara Yoga*, Yoga Publication Trust, Munger, 1984, p. 56

capacities are suspended. If you find while driving that your middle *svara* starts to flow, pull over and start meditating.

But this suspension of mind is exactly what powers the mystical state. Through *pranayama* you can learn when to bring on the mystical state in an appropriate moment and to leave it behind when using the left or right *svara* seems more appropriate. Mind and the five senses operate through the left nostril. *Prana*, the creative life force, and the five organs of action (locomotion, grasping, speech, procreation and defecation) express themselves through the right nostril. Consciousness, the true self, is activated and accessed through the central channel. Use each one at appropriate times.

HOW TO ALTER SVARA

Having talked at length about selecting the appropriate *svara*, I will describe here a selection of methods to change the *svara*, i.e. to change from left to right or right to left nostril respectively. Please note that a side effect of *pranayama* practice will be that you become aware at all times where your *svara* is, and this will generally enable you to postpone activities that are inappropriate for that *svara*. *Pranayama* will also condition your nervous system in such a way that certain activities will tend automatically to bring on a switch to the appropriate *svara*. Not surprisingly, this tendency exists naturally in highly successful people.

In order to change the *svara* we need to first be aware on which side it is. For this purpose close one nostril and breathe through the other and then change sides. You will notice that on one side there is much more friction while the opposite nostril is wide open. The *svara* is on the side of the open nostril. Experienced yogis are aware at all times on which side the *svara* is.

An easy method consists of simply lying on your right side, and after a few minutes you will feel how the upper nostril opens and most air will pass through it. Another common method is to press a trigger point in one's armpit to suppress the nostril on the same side and to open or activate the nostril on the other side. For example you would press the trigger point in your right armpit to suppress Pingala, the right nostril, and open Ida, the left nostril. You can use your hand to do so but you may also use the backrest of a chair. Traditionally yogis used a so-called *yoga danda* (yogic staff), which is a short crutch-like device to change the *svara*. Images of Lord Shiva, the divine yogi, often depict him resting his arm on such a *yoga danda*.

You may also use your knee as a substitute for the *yoga danda*. Assume a *Marichyasana A*-like posture and then press the knee into the armpit to open the opposite nostril. Advanced yogis may use a posture called *Ekapada Yogadandasana* to achieve the same end. Here the thigh is extremely rotated externally and the foot placed into the corresponding armpit to change the *svara* to the opposite nostril. Be careful: Do not attempt this posture unless you have exceptional levels of external hip rotation. Another simple method for effectively changing the *svara* would be plugging with cotton wool the nostril opposite to the one that you want to have open.

You may also, for example, change the *svara* to the right by pressing the left elbow into the left abdomen with fingers outstretched. Additional techniques are described in Jayatarama's *Jogapradipyaka*.[119]

As easy as it is to change from the left to the right nostril and vice versa, accessing the middle *svara* – apart from the few minutes when it automatically flows between changing brain hemispheres – is much more difficult. Apart from an act of grace through the Divine, the middle *svara* can be permanently and voluntarily accessed through the process of purifying the *nadi*s, generally called *Nadi Shuddhi* and *Nadi Shodhana*. These almost synonymous terms stand for alternate nostril breathing. Done without *kumbhaka*, it constitutes the definite prerequisite to start *kumbhaka* practice. If done with *kumbhaka*, it comprises *pranayama*'s quintessential technique. You will find a detailed account of the technique for both methods in the chapter on *nadi* purification. *Sushumna* can also be accessed by using

119. *Jogapradipyaka of Jayatarama,* ed. Swami Mahesananda et al., Kaivalyadhama, Lonavla, 2006, p. 15

two *yoga danda*s at the same time, thus suppressing Ida and Pingala simultaneously. If you do not happen to have two *yoga danda*s at hand, a rather trying method to access *sushumna* would be to enter *Dvipada Yogadandasana.* In this posture the left foot is inserted into the left armpit and the right foot into the right armpit. This makes for a very uncomfortable position, and I doubt that one would enjoy *sushumna* for long using this access method.

KUMBHAKA

Kumbhaka (breath retention) is so central to *pranayama* that many ancient texts use the term *kumbhaka* instead of *pranayama*. The *Hatha Yoga Pradipika*, for example, mentions eight types of *kumbhakas* and does not consider techniques that do not contain breath retentions as *pranayama*. The *Vasishta Samhita* clearly defines *pranayama* as involving *kumbhaka*, and any technique that consists of just *puraka* (inhalation) and *rechaka* (exhalation) as not *pranayama*.[120]

Alternate nostril breathing without *kumbhaka* is treated by Vasishta as a prerequisite to *pranayama* that everybody has to go through. Vasishta precisely defines *pranayama* as (internal) *kumbhaka* with mental concentration on focal points such as the navel, toes, third eye.[121] The *Mandala Brahmana Upanishad*, too, defines *pranayama* as consisting not only of inhalation and exhalation but of *kumbhaka* as well.[122] Patanjali's *Yoga Sutra* defines *pranayama* as smoothing the flow of inhalation and exhalation,[123] internal, external, mid-way[124] and spontaneous suspension of breath.[125] Summarizing, there are authorities who equate *pranayama* with *kumbhaka* and there are those who say *kumbhaka* is *pranayama*'s most essential ingredient. What both groups have in common is that they hold *kumbhaka* in high regard.

DISAMBIGUATION OF KUMBHAKA FROM HOLDING ONE'S BREATH

Kumbhaka has as little to do with holding one's breath as *asana* is limited to stretching. Outsiders to yoga sometimes say they cannot see themselves practising yoga because they are not flexible, and as an *asana* teacher one often gets confronted with tales of gymnasts,

120. *Vasishta Samhita* III.28
121. *Vasishta Samhita* III.34
122. *Mandala Brahmana Upanishad* I.1
123. *Yoga Sutra* II.49
124. *Yoga Sutra* II.50
125. *Yoga Sutra* II.51

dancers or contortionists who would do really well at yoga. But the people who suggest this miss the point. Excess flexibility is an obstacle to yoga, and *asana* is not about getting into more and more distorted-looking postures, but about the transformation of body and mind in the process of getting there. Similarly, when one teaches *pranayama* invariably one is confronted with tales of free divers who can hold their breath for an eternity, and again this misses the point of yoga. Holding the breath is only the coarsest and most superficial layer of the process of *kumbhaka*, albeit the one most visible to the non-discerning observer. Let me list here the conditions that must be met for breath-holding to constitute *kumbhaka*. The practitioner needs to sit in a traditional meditation *asana*, such as *Siddhasana* or *Padmasana*.

When *kumbhaka* exceeds 10 seconds, the *bandha*s, i.e. *Jalandhara*, *Mula* and *Uddiyana bandha*, need to be applied. The eyes need to be closed and internally focused on a particular spot and the mind must be focused on a suitable yogic (sacred) object. Alternatively the eyes may be half-closed and either locked in *Shambhavi Mudra* or gazing at a sacred object in front of the yogi. The length of all inhalations, retentions and exhalations must be counted to such an extent that their ratio to each other follows precisely a predetermined count (such as 1:4:2) and a predetermined number of rounds is practised. For example if a *kumbhaka* of a certain length is practised and the yogini is not capable of completing the related exhalation because she has to gasp for air, then any yogic merit is lost as no fixation of *prana* can take place. In *kumbhaka* the practitioner learns to extract large amounts of *prana* by becoming receptive to subtle energy streams in the body, by concentration and by *bandha*s. Without this sensitivity, *pranayama* cannot succeed. *Kumbhaka* is a tool to slowly gain mastery over *prana* and with it eventually mastery over mind, because it is *prana* that powers mind. *Kumbhaka* is not athletic breath-holding for the mere sake of it. I repeat: *kumbhaka* takes place only if its length and count can be repeated over and over again and each exhalation can be sustained to exactly the predetermined length.

PURPOSE OF KUMBHAKA

According to Patanjali, the practice of *pranayama* makes the flow of *prana* smooth and even, which correlates with a calm and collected mind. Practice of volitional *pranayama* techniques eventually leads to *Kevala Kumbhaka*, called *Chaturtah* by Patanjali, which automatically leads to *samadhi*. He adds, however, that, long before that state is reached, *pranayama* enables the mind to achieve *pratyahara* (withdrawal of the senses, fifth limb)[126] and prepares it for *dharana* (concentration, sixth limb).[127]

The medieval *Hatha* texts see additional effects of *kumbhaka*. Sundaradeva states in his *Hatha Tatva Kaumudi* that *kumbhaka* is instrumental in rousing Shakti, i.e. Kundalini.[128] As previously explained, Kundalini is nothing but the motor for *dharana*. The ancient sages were silent about Kundalini because during their ages (i.e. *Satya*, *Treta* and *Dvapara yuga*s) practitioners were still able to access *dharana* without taking recourse to Kundalini methods. Due to attachment to the body and the functions of the lower *chakras* during the current *Kali Yuga*, the powerful force of Kundalini has to be utilised to lift awareness to the higher *chakras*, which enable *dharana*.

Sundaradeva also states that time has no pertinence in *kumbhaka*,[129] a fact that is already outlined in the *Hatha Yoga Pradipika*. This indicates that the yogi in *kumbhaka* is in a timeless and hence deathless state. Sundaradeva and many other authors say that, if during the predetermined time of a yogi's death he is in *kumbhaka*, death cannot reach him. Time is created by the mind in the form of Ida and Pingala, and if both are suspended time is suspended too.[130]

Kumbhaka may also be used for absorption and fixation of *prana*. The fixated *prana* can then be distributed to areas of chronic depletion. For this reason it has great health benefits. The *Hatha Yoga Pradipika* states that, during internal *kumbhaka*, *prana* should be

126. *Yoga Sutra* II.54
127. *Yoga Sutra* II.53
128. *Hatha Tatva Kaumudi of Sundaradeva* XLIV.61
129. *Hatha Tatva Kaumudi of Sundaradeva* XL.55
130. *Hatha Yoga Pradipika* IV.17

fixated in a diseased organ to cure that organ from its ailment.[131] The *Yoga Rahasya* goes even further by declaring that *prana* must be directed into the *chakra*s to increase the span of life and reduce the likelihood of illness.[132]

TYPES OF KUMBHAKA

Kumbhaka is firstly divided into *Sahita* and *Kevala*. *Kevala Kumbhaka* is the goal of *pranayama*. It is a spontaneous suspension of *prana*, which accompanies or invokes *samadhi*. It is described towards the end of this book in a chapter of the same name. *Kevala Kumbhaka* occurs once *Sahita Kumbhaka* is mastered. *Sahita Kumbhaka* means the wilful and formal effort to time *kumbhaka* in relation to inhalations and exhalations. *Sahita Kumbhaka* is then again subdivided according to where the breath is retained, that is outside, inside or midway, with the latter being much more uncommon nowadays. Suspending the breath after an exhalation is called external (*bahya*) *kumbhaka* whereas suspending the breath after an inhalation is called internal (*antara*) *kumbhaka*.

Some teachers hold that internal retention needs to be mastered first, while others teach first external retention. Many yogic treatises such as the *Vasishta Samhita* talk only about internal *kumbhaka*.[133] However, it is *bahya kumbhaka* that is explicitly mentioned in Patanjali's *Yoga Sutra* as a means of clearing the mind.[134] Both the *Hatha Yoga Pradipika*[135] and the *Hatha Tatva Kaumudi*[136] ascribe mastery of Raja Yoga (i.e. objectless *samadhi*) to external *kumbhaka*. Both types of *kumbhaka* are also mentioned in the *Brhadyogi Yajnvalkya Smrti*.[137]

Nathamuni's *Yoga Rahasya* advises the practice of both types of

131. *Hatha Yoga Pradipika*, Kaivalyadhama edn V.19–23
132. M.M. Gharote et al. (eds), *Therapeutic References in Traditional Yoga Texts*, Lonavla Yoga Institute, Lonavla, 2010, p. 192
133. Swami Digambarji et al. (eds) *Vasishta Samhita (Yoga Kanda)*, Kaivalyadhama, Lonavla, 1984, p. 21
134. *Yoga Sutra* I.34
135. *Hathapradipika* (10 chapters) IV.67
136. *Hatha Tatva Kaumudi of Sundaradeva* XLIV.60
137. *Brhadyogi Yajnvalkya Smrti* VIII.20–21

kumbhaka,[138] but states that certain benefits such as purification and activation of the 2nd and 3rd *chakras*, *Svadhishthana* and *Manipura*, can be obtained only through *bahya kumbhaka*.[139] The importance of this information cannot be overstated. Other texts like the *Brhadyogi Yajnavalkya Smrti* also talk about the importance of *bahya kumbhaka*. According to Swami Niranjanananda, one of the important differences between internal and external *kumbhaka* is that internal *kumbhaka* (especially when practised with *Mula* and *Jalandhara bandhas*) triggers the parasympathetic nervous system, whereas the external *kumbhaka* (particularly when practised with full external *Uddiyana*) brings the sympathetic nervous system to the fore.[140] Parasympathetic activity, however, slows down the heartbeat and lowers blood pressure and thus oxygen consumption, whereas sympathetic activity does the opposite. This is one of the reasons why external *kumbhaka* is more difficult to master. To practise both forms of *kumbhaka* in the same round of *pranayama*, however, leads to a balance between both branches of the nervous system. External *kumbhaka*s are also more difficult than internal ones as, during internal *kumbhaka*, your lungs are full of oxygen and *prana* can still be extracted. During external *kumbhaka*, your lungs are empty and therefore ask for an inhalation earlier.

I suggest the following approach: Learn first external *kumbhaka* with full external *Uddiyana Bandha* (*Bahya Uddiyana*) in *mudra*s such as *Yoga Mudra* and *Tadaga Mudra* and during *Nauli*. The advantage here is that you don't have to observe count. This means you can familiarise yourself with the technique without having to stay in *kumbhaka* for a predetermined time. The instruction for *kumbhaka* within a particular *mudra* is 'Hold to capacity'. That means you can come out of *kumbhaka* whenever your capacity is met. Then go on to learn internal *kumbhaka* within a *pranayama* setting, where you do have to observe count.

138. *Yoga Rahasya* II.49
139. *Yoga Rahasya* II.50
140. Swami Niranjanananda, *Prana and Pranayama*, Yoga Publications Trust, Munger, 2009, p. 146

Count means, for example, that you may inhale for 10 seconds, hold *kumbhaka* for 40 seconds and exhale for 20 seconds. Once you have attained a certain level of proficiency in internal *kumbhaka*, add external *kumbhaka*s into your *pranayama*. They will now pose less difficulty, as you have practised them already in *mudra*s. Additionally, external *kumbhaka*s may be learned in conjunction with *Bhastrika*. Due to the massive supply of oxygen that *Bhastrika* delivers, it appears more acceptable to suspend the breath with empty lungs. Once external *kumbhaka*s are mastered here, they can then be integrated into *Nadi Shodhana*. Either way, both *Bhastrika* and external *kumbhaka*s are not beginner techniques and must be learned under the guidance of an experienced and qualified teacher.

LENGTH OF KUMBHAKA

No book on *pranayama* would be complete without a discussion of *kumbhaka* length and its purpose. I have to admit that initially I was stupefied myself about descriptions of *kumbhaka*s lasting several minutes and even far beyond this, but it is surprising what worlds open up when one practises diligently for long enough. Analysing modern literature on the subject and the ancient yogic treatises, I found three different ranges of *kumbhaka* length. Modern authors who deal mainly with the health aspects of *kumbhaka* describe *kumbhaka*s up to 40 to 50 seconds in length. These *kumbhaka*s are accessible to all.

Serious modern spiritual adepts and the yogic scriptures describe *kumbhaka*s of around 2 or even 3 minutes. Such *kumbhaka*s are used to raise Kundalini, thus empowering meditation. Those employing them need to be firmly established in *asana*, *bandha*, *mudra*, *mitahara* (moderate diet), *yama*s and *niyama*s on a daily basis over a long time frame.

There is a third range of *kumbhaka* length, which extends to one or multiple hours or even far beyond that. These *kumbhaka*s not only are described in yogic scriptures but were also practised by some modern yoga masters, such as Trailanga Swami and Pilot Baba. They are used to lock the mind in *samadhi*. Please note, such *kumbhaka*s are not the only way to attain *samadhi*, but for some they are the method of choice. Let us have a closer look at these three ranges of *kumbhaka* length.

Firstly it needs to be said that considerations regarding *kumbhaka* length apply to all people evenly. The *Yoga Rahasya* ascribes the same respiratory rate to all people.[141] However, many different aspects concerning the environment and the individual need to be taken into consideration. Altitude will decrease the possible time spent in *kumbhaka*, as less oxygen is available. Increased humidity also decreases *kumbhaka* time, as it decreases oxygen uptake. High temperatures make it more difficult to cool the organism, which heats up in *kumbhaka*; hence in cold climates *kumbhaka* can be extended.

This is one of the reasons why yogis ascended into the crispy cold altitudes of the Himalayas. In the mid-1980s I trekked with an Indian Shaivite *sadhu* (religious ascetic) through the Himalayas towards the holy site of Muktinath, which has great significance for *sadhu*s. As we ascended higher and higher into the mountains every day, the nights grew increasingly crisp. A *sadhu* is not allowed to stay in closed human habitations and is also not allowed to wear the garments of civilization such as trousers. The only protections my *sadhu* had to shield him from the freezing Himalayan air was a thin cotton robe and a large shawl made from the same material. Come evening, we approached a human habitation within reach and asked for some food and permission to sleep on the veranda. After a while, not being bound by a religious vow I forsook my pride and joined the locals inside their house in the vicinity of a smouldering campfire.

Despite this – and my expensive Western-made doona sleeping bag – I was woken by the freezing cold. Sheepishly I ventured out into the open, half expecting to find my *sadhu* either frozen to an ice block or at least suffering from pneumonia. I was surprised to find he was absolutely fine. He told me he was used to keeping his body temperature stable overnight by use of *kumbhaka*. The colder the temperature, the longer *kumbhaka* needs to be to stabilise body

141. *Yoga Rahasya* I.57

temperature. At the same time these long *kumbhaka*s can be used to power meditation.

Other factors that need to be taken into consideration in regard to *kumbhaka* length are emotions and stimulants. Being emotional does expel *prana* and makes fixation of *prana* more difficult; hence it can entirely prevent practising *kumbhaka* or at least shorten its duration. Similarly, the consumption of stimulants such as coffee and alcohol expels *prana* and prevents long *kumbhaka*s. Stress, anxiety, anger, pain, guilt and shame also decrease *kumbhaka* length.

Thus it is very difficult, even for an experienced teacher from the outside, to determine the right length of *kumbhaka* for a student. However, these facts drive home the necessity for such a teacher to have the competence to give advice should a student ask for it or should adverse symptoms present themselves. *Pranayama* and *kumbhaka* cannot be learned from a book, and this book is not intended to replace a teacher, but is offered as additional support for teachers and students.

Even Sundaradeva, one of the most learned experts on *pranayama*, admits in his *Hatha Tatva Kaumudi* that it is difficult to say how long one needs to stay in *kumbhaka*. He suggests it can be determined by a wise person with keen intelligence by means of firm judgment.[142] In other words even a generally wise person with moderate intelligence and impaired judgment will not necessarily be up to the job. Nor will a person who is very intelligent, but who lacks wisdom and judgment, be able to determine it. The idea here is to proceed prudently and slowly until you are completely satisfied that you have thoroughly digested your current level of practice before you intensify it.

I have frequently heard advanced or established *asana* practitioners say that they just cannot practise *kumbhaka*. Inevitably this impression arose because *kumbhaka*s of excessive length were chosen too early. If such practitioners were to reduce their breath count by half and practise daily, they would suddenly find themselves able to

142. *Hatha Tatva Kaumudi of Sundaradeva* XXXVIII.75

perform *kumbhaka*s. But often this path is not chosen due to pride. The attitude here seems to be 'either really long *kumbhaka*s or none at all'. This is a shame, as it prevents us from harvesting the incredible gifts of *pranayama*. It is important to find a level of practice where you personally can be at ease and not one that is imposed from the outside by a teacher who forces you ahead too quickly. This will always backfire. Choose a teacher who does not have expectations about how long you should be able to hold *kumbhaka*.

The failure to continue one's *kumbhaka* practice comes from the inability to start slowly and stay with shorter *kumbhaka*s for longer. This ambition, which is considered normal in modern *asana* practice, will prevent any progress in *pranayama*. It is not by chance that *pranayama* is the fourth limb of yoga and thus seen as more advanced than *asana*.

The *Hatha Tatva Kaumudi* states that short *kumbhaka*s are used for the removal of demerit whereas long *kumbhaka*s are used for attaining emancipation.[143] This means that we will go through a purification process of a certain length during which shorter *kumbhaka*s are used to burn accumulated demerit such as *karma*. Once some progress is achieved in this process, *kumbhaka*s will automatically lengthen.

Noted yoga scholar Dr M.L. Gharote tells us that during normal breathing the respiratory rate is 15 per minute, which amounts to 4 seconds for each breathing cycle. This should be lowered in *pranayama* to 2 or 3 per minute, which can be achieved for example by inhaling for 5 seconds, retaining the air for 20 seconds and exhaling for 10 seconds.[144] The main technique of *pranayama* is to reduce one's respiratory rate slowly over time. After some years of daily practice, intense *kumbhaka*s are then reached, in which deep transformation is possible.

Ranjit Sen Gupta, author of *Pranayama: A Conscious Way of Breathing*, considers that *kumbhaka*s of 40 seconds are the maximum, but difficult

143. *Hatha Tatva Kaumudi of Sundaradeva* XXXVIII.136
144. M.L. Gharote, *Pranayama: The Science of Breath*, Lonavla Yoga Institute, Lonavla, 2003, p. 23

to achieve.[145] Andre Van Lysebeth considers *kumbhaka*s in excess of 40 seconds so intense that one should do them only straight after one's *asana* practice.[146] Dr K.S. Joshi, author of *Yogic Pranayama*, considers 50 seconds to be the maximum.[147]

These numbers are for a general audience, and they contrast with those given for initiates in the bulk of yogic texts – 48 seconds for inferior (*kanishta*) practice, 64 seconds for intermediate (*Madhyama*) practice and 80 seconds for intense (*uttama*) practice.[148] The notion of 80-second *kumbhaka* as the reasonable upper boundary is confirmed by Swami Niranjanananda, who suggests extending internal *kumbhaka* in *Nadi Shodhana* to 80 seconds before any other *pranayama*s are tackled.[149] He also advises practising *Nadi Shodhana* with an internal *kumbhaka* of 80 seconds and additionally an external *kumbhaka* of 40 seconds four times per day for at least 3 months before continuing on to other *pranayama*s.[150] This is quite a formidable practice and, if it were followed, only a handful of people would ever go past *Nadi Shodhana*. If we add up the lengths of time given by Swami Niranjanananda for both *kumbhaka*s we arrive at 120 seconds. Roughly the same number is suggested by Yogeshwaranand Paramahamsa, who talks of *kumbhaka* lengths of 120 seconds[151] and 128 seconds.[152] Almost the same length, 124 seconds, is given by the *pranayama* research author Shrikrishna as necessary to raise Kundalini.[153]

145. Ranjit Sen Gupta, *Pranayama: A Conscious Way of Breathing*, New Age Books, Delhi, 2000, p. 58
146. Andre van Lysebeth, *Die Grosse Kraft des Atems*, O.W. Barth, Bern, 1972, p. 98
147. Dr K.S. Joshi, *Yogic Pranayama*, Orient Paperbacks, Delhi, 1982, p. 80
148. *Jogapradipyaka of Jayatarama*, ed. Swami Mahesananda et al., Kaivalyadhama, Lonavla, 2006, p. 82
149. Swami Niranjanananda, *Prana and Pranayama*, Yoga Publications Trust, Munger, 2009, p. 224
150. Swami Niranjanananda, *Prana and Pranayama*, Yoga Publications Trust, Munger, 2009, p. 220
151. Yogeshwaranand Paramahamsa, *First Steps to Higher Yoga*, Yoga Niketan Trust, New Delhi, 2001, p. 358
152. Yogeshwaranand Paramahamsa, *First Steps to Higher Yoga*, Yoga Niketan Trust, New Delhi, 2001, p. 320
153. Shrikrishna, *Essence of Pranayama*, Kaivalyadhama, Lonavla, 2nd edn, 1996, p. 65

We thus can recognise two clusters of numbers, one group with a recommended *kumbhaka* length of around 40 to 50 seconds and a second group extending the time to around three times that length, around 120 seconds. It is obvious that the first group are modern authors who wrote primarily for a health-conscious general audience, and for this purpose *kumbhaka*s can be limited to around 40 to 50 seconds. The second group consists of accomplished spiritual adepts who are and were ready to teach *pranayama* to serious spiritual seekers. In this case *kumbhaka* is used to raise Kundalini, and may need to be extended to around 2 minutes or beyond.

A third range of *kumbhaka* length extends far beyond the 2-minute stage. Reading about these super-long *kumbhaka*s in yogic scripture, it is easy to be discouraged because you may think you will never attain them. But this is akin to refusing to take up *asana* practice because you saw a book with a yogi performing sickening contortions, or refusing to learn the violin because you heard Paganini play. Yet for some reason this attitude is widespread in relation to *pranayama*.

I will not discuss these *kumbhaka*s here in detail, as I don't think their descriptions are very helpful for the fledgling practitioner, but rather an obstacle. If you want to read about them please consult Raghuvira's *Kumbhaka Paddhati* or Theos Bernard's *Hatha Yoga*.

What is important for the student is that all *kumbhaka*s bring effects, but the longer ones more so, and what authors like Raghuvira want to achieve is that practitioners do not become complacent but keep extending their capacity in *kumbhaka*. He recommends over and over again increasing the length of *kumbhaka*,[154] and explains the link between length of *kumbhaka* and *samadhi*.[155] The longer your *kumbhaka*, the more likely you are to fall into *samadhi*. With longer *kumbhaka*s, more exalted *samadhi*s can be reached. Raghuvira is far from talking about an ambitious athletic pursuit for its own sake, because almost every time he talks about extending the length of *kumbhaka*s he

154. *Kumbhaka Paddhati of Raghuvira* stanzas 176, 177, 205
155. *Kumbhaka Paddhati of Raghuvira* stanza 218

adds that this has to happen with utmost devotion to God, for yoga without *bhakti* is dead.

The problem with modern yoga is that in many instances it has already been transformed into a circus in which whoever can perform more scintillating contortions is afforded more self-worth. The last thing we want to do with *pranayama* is turn it into a rat-race in which students with tongues hanging out strive after longer and longer *kumbhakas*. Much more important in terms of yoga are the love that you experience for the Divine and all beings, and the quality of service that you can provide for the awakening of other beings. We also need to keep in mind that such extreme *kumbhakas* are only one of the many yogic tools for reaching *samadhi*.

RATIONALE BEHIND EXTREME KUMBHAKAS

One of the yogic tenets says that where *prana* goes there goes *chitta* (mind). If *prana* does not move, the mind does not move. If the mind does not move, the yogi automatically abides in consciousness. Mental activity in somebody who has not mastered mind is nothing but the act of projecting yourself out from your true nature, the consciousness, into the mind. This is hard to understand as long as the mind moves, but it is self-evident when the mind is arrested. When *pranayama* is mastered, any signs of life can be halted. This can be taken to the extent that some yogis have had themselves interred. When buried in the ground, no oxygen is available, and this means that, unless the yogi enters a very advanced spiritual state, he or she will die. The greatest known *pranayama* master of the last few centuries was probably Trailanga Swami. He was observed by very large crowds to submerge in the Ganges at Varanasi and stay under the water for extremely long times, many sources say for weeks on end. But the purpose of Trailanga's *tapas* was not to impress the crowds, for he lived as a naked homeless beggar in the streets of the city and was despised by many. After Paramahamsa Ramakrishna met Trailanga towards the end of his life, when he was close to 280 years old, Ramakrishna remarked that he was like a second Shiva.

What he meant was that he could not see a difference between God and Trailanga. Interestingly enough, this is a statement from a spiritual master who had no vested interest at all in *pranayama* nor in any other yogic technique. But he confirmed that the yogi Trailanga had achieved the aim of all spiritual discipline and all yogic methods, which is true unity with the Divine.

And Trailanga is not the only person for whom *prana* played an important role in attaining that state. In the Gospel of Mark we learn that, after meeting John the Baptist, the Holy Spirit descended onto Jesus Christ.[156] However, the English translation of Holy Ghost or Holy Spirit does not convey the full meaning of the Greek original in the New Testament, which is *pneuma*, a word derived from the Sanskrit term *prana*.[157] It means breath. Translated into yogic terminology, Jesus received God's *prana Shakti* after being baptised by John, and from then on it hovered like a dove over him. It is relevant here that the *Hatha Yoga Pradipika* describes *prana* as a bird.[158]

ADVANCED KUMBHAKAS AND KUNDALINI

Before exploring the connection between *kumbhaka*s and Kundalini-raising, it must be noted that there are alternative methods to achieve the same end. Some of them are divine grace, *mantra*, *mudra*s or meditating on the *chakra*s in a particular way (*Bhutashuddhi*). Advanced *kumbhaka*s are not the only method but they are an important method.

As I have previously pointed out,[159] the eight limbs of yoga are not to be practised in isolation but stacked into each other like a set of Russian dolls. The goal of yoga, liberation, can be reached by three yogic means: *pranayama*, *samadhi* and devotion to the Divine. If the first of these three options is used and spiritual freedom is directly accessed from the fourth limb, very long *kumbhaka*s are needed. The length of *kumbhaka* may be reduced somewhat if

156. Mark 1.10
157. John Carroll, *The Essential Jesus*, Scribe, Melbourne, 2007, p. 24
158. *Hatha Yoga Pradipika* III.55
159. Gregor Maehle, *Ashtanga Yoga: The Intermediate Series*, New World Library, Novato, 2009, p. xvii

consecutive limbs are stacked within *pranayama*, which itself takes place within *asana*.

In the *Gheranda Samhita* we learn that *Dharana* (concentration), the sixth limb, is to be practised within *kumbhaka*.[160] Gheranda suggests here sequential concentration on the elements within *kumbhaka*. Although we are still using *pranayama*, the practice is now called *dharana*. This makes it more time effective. Let's remember that yoga holds that mental freedom is obtained by realizing our underlying nature, consciousness. Consciousness is veiled due to mental activity. With the removal of this veil, the mind can be stilled through stilling the breath, which itself powers the mind. Alternatively the mind can be stilled through meditation. Meditation in itself can take the form of a wilful effort in stopping the mental flow, as was successfully practised by Shri Aurobindo, or the form of passive observation of mental flow in the expectation that this would over time lead to its reduction, as taught by Swami Vivekananda.

Eight-limbed yoga takes a different approach. Here concentration on a sacred object, which has in itself a stilling effect on the mind, is placed within *kumbhaka*. Thus both the mind and the breath are stilled simultaneously and the effect of both practices is multiplied. Mind ruffles *prana* and *prana* ruffles mind. The greatest effect is reached when we enter stillness from both sides simultaneously. However, *pranayama* must be learned first, as it is much easier to still the breath than still the mind. Similarly, before practising *pranayama* the body must be stilled through *asana*, which is again easier. Calming an agitated mind by going straight to meditation is like trying to mollify an angry tiger by grabbing its tail.

We have learned already that awakening the Kundalini means to empower oneself for *dharana* and that *pranayama* is the prime means of raising Kundalini. The subtle life force, without being raised, expresses itself through the lower urges. Once it is raised, the practitioner is inclined towards the sacred. Kundalini is not a phantom but a phenomenon that can be seen and felt in the rapture of mystical states.

160. *Gheranda Samhita* III.70

Since the *siddhas* have left behind precise descriptions of Kundalini, it is easy for contemporary practitioners to visualise Kundalini, and this in itself, when done with great intention and precision by a focused mind, will in due time raise Kundalini. Yogeshwaranand Paramahamsa recommends visualising Kundalini during *kumbhaka*.[161] This is confirmed by Theos Bernard, who describes how, during each *kumbhaka*, he awakend Kundalini by conducting it by means of concentration through the *chakras*, unifying it with consciousness at the crown *chakra*.[162]

The link between *kumbhaka*, Kundalini and mental focus is also confirmed by the great Shankaracharya. In his *Yoga Taravali* he states that focus on the *Ajna Chakra* during kumbhaka lets *prana* enter into the central energy channel.[163] He adds that once it rises upwards it is referred to as Kundalini[164] and when it has reached the top it enables one to effortlessly reach *dharana* (concentration) and *dhyana* (meditation).[165] In three short stanzas the great master has here explained the intricate link between *kumbhaka*, mental focus and meditation. The emphasis here is on 'effortlessly'. By applying Kundalini, the higher limbs can be achieved with relatively little effort whereas, without the tool of Kundalini, meditation can end in decades of empty, meaningless drudgery.

However, Kundalini-rising should not be attempted without mastering *asana* and *pranayama* beforehand.[166] Once the yogi is established in both, the primary *mudras* (energy seals) need to be learned, whereas basic *mudras* like the *bandhas* and *asana mudras* are to be learned before *pranayama*. The *Yoga Sutra* does not explicitly mention the *mudras*, but they are implied under the headings *asana*

161. Yogeshwaranand Paramahamsa, *First Steps to Higher Yoga*, Yoga Niketan Trust, New Delhi, 2001, p. 359
162. Theos Bernard, *Hatha Yoga*, Rider, London, 1950, p. 95
163. *Yoga Taravali of Shankaracharya* stanza 11
164. *Yoga Taravali of Shankaracharya* stanza 12
165. *Yoga Taravali of Shankaracharya* stanza 14
166. Swami Niranjanananda, *Yoga Darshan*, Sri Panchadashnam Paramahamsa Alakh Bara, Deoghar, 1993, p. 359

(such as *Yoga Mudra, Tadaga Mudra*), *pranayama* (such as *Uddiyana Bandha Mudra*), *pratyahara* (such as *Viparita Karani Mudra*) and *dharana* (such as *Shambhavi Mudra, Shanmukhi Mudra*). In other words all *mudra*s can be assigned to a particular limb.

Important here is that *kumbhaka* length on the one hand is extended to enable a more precise visualization of Kundalini in all its details. On the other hand, such visualization steadies, concentrates and purifies the mind and makes longer *kumbhaka*s possible.

The *Hatha Yoga Pradipika* determines the link between *pranayama* and the higher limbs in the following way:[167] 12 *pranayama*s make one *pratyahara* (the fifth limb), 12 *pratyahara*s make 1 *dharana* (the sixth limb), 12 *dharana*s make 1 *dhyana* (the seventh limb) and 12 *dhyana*s make 1 *samadhi* (the eighth limb and culmination of yoga).

---

167. *Hatha Yoga Pradipika* (10 chapters) I.36–37

GENERAL GUIDELINES FOR PRANAYAMA

WHEN TO PRACTISE PRANAYAMA

When to start one's practice

Guidelines for timing the start of one's *pranayama* practice differ wildly due to the fact that the idea of what constitutes *pranayama* differs greatly from one teacher to another. For example Swami Sivananda says that preparatory *pranayama* may be practised by anyone without any prerequisites.[168] He also suggests not postponing the start of practice until one finds a guru, but to begin immediately using the directions he gives in his book.[169] The Swami was referring here to a very simple and basic form of practice. He was aware that there are not a lot of *pranayama* experts left in the world, and the chances of finding one are not great. Another consideration is that one never knows what will happen with the novice, and current enthusiasm might have evaporated by the time the teacher finally appears. However, there is a downside to going ahead without a teacher. When a student learns *asana* solely from books and DVDs they usually end up with such a stunted practice that it can be very difficult to change their bad habits. I would be surprised if the case with *pranayama* were any different.

As quoted earlier, Swami Ramdev said that *pranayama* was so harmless that it could be practised even by children. He also has outlined an introductory form of practice. T. Krishnamacharya taught *pranayama* to some patients who were too sick to practise *asana*, in this case using a gentle therapeutic *pranayama*.

In contrast to that, K. Pattabhi Jois, a student of T. Krishnamacharya, introduced *pranayama* as an intense *sadhana* containing long *kumbhakas*, and so required a very high level of *asana* proficiency in his students. Used as a spiritual *sadhana*, *pranayama* requires that the state of *asana*

168. Swami Sivananda, *The Science of Pranayama*, BN Publishing, 2008, p. 98
169. Swami Sivananda, *The Science of Pranayama*, BN Publishing, 2008, p. 100

siddhi (perfection in *asana*) in certain meditation postures (preferably *Padmasana*) be gained. This means you need to be able to sit comfortably in your meditation posture for the duration of your *pranayama* session with both knees and both sit bones on the floor. Do not sit for spiritual *pranayama* on a chair or in the so-called *Sukhasana* (easy posture), where one simply sits cross-legged without the knees being able to descend all the way down to the floor. Neither in *Sukhasana* nor while sitting in a chair or leaning against a wall or slouching on a sofa are you likely to divert the pranic current upwards, which is necessary for spiritual liberation. This subject is explored in detail in the chapter on *asana*.

One of my *pranayama* teachers, B.N.S. Iyengar, another student of T. Krishnamacharya, said that *pranayama* generally should be started after 6 months of *asana* practice, and meditation should start within a year of commencing *pranayama*. Otherwise one would waste one's incarnation. He introduced *pranayama* at a medium level of difficulty but intensified this quickly when he had the impression that the student could digest it. He expected that a full *asana* practice would be performed twice a day and recommended that *pranayama* be practised four times a day ideally, but with an absolute minimum of twice a day. Iyengar belonged to a generation of Brahmins who grew up sitting on the floor, not on chairs. This leads to the hip joints opening completely and, by the time you start formal yoga practice, it is a relatively small step to perform *pranayama* sitting in *Padmasana* or at least *Siddhasana*.

Jayatarama, the author of *Jogapradipyaka*, reasons that *pranayama* should be done only after *Shodhana karma*,[170] i.e. the purifications processes known as *kriya*s. Gheranda Samhita supports this view, but doubt was cast on it by Swatmarama in his *Hatha Yoga Pradipika*. Gheranda taught the *kriya*s to all yogis, whereas Swatmarama said that only those with impurities need to practise them.

Living in our modern industrial society, with many types of pollutants present, I would recommend to all those who want to start

170. *Jogapradipyaka of Jayatarama* stanzas 463–465

pranayama that they first regularly practise *Nauli*, *Kapalabhati* and *Neti kriya*s. These are described in detail in the chapter on *kriyas*.

Summarizing, the question of when *pranayama* practice should be started has been treated very differently by different teachers, reflecting the different degrees of difficulty of the *pranayama* they taught. You may start easy *pranayama* early on or difficult *pranayama* later. The outcome is probably similar, as in the first case your capacity to perform *pranayama* will slowly grow as your *asana* practice matures. Understandable also is Swami Sivananda's concern that a student might ask for *pranayama* at a pivotal moment in her life and, if it is withheld, she may then turn in a more materialistic or downward direction. Similarly, Swami Ramdev looks at *pranayama* as a tool for health education for the masses that makes them less dependent on expensive medicines. T. Krishnamacharya seems to have trodden a middle path by teaching desiring students a level of *pranayama* that was appropriate to their current level of *asana* practice, whether at the novice level or advanced.

Season

Medieval texts say that *pranayama* should not be commenced in winter or summer, but only in spring or autumn. *Pranayama* can affect the temperature management of the body and one may feel hot or cold when commencing it. In the olden days yogis had no modern apartments with heating and air-conditioning, nor did they have insulated roofs, windows or warm clothing. If you do live in a thatched-roof hut with the traditional cow-dung floor you should follow the above advice relating to seasons; otherwise you can look at it as dated.

Time of day

You need to leave 4 hours after a meal before you start practising *pranayama*. The *Yoga Rahasya* even talks of 6 hours. The emptier the alimentary canal the easier *pranayama* practice will be. In essence this means that you need to practise before meals, not after them. However, half an hour after completion of *pranayama* should pass before one takes food. The exception is a cup of milk, which can be taken right after and even before *pranayama*.

The *sandhi*s, the so-called junctions of the day, are considered auspicious for *pranayama*. *Sandhi*s are the times when the night merges into the day, i.e. dawn, when morning merges into afternoon, i.e. mid-day, and when day merges into night, dusk. The best time for *pranayama* is sunrise, as Brhadyogi Yajnavalkya Smrti confirms.[171]

After asana

If you practise *pranayama* once a day, then ideally it is to be practised right after *asana*. In his commentary on the *Yoga Sutra* the rishi Vyasa said 'sati asana jaye', meaning 'once victorious in *asana*'. Many authorities interpret that as 'Gain victory in an *asana*, only then practise *pranayama*'. This makes sense because, if you cannot sit in an *asana*, *pranayama* is difficult. However, some authorities think Vyasa's dictum means 'Right after *asana*, practise your *pranayama*'.

Certainly the body is ideally prepared after *asana*. You will be able to go much deeper into *kumbhaka* and absorb more *prana* if you have prepared your body with *asana*. Your neck will be thoroughly prepared for *Jalandhara Bandha* (chin lock) if you have practised *Sarvangasana* (shoulder stand). If you practise *pranayama* twice a day, with the first session right after your *asana* practice and the second not preceded by an *asana* session, you will easily notice that during your second session you cannot keep up with the progress made in the session that was preceded by *asana*.

If you do practise *pranayama* without immediate preparation through *asana*, limit your *kumbhaka*s to about 40 seconds, unless you are a very experienced practitioner or are being taught and supervised by such a practitioner.

---

171. *Brhadyogi Yajnavalkya Smrti* VIII.38–40

Phase of life

The *Yoga Rahasya* calls *pranayama* the principal practice for *Grihasthas* (householders)[172] and says that the primary time to apply it is from approximately 25 to 75 years of age.[173] The *Yoga Rahasya* teaches that before 25 the main focus should be on *asana* and after that on *pranayama*. However, if you have not focused on *asana* prior to your 25th year, you cannot jump the queue: you will still have to go through such a phase later in life for reasons outlined above. *Yoga Rahasya*, though, gives us a definite sequence, which, as the yogi matures, leads from *asana* on to *pranayama* and then to *dhyana* (meditation). This sequence guarantees that we harvest the fruit of our toil, but only when the previous stages are maintained. The guardian of *Yoga Rahasya*, T. Krishnamacharya, maintained his *asana* and *pranayama* practice into his 90s. The important message of the *Rahasya* is to keep stepping up on the ladder of yogic techniques. Do not get stuck at the level of *asana*.

When not to practise pranayama

Pranayama should not be practised when tired, overcome by worries, unclean of body or overworked.[174] When you are tired, first practise *Shavasana* (corpse posture). If you are tired from your *asana* practice, then spend more time on your inversions to recharge. Following that, do a short *Shavasana* and then spend several minutes with *Kapalabhati* to recharge before going into *pranayama*. Try it out. *Kapalabhati* works miracles. More advanced practitioners may use both *Kapalabhati* and *Bhastrika* together for the same purpose.

   If you are unclean, first take a shower. Do not practise when you have a headache. If *pranayama* gives you headaches, change what you are doing. Your *Jalandhara Bandha* may be incorrect or too loose. *Pranayama* can give you a headache if *prana* rises into the brain. This is a sign that your technique is wrong or your *kumbhaka* too long.

172. *Yoga Rahasya* II.45
173. *Yoga Rahasya* II.37
174. *Hatha Tatva Kaumudi of Sundaradeva* III.14

76

Do not practise *kumbhaka* during pregnancy, as it increases intra-abdominal pressure, or when suffering from a heart disorder, as it increases intrathoracic pressure. *Kumbhaka* should not be practised with high blood pressure as it may initially raise it. In the long term *pranayama* is beneficial for high blood pressure, but you need to find a strategy for dropping the blood pressure before you embark on *kumbhaka*s. For example, breathing with a ratio of 1 to 2, i.e. 1 count inhalation to 2 counts exhalation, lowers blood pressure. Slowly, over weeks and months, extend this count until 1 breath takes 1 minute. Before commencing *kumbhaka*, get medical advice and seek a qualified *pranayama* teacher or yoga therapist.

Do not practise *kumbhaka* during a thunderstorm, as it is a powerful pranic phenomenom. Do not practise *kumbhaka* when emotionally upset. When emotional, one depletes one's *prana*. To be emotional can mean either the pathological bottling up of emotions or their constant venting. Whereas our society for centuries demanded of its members that they bottle up emotions and suppress them, it is now *en vogue* to display emotional behaviour. From yoga's view, both the suppressing of emotions and the attachment to their expression leads to more emotion in the future. However, being emotional means that you have subconsciously imprinted a certain reaction, in yoga called *samskara*. When the stimulus of the *samskara* reappears, a more powerful reaction surfaces than would be explainable from the situation.

For example let's say your partner tells you that they would prefer you not to take a certain action but leave it to them because they deem themselves better equipped than you. You reflect for a moment on whether this is the case and then calmly accept the suggestion or reject it. If, however, a similar situation had repeatedly occurred in your childhood and your parents always told you that you couldn't do certain things because you were incapable, then a *samskara* (subconscious imprint) would have formed. The present-day suggestion of your partner, which might have been completely reasonable, may then trigger the *samskara* and a lifetime charge of suppressed unworthiness may surface with it. This is now an emotion, a present reaction

77

based on a past imprint. Emotions expel *prana*, in a not dissimilar way to cocaine and coffee. They also make your breath short. When emoting do not practise *kumbhaka* but, as in the case of high blood pressure (which may anyway accompany emoting), simply breathe with a ratio of 1:2 and slowly extend your count.

Emoting is different to feeling. A feeling is a present sensation, authentically experienced for the first time. An emotion is a stored feeling, which is triggered by a present-time stimulus and makes you relive the past feeling. Feeling is hence something that makes you arrive in the present moment, whereas emoting draws you out of the present moment and back into your past conditioning. It decreases through the use of *pranayama*.

WHERE TO PRACTISE PRANAYAMA

The *Hatha Yoga Pradipika* considers that location is important for the practice of both *asana* and *pranayama*, whereas the *Gheranda Samhita* and the *Jogapradipyaka* consider it important only for *pranayama*.[175] They all agree, however, that the place where one practises needs to be carefully chosen, as it deeply influences the outcome. Most yogic texts mention the importance of a hermitage (*ashrama*, *tapovanam*) in a beautiful spot close to a river with lots of fruit and root vegetables close by, located in a peaceful country. Goraksha Natha, for example, recommends that one's place be secluded.[176] Sage Vasishta advises that it should be in a forest by the side of a river.[177] In modern days this suggestion was picked up by Swami Ramdev, who also recommends practising near a body of water.[178] Such places generally fulfil the following requirements:

Closeness to water
Bodies of water, especially moving bodies of water such as waterfalls, charge the air with negative ions, which is very empowering in *pranayama*. Swami Niranjanananda writes that the pranic value of

175. *Jogapradipyaka of Jayatarama*, stanzas 365–367
176. *Goraksha Shataka* stanza 41
177. *Vasishta Samhita* II.57
178. Swami Ramdev, *Pranayama*, Divya Yog Mandir Trust, Hardwar, 2007, p. 18

metropolitan air is a fraction of that of air in the mountains or in proximity of a waterfall.[179]

Beautiful, peaceful spot in nature

The ideal place for *pranayama* is a cabin or habitation in a beautiful spot in nature, as it enables us to gain inner strength, which motivates us for practice.

Clean air

It is important that *pranayama* be practised in a place away from the smoke, dust, air pollution and electrosmog of the cities. O.P. Tiwari, for example, says that *pranayama* in a polluted city may not be effective. One may need to use common sense and an air purifier.[180] An ioniser, for example, will improve the effectiveness of *pranayama* in a city. If you do live in a city, have a look at the generally prevailing wind direction. There may be a vast difference in air quality at the side of the city that faces the wind. Swami Ramdev suggests to city dwellers that they purify the air prior to *pranayama* by burning incense or using a ghee lamp.[181]

Pranayama also should not be practised in excessive dampness; the place must be free of insects such as mosquitoes; it must be sheltered from direct sunlight, which would make you overheat in *kumbhaka*, and protected from draught, which interferes with the fixation of *prana* during *kumbhaka*. This calls for practising not in the open but in some form of dwelling with a roof and walls.

Seclusion

The *Hatha Tatva Kaumudi* leads the charge here. It advises that *pranayama* be practised alone while remaining silent,[182] in an isolated countryside,[183] staying in a lonely place,[184] living in an isolated place[185]

179. Swami Niranjanananda, *Prana and Pranayama*, Yoga Publications Trust, Munger, 2009, p. 15
180. O.P. Tiwari, *Concept of Kundalini*, DVD, Kaivalyadhama, Lonavla
181. Swami Ramdev, *Pranayama Rahasya*, Divya Yog Mandir Trust, Hardwar, 2009, p. 82
182. *Hatha Tatva Kaumudi of Sundaradeva* XXXVI.70
183. *Hatha Tatva Kaumudi of Sundaradeva* XXXV.6
184. *Hatha Tatva Kaumudi of Sundaradeva* XXXVIII.13
185. *Hatha Tatva Kaumudi of Sundaradeva* XXXVIII.44

or a secluded place.[186] This may sound surprising from a citizen of Varanasi, which even in Sundaradeva's times was a metropolis in relative terms. Sundaradeva was obviously not averse to city dwelling, but he recommends seclusion for intense bouts of practice such as are required to raise Kundalini.

The *Yoga Kundalini Upanishad* names excessive social intercourse as one of the six causes of disease.[187] Swami Niranjanananda explains that gossiping, criticising and pandering to emotional demands leads to dissipation of *prana*.[188] This explains why aloneness during intense phases of *pranayama* was considered important. Swami Muktibod-hananda similarly holds that pranic flow in our bodies is influenced by the people we socialize with.[189] One needs, then, to choose one's company very wisely or be alone. This is particularly important for the beginner. The yogic texts often point out that restrictions apply mainly to beginners; once mastery is achieved no restrictions apply.

The beginner in *pranayama* is most sensitive to *prana* going astray. Often beginners are so enthusiastic about their new-found practice that they go out and talk to everybody about it. When they meet a wall of non-understanding they then become insecure and discontinue their practice. That is why some texts suggest practising in secret until you are firmly established and not inclined to waver any more. The more established the practitioners the more they are able to absorb adverse conditions.

It is important to understand that the above injunctions are related to a multi-hour per day *pranayama* practice to raise Kundalini. They are certainly not applicable to practising 30 minutes of *pranayama* after daily *asana* practice. Let's remember here that the *Yoga Rahasya* con-siders *pranayama* the main practice for householders, that is people who have a partner and children, maintain a profession and / or run a business. The *Yoga Yajnavalkya* and *Yoga Vasishta* insist that yoga

186. *Hatha Tatva Kaumudi of Sundaradeva* XXXIX.2
187. *Yoga Kundalini Upanishad* I.56–57
188. Swami Niranjanananda, *Prana and Pranayama*, Yoga Publications Trust, Munger, 2009, p. 221
189. Swami Muktibodhananda, *Swara Yoga*, Yoga Publication Trust, Munger, 1984, p. 73

should always be practised along with performing one's duty to family and society and never as a dropout gambit.

Very illuminating in this context is Goraksha Natha's call for practising in seclusion, already quoted above. Goraksha recommends in the same breath devoting oneself to God.[190] This is reminiscent of Paramahamsa Ramakrishna's frequent calls to regularly go alone into nature and listen to God.[191] When talking much, one projects *prana* out of the mouth, which weakens the spirit. When alone in nature, it becomes more likely that one will listen to the Divine. It is not by chance that the founders of our great religions – the Vedic rishis, Mahavira, Buddha, Moses, Jesus and Mohammad – spent long phases in solitude, where they received insight.

For many practitioners a place that has all of the aforementioned characteristics is not readily available. In this case consider a retreat situation. If you can go alone once in a while to a beautiful spot in nature for a few days, your success in practice there may carry you through the rest of the year. Also try to reproduce such a place in your home. Most people cannot put an entire room aside for practice. Create a corner that has no rajasic or tamasic elements. Use an ioniser or air filter to improve air quality. Ideally practise early in the morning when your house and suburb are still quiet. The humming and vibrating of a city has a very rajasic influence on the mind.

HOW MANY ROUNDS IN HOW MANY SITTINGS HOW OFTEN PER WEEK?
One of the aims of *kumbhaka* is to increase the *prana* concentration and pranic pressure within the body. You are pumping up the body with *prana*, which slows down the mind and turns it away from the material. To be spiritually fully effective you need to practise *pranayama* daily, with *kumbhaka*s exceeding 40 seconds, for approximately 25 to 30 minutes within a 24-hour period. Health effects can be gained with significantly less than that.

190. *Goraksha Shataka* stanza 41
191. Swami Nikhilananda (transl.), *The Gospel of Ramakrishna*, Ramakrishna Math, Madras, 1942, pp. 81, 246

Before we delve into the way to measure each individual
kumbhaka and its suggested length, let us determine how many rounds
should be practised in how many sessions over a 24-hour period.
It is important that you do as many rounds as you are comfortable
with over the long term and not more. If you start straining in
kumbhaka due to the duration of your practice, you are likely to
develop adverse symptoms such as headaches, stress, anxiety or
ear pain. In such a case you might abandon your practice altogether
and not enjoy its many benefits. Therefore never overdo it. If in
doubt underdo it, meaning err in the direction of practising slightly
too little.

Swami Ramdev suggests starting with 5 to 10 minutes a day and,
once established, to extend the time up to 30 to 60 minutes.[192] Certainly,
you can't do much wrong practising for 10 minutes, but into this time
frame would fit not much more than, say, a few rounds of Vasishta's
Nadi Shuddhi without breath retention.

If you were to extend your practice over a time frame of 6 months
to reach a length of 30 minutes and over a period of 12 months a full
hour, you would need at the same time to make sure that:
• you maintain an uninterrupted daily *asana* practice
• you maintain an uninterrupted daily *pranayama* practice
• you accept certain dietary restrictions as listed in the diet chapter
• you have established a sound practical knowledge of the *bandhas*
as described in the respective chapter
• you have practised certain *shatkarmas* as described in their respective
chapter. In other words you practise initially as little as you like, but
if you intensify your practice you must also intensify your efforts in
the auxiliary and supporting limbs of *pranayama*.

Sundaradeva suggests starting practice with 10 rounds in the first
month, 20 in the second and so on.[193] This constitutes a very steep
incline in practice. Sundaradeva lived in the 18th century in the holy
city of Varanasi, and he probably met some of the most advanced

192. Swami Ramdev, *Pranayama*, Divya Yog Mandir Trust, Hardwar, 2007, p. 18
193. *Hatha Tatva Kaumudi of Sundaradeva* XXXVIII.82

pranayama practitioners of the subcontinent, such as Trailanga
Swami, who frequented Varanasi at that time. It would be wise for
modern yogis to increase their practice at a much slower pace.

The yogic scriptures recommend practising *pranayama* 3 to 4 times
a day. The *Hatha Yoga Pradipika* suggests that one should increase
kumbhaka practice gradually to 4 sittings per day, i.e. morning, noon,
evening and midnight.[194] With 80 being the suggested number of
kumbhakas per sitting, this would bring the total number of *kumbhakas*
per day to 320. However Brahmananda, in his commentary Jyotsna
on the *Hatha Yoga Pradipika*, relents to the extent of declaring that it
is inconvenient to practise at midnight, thus limiting the number of
kumbhakas to only 240 per day.[195] I was glad to read that, for it is certainly
inconvenient to get up at midnight to practise *pranayama*, although I
tried it for a while because B.N.S. Iyengar recommended it to me.

Nathamuni's *Yoga Rahasya* agrees that *pranayama* should be practised
4 times a day.[196] Theos Bernard, quite likely one of the most sincere Western
pranayama practitioners, also speaks of 4 sessions a day, but his teacher
told him that such strenuous practice needs to be maintained only for a
certain time, in his case for at least 3 months.[197] Any *pranayama* practice
consisting of that many sessions per day is generally dedicated to
Kundalini-rousing, and must be supplemented by other forms of
practice.

The *Brhadyogi Yajnavalkya Smrti* speaks of a single session of 100
rounds of *pranayama* at sunrise to delete all karmic demerit.[198] Again,
for such a powerful effect to ensue you need to practise intensely.

The ten-chapter edition of the *Hatha Yoga Pradipika* offers us a less
demanding scenario for the practice of *Nadi Shodhana*. Here we find
that 12 rounds are suggested for inferior yogis, 24 for moderate and
36 rounds for advanced yogis.[199]

194. *Hatha Yoga Pradipika* II.11
195. *Hatha Yoga Pradipika with Commentary Jyotsna*, Adyar Library, Madras, 1972, p. 24
196. *Yoga Rahasya* II.57
197. Theos Bernard, *Heaven Lies Within Us*, Charles Scribner's Sons, New York, 1939, p. 181
198. *Brhadyogi Yajnavalkya Smrti* VIII.38–40
199. *Hatha Yoga Pradipika* (10 chapters) IV.17

T. Krishnamacharya sustained a *sadhana* of 3 *pranayama* sittings per day to a very great age, but let's not forget that he did this after his children were grown up and had left the house. Many yogic texts insist that responsibility for family and society should not be neglected by immersing oneself into yoga too deeply too early. It is a process that slowly needs to be faded into one's life. During each successive stage of life, daily time spent in yoga practice should slowly be increased. If this model were followed in our society the bingo halls would be somewhat emptier, but on the other hand the elderly would be much more sought after as spiritual guides. This was the case in ancient society and still is to some extent in indigenous societies around the world.

PROCEED CAUTIOUSLY AND PRUDENTLY

This is likely to be one of the most important chapters in this book. The great *siddha* Goraksha Natha recommends not overdoing *kumbhaka*s and always to exhale slowly.[200] If you aggressively push your *kumbhaka*s to the maximum you can damage lung tissue, primarily that of the alveoli. It is exactly the same principle as with *asana* practice. If you practise *asana* egotistically you may end up with all sorts of physical damage, as is the case with sports, gymnastics or any physical pursuit. Apart from holding *kumbhaka* for too long, you also can inhale too deeply, which also may damage the alveoli. If you find that at the beginning of *kumbhaka* your chest almost bursts, then briefly release your *Jalandhara Banda*, exhale a small quantity of air and then resume your *kumbhaka*.

Similarly, you can exhale for too long. This will put a lot of pressure on the heart and has the potential to damage it. As with an inhalation that makes your lungs hurt, an exhalation that is too long creates pain in your heart. This is a warning signal that you need to shorten your entire breathing cycles. Do not ignore it.

In *pranayama* you need to proceed even more slowly and cautiously than in *asana*. Proceed according to your own abilities and, as in *asana*,

200. *Goraksha Shataka* stanza 51

never compare yourself to anybody else. When you are gasping for air, your *kumbhaka*s are too long.

Never, ever strain; always practise according to your capabilities. You need to start *pranayama* with a simple count that does not tax you at all. The next day extend your count by 1 second and see what happens. If you still feel under-challenged then extend your count again the next day. You will quickly come to a point where, without straining, you feel that the practice suddenly becomes more engaging, more rewarding. Stay at this point for days, weeks or months until again you find that your mind tends to wander because it feels that you are not doing any work. Then again increase your cycle by 1 count. Finally you will come to a point that I call the raw, unrefined potential of your body for *kumbhaka*. Up to this point progress is relatively straightforward, but from here on you will have to work. In my case this point appeared at around 44 seconds of internal *kumbhaka*, but this is probably already taking into account my long-term relatively intense *asana* practice. You may have to stay at this count for several months, before you can increase it again. If you increase too quickly, two things may happen. Either you realize that you overdid it and you again reduce your count; or you are too ambitious and keep struggling until you are so thwarted by adverse symptoms that you drop out and stop your practice altogether. The trick is to keep your practice so simple that you never strain and will continue, and on the other side to make it challenging enough to keep yourself interested and to notice the changes taking place in you. To succeed in *pranayama* you need to stay on course and not get sidetracked. Be prepared to continue this practice for the rest of your life and do not run out of steam.

The *Hatha Tatva Kaumudi* warns that imprudent *pranayama* may cause swelling, pain, fever and other problems.[201] Symptoms such as swelling are believed to be caused by *prana* going astray. If the yogi does not take the time needed to learn *pranayama* properly and to progress slowly, then *prana* may go astray by faulty practice. Faulty

201. *Hatha Tatva Kaumudi of Sundaradeva* III.31

practice means for example faulty *bandhas*, exhaling too quickly, sucking in air too fast, holding *kumbhaka* too long, trying to progress too fast, unsuitable diet, not sitting in the proper *asana* or slouching, having a tamasic or rajasic mind when practising, continuing to intoxicate although having taken up the practice of *pranayama*, or combining *pranayama* with drugs, alcohol or coffee, not practising with an attitude of devotion to the Divine, not supporting *pranayama* enough through appropriate practice of *asana* and *kriya*, etc., etc.

It becomes apparent how important a competent teacher is. Where are you to turn if nobody can look at your practice from the outside and give advice? In the movie *Meetings with Remarkable Men* the Armenian mystic George I. Gurdjieff approaches an Indian yoga master and describes his breathing method. The master studies him with a long glance and then with great compassion says 'I recommend to you to stop all of your exercises'. He realizes that without proper guidance Gurdjieff is likely to do more harm than good. Gurdjieff then walks off in a dejected mood, validating the master's judgment that he was not ready to do whatever it took to rectify his mistakes.

During *pranayama* one should experience neither strain, nor discomfort, nor ambition, as otherwise damage to the *nadis* may occur. This sums up neatly what this chapter is trying to convey. Strain, discomfort and ambition will make you go backwards. In many life situations we have learned that this trio will get us forward. Not so here: When the subject is our soul, strain, discomfort and ambition will get us nowhere. This trio is caused by our conditioning, and *pranayama* is a method for loosening and deleting negative conditioning so that we may experience life and the world as they truly are and not according to the painful imprints of our past.

Swami Ramdev says that when suffering from hypertension or heart disease only gentle *pranayama* should be applied.[202] *Pranayama* is not completely ruled out in these cases, but one needs to be even more cautious and consult a yoga therapist. The *Hatha Yoga Pradipika*

202. Swami Ramdev, *Pranayama Rahasya*, Divya Yog Mandir Trust, Hardwar, 2009, p. 85

declares that even as elephants, lions and tigers are tamed step by step, so *prana* is controlled slowly and steadily.[203] If you rush, according to the *Pradipika*, the *prana* may kill you even as a wild beast may kill you if tamed in too much of a hurry. Although *prana*, the life force in our body, may seem insignificant, it is identical with *prakrti*, the force that created and maintains this entire universe. It is a force incredibly larger than us and can destroy us in an instant if we do not respect it, understand it and use it responsibly.

The *Pradipika* then goes on to proclaim that, if *pranayama* is practised in a wise fashion, it removes the causes of all diseases, but if practised imprudently it will have the opposite effect – creating diseases.[204] This stanza describes the situation of an individual but it is also valid, and perhaps currently more pressingly so, on a global scale. The power of nature (*prakrti*) can be harnessed prudently and peacefully and used for the good of all, or it can be misused and then come back to haunt us in the form of monster cyclones and hurricanes, mega-earthquake clusters and tidal waves of a power yet inconceivable.

The next two stanzas of the *Pradipika* list asthma, emphysema, headache, ear pain, glaucoma and heart disorders as problems that can be created through disturbance of *prana*, and that these are to be avoided by practising with great skill and subtle intelligence.[205]

The listed respiratory problems can only occur when one inhales too deeply or holds *kumbhaka* for too long. Heart problems may occur if one draws out the exhalation for too long (that is if one has chosen a count beyond one's capacity). Cranial, ear and eye problems may occur if *Jalandhara Bandha* is not properly applied. None of these problems can occur if one practises properly, following the rules.

There is talk of a great skill here, which develops into mastery slowly when one practises patiently over a long time. The attitude required is that of the owner of a timber plantation. Timber is a crop

203. *Hatha Yoga Pradipika* II.15
204. *Hatha Yoga Pradipika* II.16.
205. *Hatha Yoga Pradipika* II.17–18

that can be harvested only after a long time, in some cases only by future generations. However, if it is not planted, nobody will ever get to harvest it. One may also cut it down too early in an attempt to make a fast gain. *Pranayama* cannot succeed if we ask for fast success and reward. The skill it asks for is acquired only when the need for swift gain and success is surrendered. Then one is able to arrive in the moment and the breath will reveal its great secrets.

ATTITUDE OF DEVOTION AND MENTAL FOCUS

The *Mahabharata* narrates a story about the importance of focus.[206] The martial arts teacher Acharya Drona had an artificial bird placed on a tall tree to serve as a target. He assembled all of the Pandava and Kaurava princes to have a shot at the target in turn, with the goal of shooting off the head of the bird. However, before he got them to shoot he asked each of them the same question, 'What do you see?' One by one they answered, 'I see you, I see myself and the other bystanders, I see the tree and I see the bird'. Drona told the respective princes to stand back because they were not ready to shoot. Arjuna was the last to take his turn. When asked what he saw, he said 'I see the bird only'. Drona then asked him to look more precisely and Arjuna answered, 'I see only the head of the bird'. When asked to release his arrow, Arjuna cleanly shot off the bird's head.

This story illustrates the importance of mental focus in yoga, for the arrow of our mind will hit its target only if we clearly see the target and are not distracted by the many interferences that the world will offer us. But what exactly is the target in *pranayama*?

In sutra III.1 Patanjali describes concentration (*dharana*, the sixth limb) as binding the mind to one place. The Sanskrit word for place that he uses is *desha*. The term occurs also in sutra II.50, where Patanjali says that the breath becomes long and subtle through performing the various *kumbhaka*s if place (*desha*), time and count are observed studiously. *Desha* is one of the three parameters that will determine our progress. The more sattvic the place or object to which we bind the

206. *Mahabharata, Adi Parva,* CXXXV

mind during *kumbhaka*, the faster our progress to mystical insight will be. The ideal meditation object or place to which the mind is bound during *kumbhaka* is the Divine.

In fact a practitioner who has complete and absolute love for the Divine does not need *pranayama*. The *nadis* can be purified and Kundalini can be raised through an act of grace of the Divine.[207] Other than through *pranayama*, such grace may be obtained by intense and total devotion (*bhakti*). For those who cannot bring themselves to devotion of such intensity, *pranayama* is of great help, as it slowly and gradually purifies the subconscious (*vasana*). However, even then, during such gradual purification, the extent of devotion and love towards the Divine that is felt is paramount.

The *Yoga Kundalini Upanishad* proclaims that *pranayama* needs to be performed daily with the mind firmly focused on the Divine.[208] The same was already stated in the ancient *Brhadyogi Yajnavalkya Smrti*.[209] *Pranayama* performed with the mind on tamasic (materialistic) objects will make the mind more tamasic. If it is set on rajasic (sensual, desirous) objects during *pranayama*, the mind will amplify the rajasic quality of the object. The most sattvic meditation object of all is the Divine. If the mind is firmly set on the Divine during *pranayama* one will succeed swiftly.

The *Kumbhaka Paddhati of Raghuvira* declares that *pranayama* should never be practised without being devoted to the Divine.[210] *Kumbhaka* gives great power. There is almost nothing that cannot be achieved if *kumbhaka* is mastered. It is absolutely essential that this power be laid at the feet of the Divine and nowhere else. It belongs to the Divine, as does everything else in the universe. There are paths that do not deal with the power of *prana*, such as the *Samkhya* and Buddhism. On these paths it is not essential to devote oneself to the Divine. Yoga and *pranayama* are different. Yogis who do not

207. *Kumbhaka Paddhati of Raghuvira* stanzas 181–182
208. *Yoga Kundalini Upanishad* I.62.
209. *Brhadyogi Yajnavalkya Smrti* IX.192–194
210. *Kumbhaka Paddhati of Raghuvira* stanza 179

sincerely devote themselves to the Divine risk devoting themselves to their egos and minds instead. The problem is that, if you leave a vacuum, the mind will fill it with something else beyond your conscious choice. The choice is then made by your conditioning and subconscious. For this reason it is better to give the mind an object to rest on that is chosen by the heart rather than let the mind make its own choice.

The final aim of *kumbhaka* is to make the mind objectless. When the mind does become objectless, the underlying deep reality will shine through. That deep reality is the Divine. Before the mind becomes objectless, the Divine is veiled by those objects to which the mind subconsciously gravitates. The *Yoga Sutra* states that the power of *samadhi* is obtained through the grace of the Divine.[211] With or without *kumbhaka*, *samadhi* is easily attained during the time when the mind is firmly fixed on the Divine.

The *Kumbhaka Paddhati* also suggests increasing the length of breath retentions with awareness of the movements of *prana* while being devoted to the Divine.[212] The movements of *prana* are manifestations of Shakti, the power of the Divine. *Pranayama*, if practised with devotion to the Divine, can give us the awareness that all movements of *prana* are in truth performed by the Divine. This means that through the mechanism of *prana* we are moved and maintained by the Divine. We are not the doer; we are only looking on. This is stated exactly in the *Bhagavad Gita* where Lord Krishna says 'All actions are in truth only performed by my *prakrti*. Only fools believe that they are the doer.'[213]

Brahmananda's commentary on the *Hatha Yoga Pradipika* states that one should begin the practice of *pranayama* by saluting God, by calling upon the Divine.[214] He goes on to say that the fruits and results of one's practice should then be surrendered to the Divine.[215] After

211. *Yoga Sutra* II.45
212. *Kumbhaka Paddhati of Raghuvira* stanzas 205–206
213. *Bhagavad Gita* III.27
214. Brahmananda's commentary on the *Hatha Yoga Pradipika* II.7.
215. Brahmananda's commentary on the *Hatha Yoga Pradipika* II.14

the practice is concluded, one should repeat the name of God and read sacred scriptures.[216] The idea here is that one should declare at the outset of the practice that it is our intention to reach the *darshana* (view) of the Divine to attain the divine aspect of our soul. At the end of the practice we consciously surrender the good created through it back to the Divine rather than want to hoard it for ourselves. Little is gained, however, if after all such noble intentions we return to the usual tamasic torpidity and rajasic frenzy of the mind. Brahmananda reminds us to stay in the sacred atmosphere of *pranayama*, once it is concluded, by repeating a name of the Divine and by reading sacred texts.

The *Hatha Tatva Kaumudi* declares that the yogi in a secluded place with a sparse diet, surrendered to God, should purify body and mind.[217] Purification of the body is useless if one eats a rich diet. A rich diet will produce a lot of metabolic toxins, which counteract purification of the body. If one eats little, the body will absorb most of it and few waste products remain. The more one eats the more toxins will clog up the body. Purification of the mind is, of course, aided by adding the component of surrender to the Divine. Surrendering to the Divine will prevent and remove mental toxins. Surrender to the Divine aids in removing vindictiveness, ambition, competitiveness, jealousy, bitterness, cynicism and hatred. These and other toxins of the mind are made up of *rajas* and *tamas*. If plagued by them we need to ask the Divine to make our mind peaceful, content, forgiving, compassionate and above all wishing to give and contribute to the life of others and enable their healing. This is the suitable mindset for *pranayama*.

Goraksha Natha called upon us to practise *pranayama* in a hidden place while sitting in *Padmasana* with our gaze fixed to the nose and being devoted to the Divine.[218] He suggests the place to be hidden so that nobody can find us and distract us from our work. *Padmasana* is ideal, because of its natural upward flow of *prana* while feet and

216. Brahmananda's commentary on the *Hatha Yoga Pradipika* II.18
217. *Hatha Tatva Kaumudi of Sundaradeva* XXXIX.1–2
218. *Goraksha Shataka* stanza 41

91

hands are turned towards the sky. *Padmasana* is the perfect physical expression for our longing for the Divine and turning away from the lower urges of our animalistic past. Directing the eyes to the nose (*nasagrai drishti*) encourages application of *Mula Bandha*, which awakens *Muladhara Chakra*, turns *apana vayu* (the vital downward current) upwards and aids in awakening of Kundalini. Devotion to the Divine is thus the natural result and fruition of the other aspects of meditation. It is the core and essence of *pranayama*.

Which form of the divine?
After talking so much about the Divine it is now important to clarify yoga's idea of God. The *Yoga Sutra* states that there is one God only, Ishvara. Ishvara means nothing but God, but the *Yoga Sutra* doesn't specify which God it is. Because God is difficult to fathom, the concept of *ishtadevata* is used, that is one's meditation-deity. Meditation-deity means that we choose an image or concept of God, which is the most likely for us to succeed with. There is no point in choosing a concept that is alienating to you, because you cannot fall in love with the Divine if you see God through an alienating concept. For this reason it has to be suitable for you, even if that means it is a concept that is not suitable to anybody else on earth.

The other really important notion contained in the term *ishtadevata* is that no *ishtadevata* has exclusive rights to be the one Godhead, the one Supreme Being. We can say that there is only one God, but we cannot say that this one God is my *ishtadevata* and not somebody else's. If my *ishtadevata* is right for me it just means that I understand the one and only Supreme Being best by using this particular *ishtadevata*. It can never be more right than the *ishtadevata* of the person next to me.

Yoga has developed out of the Hindu tradition, but has gone beyond it. Within Hinduism there are approximately 33,000 deities, which are only faces or aspects of the one Brahman (infinite consciousness). There is no wrong or right God, as all deities lead to the one Brahman. In the *Bhagavad Gita* Lord Krishna says that through whatever path you worship, you will always come to him.[219] Where else would you go? There is only one God. Krishna also says to us that, whichever aspect of the Divine we worship, he will make that faith unshakable.[220] It is the one Supreme Being that has inspired and caused the sacred traditions on all continents and cultures. But, since nations, cultures and individuals are so different, our ideas of the one Divine differ. But it is still the same Divine, only seen through different glasses. It does not matter which form of the Divine you worship. What matters is that you do worship the Divine.

Yoga also does not believe in converting people to Hinduism, nor does Hinduism believe that. In fact an authentic yoga teacher would, as T. Krishnamacharya has done, recommend students to first seek out the tradition of the ancestors of their own culture. This is due to the fact that it will be easier to connect to an *ishtadevata* if you have subconscious imprints (*samskaras*) relating to it. So a yogi coming from the Judeo-Christian-Islamic tradition will be advised to meditate on the Divine according to their own culture. For a yogi the concept of the Divine through which you attain to the Divine is not important. What is important is that you do.

If you do not have a tradition to look back to and do not have yet an *ishtadevata*, the method for finding yours is simple and straightforward. Patanjali says 'svadhyayat ishtadevata samprayogah', meaning to find your meditation-deity read the sacred books.[221] Pick up sacred books in any order you prefer and start studying them, and soon enough it will become clear to you which form, manifestation or avatar of the Divine is the most suitable to you. You attract and become that which you think of. If you keep reading the real estate pages your real estate portfolio will grow. If you read fashion magazines your wardrobe will burst and if you read sacred books you will be attracted to the form of the Divine that is suitable for you.

The scenario described so far is the one pertaining to the so-called

---

219. *Bhagavad Gita* IV.11
220. *Bhagavad Gita* VII.21
221. *Yoga Sutra* II.24

saguna-Brahman, that is God with form. God (Ishvara) is a person-alized form of the formless absolute, *nirguna*-Brahman. There are yogis who have as an *ishtadevata* the formless absolute. However, those people generally do practise Jnana Yoga and not Raja Yoga or Karma Yoga. That means they are only reflecting on the nature of absolute reality, and do not practise *asana, pranayama* and *mudra*. This is considered the most difficult form of yoga, simply for the reason that our mind is designed to attach itself automatically to form. It cannot comprehend the formless. It is only once the intellect is completely purified from any attachment to forms such as material wealth or beautiful manifestations of the opposite sex (or the same sex) that it gravitates to the formless absolute. Traditionally this re-quires from Jnanis that they are celibate and without any property / belongings. For obvious reasons this path is not suitable for the vast majority of people and, if a large group of yogis chose it, society would become dysfunctional. Yoga, however, holds that society is good and part of Divine expression, and therefore its perpetuation is a noble pursuit.

Lower yoga and Raja Yoga
The *Hatha Ratnavali* states that the lower yogic techniques like *asana, pranayama* and *mudra* are useless without having the goal of Raja Yoga in mind.[222] Raja Yoga means royal yoga. It is a term that denotes the 'high road' of yoga, generally used to indicate the *antaranga*s (inner limbs) of *dharana, dhyana* and *samadhi* (the sixth through to the eighth limb). Through *asana, pranayama* and *mudra* you may obtain a perfect body, perfect health and maybe even some occult powers to manipulate people, but all this will still let you die ignorant of the Divine hidden within your heart, your own true nature.[223] Raja Yoga and devotion to the Divine are those aspects of yoga that actually do make a difference on your deathbed. People nowadays are attracted to yoga to harvest its health benefits. You may hope that, if you obtain

222. *Hatha Ratnavali of Shrinivasayogi* I.19
223. *Bhagavad Gita* X.20: 'I am the self resting in the heart of every being.'

94

perfect health and a perfect body, you can experience pleasure and comfort for longer and subconsciously push away the hard fact of your own death and the day of reckoning. In some regards this is right, but even 20 to 30 years' life extension through yoga is really just a blip compared to the eternity of your existence. In the *Bhagavad Gita* Lord Krishna says – and he addresses not just Arjuna but every single one of us – 'You and I are ancient beings. The difference between us is that you do not know your past but I do.'[224]

The few decades of life extension gained through yoga will rush past like a second, after which the great moment arrives when you must forsake your body. Then the pleasure and comfort you managed to gain through yoga will provide no solace in an old dying body when you ask yourself what your life was about and whether you came from an attitude of giving, whether you contributed any good to this world and fulfilled your destiny. Think about it for a moment: To make your body perfectly proportioned and healthy may just give you the opportunity to ignore the reality of your death for longer. But even then you will die, and, if you ignore that fact longer, you may actually die a bigger fool than if you hadn't been involved in life-extending yoga practices at all. By 'bigger fool' I mean even more attached and identified with body and mind and even less appreciative of your eternal, spiritual nature. Not long ago I talked to a yoga student about yoga being about a school of preparation for death. She got really upset with me and told me she had just figured out her body through yoga, had attained health and was enjoying her body, and didn't want to hear anything about death. This is very concerning. In this case the student had actually successfully used yoga to push further away from her the most burning and important issue of life, the moment of truth, and yoga enabled her to live longer as if she would live forever – to live a lie. Here yoga has actually been used to lead somebody further into the darkness.

It is not the case that from mere practice of postures you will

224. *Bhagavad Gita* IV.5

automatically grow spiritually. You may actually spiritually shrink
as in the case of this student, who used postures to become even
more obsessed with her body – her material aspect – than she already
had been. Traditionally yoga postures are not to be engaged in to
gain health (although they will have that effect) but they are to be
done with an attitude of prayer to the Divine. Postures are prayer in
movement. That is why K.P. Jois called his book *Yoga Mala*:[225] you
use the postures like the beads of a *mala* to remember the Divine. The
Bhagavad Gita says that, unless they are performed as an offering to
the Divine, all actions lead to bondage.[226] This is also the case for
asana and *pranayama*.

Such are the dangers of modern postural yoga. The intention of
yoga is to fix your health only so that your mind becomes clearer
and you have more energy to focus it on the big questions of life.
The true purpose of yoga is to give you the visceral experience of
something that actually holds up even at the moment of death. In
the throes of death, most/all of what we were/are is stamped out by
the intensity of dying, but there is one experience that holds up even
right through the process of dying, and that is intense love for God,
sometimes also called knowledge of the Divine. To get this knowledge is not only our birthright but also our divine duty. Only if we
fulfil this divine duty can we die in complete and perfect peace. With
this experience we can die in peace, since we know that we can leave
because we have found completion. In this regard it is much more
important to die a perfect death than to live before death in perfect
health. The new obsession of postmodern, materialistic society with
health is born out of the need to be able to compete for non-renewable
resources for longer. We just don't want to die any more – to vacate
that spot on the cappuccino strip, on the beach and in the casino for
somebody else. 'Let me live and enjoy pleasure for longer! That's
why I do yoga!'

That's why the *Hatha Ratnavali* says that *asana*, *pranayama* and

225. K. Pattabhi Jois, *Yoga Mala*, Astanga Yoga Nilayam, Mysore, 1999
226. *Bhagavad Gita* III.9

mudra are useless without Raja Yoga. By themselves, without Raja Yoga, they are a form of bodybuilding in the regard that, if done without Raja Yoga, they are only aimed at perpetuating the body. A true yogi is one who would rather be dead, having died with divine knowledge, than be alive in a perfectly healthy body only to just go on consuming resources. In that regard the new fad of using yoga solely for body beautifying and health may be more dangerous to the sacred essence of yoga than many other adversities it has encountered in its long history.

EYES / FOCAL POINT

The *Yoga Rahasya* recommends keeping one's eyes closed during *pranayama*.[227] Keeping one's eyes closed can aid in deepening concentration and shutting out distractions. It is the method of choice for a yogi who has already acquired a predominantly sattvic mind and can keep in the mind a sattvic (sacred) object. Typical sattvic objects would be a *mantra* like *OM*, the *Gayatri mantra* or the Arabic *La ilaha ilallah* (there is no God but God). Depending on your faith you could also choose *I Am That I Am*,[228] the answer that Yahweh gave to Moses on the mountain, when Moses asked by which name He should be called, or Christ's *I am the way, the truth and the life*.[229] Visual objects can be an image of your *ishtadevata* such as Lord Krishna or Jesus Christ, an image such as the *OM* symbol, the cross or the half moon, or the word *Allah* written in Arabic. What is important is the ability to sustain focus on the object in one's mind during *pranayama*.

However, if one has a very active, visual, fantasizing mind, keeping the eyes closed can actually be counterproductive. In this case closing the eyes might enable you to leave the present moment on the wings of your imagination, but this is not exactly what you want to achieve during *pranayama*. During sleep, the eyes engage in a pattern of REM (rapid eye movement). REM is linked to dreaming and thus

227. *Yoga Rahasya* I.92
228. Exodus 3.14
229. John 14.6

to activity of the subconscious (*vasana*). In the waking state as well, the subconscious expresses itself through eye movement. Seemingly erratic eye movement that is not directly linked to any conscious activity indicates that the subconscious is processing past data. In this case your subconscious will project past experiences like shame, guilt, fear, anger and pain on to the present moment. This is not conducive to *pranayama*, as it tends to create rajasic or tamasic images in the mind.

Contrary to *Yoga Rahasya*, Goraksha Natha suggests practising *pranayama* with eyes directed to the nose.[230] Here the eyes are half closed so that one can barely see one's surroundings, keeping oneself in the present moment. To prevent the eyes from wandering around, they are bound to the nose (*Nasagrai Drishti*). The *Nasagrai Drishti* is linked to *Muladhara Chakra*, which it activates similarly to *Mula Bandha*. This *drishti* should be chosen when the yogi tends to dream off with closed eyes and if *Mula Bandha* is still weak. It should also be used during times when awakening of Kundalini from *Muladhara Chakra* is attempted.

Sundaradeva recommends focusing the mind during *pranayama* between the eyebrows (*Bhrumadhya Drishti*).[231] During *Bhrumadhya Drishti* the eyes are gently raised upwards. It is important that this *drishti* remains gentle, as one can strain the optic nerves if it is forced. Slowly extend the time you spend daily in this *drishti*; do not go from 0 to 30 minutes in 1 day. The *Bhrumadhya Drishti* is very potent: it draws *prana* towards the *Ajna Chakra* (3rd eye), thus raising it upwards in *sushumna*. It is a more advanced *drishti* than *Nasagrai*. When *prana* rises to the *Ajna* and remains there for long enough, objective *samadhi* takes place. *Bhrumadhya Drishti* is suggested if one meditates on the Divine with form (*saguna* Brahman). All deities constitute *saguna* Brahman. Meditation during *kumbhaka* on Jesus Christ or Lord Krishna is ideally accompanied by *Bhrumadhya Drishti*.

Raghuvira proclaims that success in *pranayama* is obtained

230. *Goraksha Shataka* stanza 41
231. *Hatha Tatva Kaumudi of Sundaradeva* XXXVI.15

quickly when supported by *Shambhavi Mudra*.[232] *Shambhavi Mudra* is a more intense version of *Bhrumadhya Drishti*. In *Bhrumadhya Drishti* it is left to you how far up you turn the eyes. It is important that the eyes are arrested to prevent them from darting around in the eye sockets, which would enable the projection of *vasana* (conditioning, content of the subconscious).

In *Shambhavi Mudra*, however, the eyes are locked between the eyebrows and turned up all the way. The eyes are turned up so far that one is literally unaware of any visual input but the inner eye is completely turned upwards to the Divine. This is a difficult yogic technique that can only gradually be integrated into one's practice. However, once it is achieved it strongly increases proficiency in *pranayama* by enabling the yogi to keep the mind absorbed into the Divine.

The keeping of a divine image in one's mind can be made easier by placing a copy of the same divine image in front of you while practising *pranayama*. Every time you lose mental focus during *kumbhaka*, open your eyes and look at it. Once you have a clear impression of this sattvic image in your mind, again close your eyes. If you do not have a divine image to meditate on, you may simply take your holy book for this purpose. The mere presence of your holy book will make your *pranayama* more sattvic. The fixing of the eyes on a sacred object is called *Trataka*. It purifies and purges the subconscious because it interrupts involuntary eye movements. T. Krishnamacharya taught that *Trataka* will lead you easily to mastery of *Shambhavi Mudra*, which in itself is a powerful method of accessing *samadhi*.[233]

TAKING REST

It is important to take a rest after *pranayama*, sufficiently long for one to feel refreshed afterwards. If you are tired or wound up before *pranayama*, it may be helpful to have a short *Shavasana* (relaxation) even right before it. If you are still tired after that, then do not engage in the practice. It is counterproductive. Reorganize your sleeping

232. *Kumbhaka Paddhati of Raghuvira* stanza 284
233. T. Krishnamacharya, *Yoga Makaranda*, rev. English edn, Media Garuda, Chennai, 2011, p. 100

patterns so that you are not tired during your practice time. It is advised that, when practising yoga, one does not sleep too much or too little.[234]

Do not engage in a multi-hour *asana* and *pranayama* practice early in the morning without sufficient rest afterwards. It is not a good idea to try to catch up by sleeping in the afternoon. The *Hatha Tatva Kaumudi* states that sleeping during daytime causes disease,[235] and the *Yoga Kundalini Upanishad* confirms that sleeping in daytime and going to bed late have that consequence.[236] This is due to the fact that sleeping in intervals or sleeping at inappropriate times makes the *vayu* go astray. This means that it disturbs the ideal flow of *prana* in the body in a similar way to taking too much food or spending time with people who have a negative influence on you. Disturbing the sleep pattern generally has a tamasic influence on the mind. It is good to go to bed early and rise early. At 4.45 in the morning *brahmi muhurta*, the divine time, begins. That is when we are closest to God; hence it is the ideal time for spiritual practice such as *pranayama*, *asana* or meditation.

Try to get your sleep in one piece rather than sleeping in the afternoon or during the day. If you are so tired that you have to, then do it, but as a long-term project try to organize your life in such a way that this is not necessary. Swami Rama said that sleeping in daytime enlarges the three *dosha*s (impediments), *vata*, *pitta* and *kapha*, and therefore should take place under no circumstances.[237] Note the difference between yoga and Ayurveda here. Ayurveda looks towards a balance between the three *dosha*s, but yoga looks at them as disturbances and wants to transform and eject them entirely. More about that later.

Generally *pranayama* will reduce your need for sleep. It will do so automatically and slowly over time. But do not reduce your sleep time just because you have started the practice. *Pranayama* tends to

234. *Bhagavad Gita* VI.16
235. *Hatha Tatva Kaumudi of Sundaradeva* III.35
236. *Yoga Kundalini Upanishad* I.56–57
237. Swami Rama, *Path of Fire and Light*, vol. 1, Himalayan Institute Press, Honesdale, 1988, p. 33

keep us in a sattvic state, but only then if it is done with a sattvic mind. Modern life can be very frantic. The frantic (rajasic) mind loses its equilibrium and descends into torpidity (*tamas*) to regain it. Then when we wake up we are so tamasic that we need coffee or cocaine to make our mind frantic enough to shoulder that much-too-large mortgage and the three jobs needed to service it. We then run our whole day on our sympathetic nervous system, to the extent that we can't switch it off any more and need sleeping pills to counteract the rajasic mind. And so the circle turns. The sattvic state avoids the extreme energy expenditure of the rajasic state and therefore does not need to descend so much into *tamas* to regenerate.

HEAT, SWEAT AND FIRE
Exhalation is a mechanism used to externalise heat. You can easily detect that exhaled air is warmer than inhaled air unless the environmental temperature is very high. In a standard *pranayama* breathing cycle, the inhalation makes up one-third and the exhalation two-thirds of the time. This means that during this cycle you can use 66% of the time to externalise heat. If you are an established practitioner and your ratio is 1 for inhalation, 4 for *kumbhaka* and 2 for exhalation, you can utilize only 28.58% of your breathing cycle for exhalation and the externalization of heat. All other parameters being equal, you will then heat up.

This heat in yoga is seen as the ignition of your inner fire used to burn through delusion and ignorance. If you do practise in a warm environment your body will produce sweat as a cooling mechanism. Both Goraksha Natha[238] and Svatmarama[239] recommend rubbing the sweat back into the body using one's hands. However, both of these recommendations are clearly positioned in chapters and passages pertaining to *pranayama* only and not to *asana*. The sweat produced during *asana* before the body is purified is toxic, and should be washed off, as *asana* is primarily designed for the purification of the

238. *Goraksha Shataka* stanza 50
239. *Hatha Yoga Pradipika* II.13

101

gross body. This is confirmed by Swami Rama, who taught that massaging of sweat into the skin was only acceptable after the body is purified.[240]

To be able to rub sweat back into the body, you need to bare your skin. For this reason, practise *pranayama* as lightly dressed as possible. You may feel at the end of your practice much hotter than at the outset. As you cannot undress during *kumbhaka* (the movement would make the *vayu* go astray), it is helpful to cover yourself at the beginning of your practice in a blanket or shawl, which you can throw off, rather than wear too much. According to the *Hatha Tatva Kaumudi*, the rubbing of the sweat back into the skin prevents the *prana* from going astray.[241] You will notice that, after an intense *pranayama* session, the rubbing of sweat into the skin, particularly into the limbs, has a distinctly integrating effect.

During summer or during a heatwave you will find that it is very difficult to maintain your *kumbhaka* length, especially during the day. Rather than strain your heart under the excess heat load, limit your *pranayama* to the early morning or the cool of the night, or reduce your *kumbhaka*s if appropriate. Once you have gone through a year or two of constant *pranayama* you will notice that the winter is the time when you advance most in regard to *kumbhaka* length. Depending on where you live, the summer is not suitable for extending *kumbhaka* and you may struggle to maintain your level.

It is much easier to extend one's *kumbhaka*s in a cold climate such as high up in the mountains. This is one of the reasons why many advanced yogis retreated into the icy-cold recesses of the Himalayas. We know, for example, that T. Krishnamacharya was able to melt the ice to a certain diameter around his body merely from the heat generated in *kumbhaka*. Another way of managing heat is by practising *kumbhaka* in or even under water as Trailanga Swami and Pilot Baba have done.

240. Swami Rama, *Path of Fire and Light*, vol. 1, Himalayan Institute Press, Honesdale, 1988, p. 53
241. *Hatha Tatva Kaumudi of Sundaradeva* XXXIX.54

Do not practise in direct sun. It will make you heat up too quickly and thus strain your heart. Do not use wind to cool down in *kumbhaka*. You need to practise in a location without draught. Draught will make the *prana* in your body go astray. It is a cause of disease. The yogis of yore built little meditation huts with one door and one window on the side facing away from the wind direction. Do not sit in the path of the wind when practising *pranayama*.

Sweat, kumbhaka length and purification of agni
The *Hatha Yoga Pradipika* and many other texts talk about three stages of practice called *kanishta* (inferior), *Madhyama* (middling) and *uttama* (superior), which are often identified with *kumbhaka* lengths of 48 seconds, 64 seconds and 80 seconds respectively. Keep in mind that terms like *inferior* here mean inferior within the scope of a serious, dedicated, spiritual practice intended to completely transform the yogi. Such a practice is considered to commence at 48 seconds, but in absolute terms it is still a serious practice, and nobody who is not properly prepared and taught should undertake it. The three stages of *kanishta*, *Madhyama* and *uttama* are said to lead to perspiration, throbbing of *prana* and finally steadiness of *prana* respectively.[242] This final stage is a precursor to the practice of the higher limbs (*antarangas*), but the perspiration accompanying the first stage is considered essential in the purification of the *nadis* and the mind. It is *tapas* in the true sense of the word, *tapas* being derived from the verb *root tap* – to cook.

Let's recall here Sundaradeva's proclamation that pure, not impaired, *pitta* (metabolic fire) kindles the fire of wisdom, expels the impediments (*doshas*) and causes awakening of Kundalini.[243] This pure, unimpaired state of *pitta*, however, rarely occurs under normal circumstances, as under such circumstances *pitta* functions as a *dosha*. *Pitta* is returned to its pure, unimpaired state (i.e. the physical expression of *sattva*) by slowly increasing the fire of *kumbhaka* while yet maintaining purity

242. *Hatha Yoga Pradipika* II.12.
243. *Hatha Tatva Kaumudi of Sundaradeva* XXXVI.55

103

of body through *mitahara* (moderate diet) and purity of mind through surrender to the Divine (*Ishvara pranidhana*). Without these two essential supports, it is better not to take *kumbhaka* to the *kanishta* stage (i.e. 48 seconds) as *pitta* will remain impaired and therefore an impediment.

HOW LONG IS ONE MATRA?

The *Yoga Sutra* calls for making the breath long and subtle.[244] In order to do so we need to measure the breath, and this means a unit of time has to be introduced. This time unit is called a *matra*. A *matra* originally was defined quite vaguely. We hear of definitions for a *matra* such as circling one's knee with one's hand once, clapping one's hand twice or snapping one's finger three times.[245] However, even more exotic ways of measuring the *matra* were given in *Kumbhaka Paddhati*. Its author, Raghuvira, defines it as the time spent in ringing the bell to call the calf to the cow.[246] Sundaradeva, in his *Hatha Tatva Kaumudi*, is more precise in calling a *matra* the time spent ringing the bell when feeding the calf at the time of milking the cow.[247]

If you were harbouring any doubts as to the precise length of a matra surely they would be removed now. Measuring matras with an hourglass made from copper was introduced as early as Shrinivasayogi's *Hatha Ratnavali* and confirmed in the *Hatha Tatva Kaumudi*.[248]

Because practising with an hourglass proved too restrictive, *matras* were then subdivided into long and short *matras*, long *matras* being called *adimatras*. A long *matra* means that, once a certain count is mastered, the length of the *matra* itself is stretched. For our purpose we can equate a *matra* with 1 second, keeping in mind that, later on the way to mastery, we may stretch the same *matra* to 2 or 4 seconds, or even the time used for an exhalation when asleep.

244. *Yoga Sutra* II.50
245. *Brhadyogi Yajnavalkya Smrti* VIII.12
246. *Kumbhaka Paddhati of Raghuvira* stanzas 158–160
247. *Hatha Tatva Kaumudi of Sundaradeva* XXXVIII.123–125
248. *Hatha Tatva Kaumudi of Sundaradeva* X.47

RATIO AND COUNT

Let's define a breath as one respiratory cycle consisting of inhalation and exhalation. At the outset of *pranayama*, a breath or breathing cycle has two components, inhalation and exhalation. In advanced *pranayama* it may have four components: inhalation (*puraka*), internal (*antara*) *kumbhaka*, exhalation (*rechaka*), external (*bahya*) *kumbhaka*. The ratio of the individual components to each other may be either even (*sama*) or uneven (*vishama*). For example a ratio of 1 *matra* for the inhalation to 1 *matra* for the exhalation is even (*sama*), whereas a ratio of 1:2 is uneven (*vishama*). The *Yoga Rahasya* states that the even ratios need to be applied first, and only when one is comfortable with them are the uneven ratios to be used.[249] Even ratios make the mind more rajasic due to the relatively long inhalation, while uneven ratios make the mind more tamasic due to the relatively long exhalation. Rajasic and tamasic tendencies are, however, balanced once *kumbhaka* comes into play, which when done correctly makes the mind sattvic.

The total length of each breath expressed in the ratio is referred to as count. When we start practising the ratio of 1:1, we first use the length of breath that we normally take. For example, if the average respiratory rate is 15 breaths per second, each breath takes about 4 seconds. We distribute half of that to the inhalation and half to the exhalation and arrive at a count of 2:2 seconds. The ratio would then be 1:1, which would be a case of an even (*sama*) ratio.

If you see a ratio that includes three components it usually refers to inhalation, internal *kumbhaka* and exhalation. The most popular ratio is the advanced 1:4:2 ratio, which according to the *Yoga Rahasya* is very important, because it is the main method of cleaning *nadis*.[250] This is an example of an uneven (*vishama*) ratio. There are also more unusual ratios: for example the *Yoga Chudamani Upanishad* recommends a 6:8:5 ratio, which is much more forgiving than 1:4:2.[251]

249. *Yoga Rahasya* I.94
250. *Yoga Rahasya* II.59–60
251. *Yoga Chudamani Upanishad* stanza 103

The *Gheranda Samhita* states that the three grades of *pranayama* (*kanishta*–inferior, *Madhyama*–middling and *uttama*–advanced) refer to inhalations of 12 *matras* (seconds) for *kanishta*, 16 for *Madhyama* and 20 for *uttama*.[252] If we take the middle length of 16 seconds for the inhalation and convert it using the important 1:4:2 ratio, then we arrive at 16 seconds for the inhalation, 64 seconds for *kumbhaka* and 32 seconds for the exhalation. This count is so important that, for example, the *Mandala Brahmana Upanishad* proclaims that it constitutes *pranayama*.[253] The *Gheranda Samhita* likewise gives this count great importance.[254]

If you do see a ratio that has four components such as 1:1:1:1, the fourth number refers to external (*bahya*) *kumbhaka*s.

MANTRA AND DIGITAL COUNTING

In our first few *pranayama* sessions we may want to count the length (*kala*) of each breathing component by counting in our mind the number of seconds while listening to a clock ticking in the background. If there is a lot of background noise it maybe difficult to hear a clock ticking. This is particularly the case if one practises rapid-breathing *pranayama*s such as *Kapalabhati* and *Bhastrika*. For this reason it is very helpful to use a metronome that has a volume function. Alternatively, with certain modern handheld devices a metronome app can be downloaded.

After a few sessions, however, I suggest that you let go of counting numbers in your head unless you want to use your *pranayama* as an additional qualification to become an accountant, mathematician or hedge fund manager, noble pursuits as they may be. Remember that you will become what you think. For this reason the yogi chooses sattvic meditation objects, and numbers are not sattvic. The best counting method for *pranayama* is the use of *mantra*.

Mantra is a very important discipline. Success in higher yoga and

252. *Gheranda Samhita* V.55
253. *Mandala Brahmana Upanishad* I.1
254. *Gheranda Samhita* V.49–51

success in Kundalini-rousing is next to impossible if one is ignorant of *mantra*. Modern *asana* practitioners should not think that disciplines like *mantra* and *chakra* are somehow for the faint-hearted. It was not long ago that there were still yogis who could light their campfire through *mantra*, an art that seems to have fallen by the wayside nowadays.

*Mantra*s are bioplasmic soundwaves used to bring about changes in the body and/or mind of the practitioner and, in cases like the campfires, even the surroundings. The importance of *mantra* is supported by *Yoga Rahasya*, which proclaims that *pranayama* should be done with *mantra*, as only then does it bring stability of mind, freedom from suffering, a long life and development of devotion.[255] The *Yoga Rahasya* becomes more specific when declaring that *pranayama* should be measured by pronouncing *OM*, as through *OM* the *chakra*s are purified. A particular popular use of *OM* with yogis is the striking of *OM* during each *matra* into the *Muladhara* (base) *Chakra* to awaken Kundalini. Advanced practitioners may switch to the much longer *Gayatri mantra* once a certain length of count is reached.

The way to introduce *mantra* into *pranayama* is by means of digital counting. To do so, touch each phalange of your digits once with the thumb when the clock or metronome ticks. Each digit has three phalanges, multiplied by four fingers (thumb is used for counting) making a total of 12 for 1 full hand. For example if you stay in *kumbhaka* for 48 seconds you count your full hand 4 times. Each time your thumb touches a phalange pronounce in your mind your *mantra* of choice, the default being *OM*. This way you use your hand for the mind-numbing task of counting, while using your powerful mind for the uplifting task of pronouncing *mantra*. Pronouncing *mantra*s silently in your mind is considered more powerful than pronouncing them audibly.

255. *Yoga Rahasya* I.97–98

Preparation for pranayama

It has been pointed out already that *pranayama* is the preparation for the higher limbs. *Pratyahara, dharana, dhyana* and *samadhi* are prepared for and powered by *pranayama* and its essence, *kumbhaka*. The following chapters, however, deal with preparating for *pranayama* and *kumbhaka*. Without this preparation *pranayama* cannot succeed.

MITAHARA

Mitahara means a moderate yogic diet. I am not a qualified nutritionist and can give advice on diet only in regard to how it impacts on yoga. However, as you will soon come to learn, your choice of foods is what will impact your yoga more than any other activity outside your formal practice. I would prefer not to enter into the diet discussion, as there exists an enormous emotional charge around it. Many people eat whatever their tastebuds dictate or whatever impulse articles they see in commercials or supermarket displays. On the other hand we have those who have an almost religious zeal when it comes to their diet. They take immense pride in it and judge those who adhere to an 'inferior' diet. This attitude, too, is dangerous to yoga, as pride will delete a lot of merit accumulated through yoga.

The *Yoga Rahasya of Nathamuni*, a text handed down through T. Krishnamacharya, is most vocal about the need for being selective towards one's food, both quantitatively and qualitatively. The *Yoga Rahasya* says that the yogi should eat limited food and only that which is sattvic. In a nutshell, sattvic food consists of fruit, vegetables, milk (for those who are tolerant to it), ghee, nuts and seeds, and some grains. The *Yoga Rahasya* also says that to limit food intake is important when dealing with the blockages (*granthi*s) and with back bending. It also ascribes the clogging of the *nadi*s and physical blockages directly to too much food and excess fat.[256] The *Yoga Rahasya* says that *Nadi Shodhana*, the main method of cleaning the *nadi*s, will only work when combined with reduced food intake and sattvic food.[257] The author of the *Yoga Rahasya* also combines the call for limited food intake with the injunction to eat only at appropriate times,[258] these being the morning, lunchtime and evening. This rules out so-called grazing, according to which small morsels and snacks

256. *Yoga Rahasya* II.29
257. *Yoga Rahasya* II.60
258. *Yoga Rahasya* III.7

are constantly eaten. This will mix undigested and digested food in the stomach, creating *ama* (poison). The strongest injunction, however, against indiscriminate food intake is delivered by the *Yoga Rahasya* when it states that physical and mental problems 'always' arise due to undisciplined food intake.[259]

Outside *Yoga Rahasya*, T. Krishnamacharya emphasized the importance of a sparse, simple diet. According to him a yogi should eat less, avoid putting on weight at all costs[260] and reduce fat.[261] The call for a moderate diet goes as far back as the ancient *Chandogya Upanishad*, which states that in purity of food lies purity of mind.[262]

Other texts agree. The *Gheranda Samhita* declares that yoga without a moderate diet will bring about disease and will intercept any merit created by the practice.[263] The *Shiva Samhita* is almost cynical when it says that no cleverness in the world can bring success to a yogi who does not eat moderately and abstemiously.[264] As do many other texts, the *Hatha Tatva Kaumudi* counts 10 *yamas* and *niyamas*. Of the *yamas* it deems *mitahara* (moderate diet) the principal one.[265] It rules out not only large quantities of food but also any sweets, and advises a moderate diet at every turn,[266] often combined with staying silent as a prerequisite for *pranayama*. Its author, Sundaradeva, advises us that without sticking religiously to a moderate diet no success whatsoever can be attained in yoga, and he again combines this with the advice to eschew talkativeness.[267] The *Shiva Samhita*, too, suggests eating and talking little.[268] The reason why we often find the two mentioned together is that food intake means energy intake, while

259. *Yoga Rahasya* III.5
260. A.G. Mohan, *Krishnamacharya: His Life and Teachings*, Shambala, Boston & London, 2010, p. 95
261. A.G. Mohan, *Krishnamacharya: His Life and Teachings*, Shambala, Boston & London, 2010, p. 96
262. *Chandogya Upanishad* VII.62.2
263. *Gheranda Samhita* V.2
264. *Shiva Samhita* V.183
265. *Hatha Tatva Kaumudi of Sundaradeva* IV.45
266. *Hatha Tatva Kaumudi of Sundaradeva* XXXVI.66
267. *Hatha Tatva Kaumudi of Sundaradeva* LV.5
268. *Shiva Samhita* III.33

talking means energy output. Energy available for yoga can be increased by selecting the right foods, but there is little point if the same energy is expended through talkativeness and gossip.

Sundaradeva's most important advice on diet is likely to be that the yogi should consume food only to preserve his/her body.[269] The contemporary trend towards turning chefs into celebrities and artists reflects the tendency to eat as a means to deriving pleasure. The emphasis is on deriving maximum pleasure from the gustatory sense, the tastebuds. However, this leaves out the rest of the alimentary canal, which is then left with having to digest the excesses of the tastebuds. The body is very similar to the engine of your car, only much more complex. Imagine your car suddenly developed tastebuds and forced you to drive to petrol stations where you can get the most sumptuous and delicious petrols and oils. More and more spices would be added and the petrol and oil would be prepared in more and more elaborate combinations and modifications. Your car would begin to stutter along and sometimes get sick or have a hangover due to the heavy and rich foods. Most often it would guzzle too much because the petrol was too yummy. Your car would start to gather middle-aged spread and not take off at the traffic lights any more. After more and more frequent stays at the workshop it would eventually fail you completely way before its time. This is what will happen to your body if you embark on the journey to eat for pleasure.

Strangely enough, people now use spiritual vocabulary when talking about experiencing food. The say that the 'food was divine'. This is a sad projection of divinity onto sensory pleasure. Because we have lost sight of the Divine within us we are now projecting it onto the superficial and shallow pleasure derived through our tastebuds. True joy is experienced when the *darshana* (view) of the Divine is gained through the higher limbs of yoga. Until we experience this true joy, we need to keep the vehicle of our body fit to travel on the road to freedom. Only then can the body fulfil its role. Eating is meant to maintain the body and supply it with fuel. Eating is not

269. *Hatha Tatva Kaumudi of Sundaradeva* LV.5

designed to give us the experience of divine joy. Divine joy is experienced upon beholding the Divine within our hearts. For, as Lord Krishna says, 'I am the self abiding in the heart of all beings'.[270]

If we eat to maintain the body, as Sundaradeva suggests in the *Hatha Tatva Kaumudi*, we will not dig our graves with our teeth. Dig our graves with our teeth we will, however, if we select foods depending on their propensity to provide intense stimulation to our tastebuds. Gustatory stimulation now has become so important in modern society because many of its members cannot experience any more the simple joy of being alive without external sensory stimulation.

Sahajananda, author of the *Hatha Yoga Manjari* and disciple of the great Goraksha Natha, goes further than the *Hatha Tatva Kaumudi* when he says that *mitahara* (moderate diet) has no equal, not only among *yamas* but also among *niyamas*.[271] The Vedic scriptures also put emphasis on moderate diet. The *Yoga Kundalini Upanishad* states that the mind (*chitta*) has two causes: conditioning (*vasanas*) and life force (*prana*). It is necessary to control only one of them, as the other will automatically be controlled as well. According to the *Upanishad*, the control of *prana* is possible through combining the restraining of one's eating habits with practising *asanas* and rousing the Kundalini (which in itself is again achieved through *pranayama*, *mudra* and meditation).[272] The same *Upanishad* considers unwholesome food to be one of the seven causes of disease.[273]

WHAT IS MITAHARA AND WHAT TO EAT

There are three ways of looking at *mitahara*, three different aspects to it. The *Bhagavad Gita* describes *mitahara* as consuming only sattvic food.[274] On the other hand the *Vasishta Samhita* measures *mitahara* through the number of mouthfuls the yogi takes,[275] meaning a yogi

270. *Bhagavad Gita* X.20
271. *Hatha Yoga Manjari of Sahajananda* I.42
272. *Yoga Kundalini Upanishad* I.1–2
273. *Yoga Kundalini Upanishad* I. 56–57
274. *Bhagavad Gita* 17.8
275. *Vasishta Samhita* I.50

takes less than an average person. A third way of looking at *mitahara* is described in the *Hatha Yoga Pradipika*, which states that one's food needs to be offered to God before eating it.[276] The *Gheranda Samhita* combines two of these aspects when suggesting eating with love for the Divine and leaving the stomach half empty.[277] For maximum effect, a wise yogi will practise all three aspects of *mitahara* simultaneously.

Before taking one's food the wise yogi will remember God in the form that is suitable for her. We need to remember that it is not by our power that the Earth brings forth food and not by our power that our body can digest it, but it is by the power of *prakrti*, by the power of Shakti, which is nothing but the nurturing female aspect of the one Supreme Being.

After having offered our food to the Divine, we need to keep our food intake to the level that is required to maintain our body. Why not more? Why shouldn't we eat to our heart's content? Foodstuffs and the resulting faeces draw the *apana vayu* downwards. Kundalini-rousing, however, relies on an upward flow of *apana* as as one of its main motors. Hence foodstuffs and faeces have to be reduced and, during the acute phase of Kundalini-rousing, almost eliminated. This is not some lofty concept, but it can be experienced by every meditator. Meditation, and in fact any spiritual practice, should take place after defaecation. However, just for the purpose of comprehension, sit down some time after a heavy meal or prior to defaecation and try to fix your mind at the *Ajna Chakra* and its energetic source in the centre of the cranium. Unless you are a very strong meditator, you will find that your awareness is drawn downwards through the force of gravitation by the presence of digested or undigested food-stuffs in the alimentary canal. This presents a strong obstacle, and the practice of yoga is about being reasonable and stacking the odds in your favour. The absence of digested and undigested foodstuffs decreases apanic downward flow and thus increases the likelihood that you have an inspiring meditation experience.

276. *Hatha Yoga Pradipika* 1.58
277. *Gheranda Samhita* V.21

The third aspect of *mitahara* is that food should be sattvic. Sattvic food is food that has the natural tendency to let the mind gravitate towards the sacred and away from the profane. The profane comes in two categories: tamasic food makes the mind dull and heavy whereas rajasic food makes the mind fickle and agitated. Sattvic food also has the highest pranic value, as it is not denaturized.

Generally speaking the sattvic category consists of fresh vegetables, fruit, milk and ghee, grains, seeds and nuts. The *Hatha Yoga Pradipika* says that food wholesome for yogis consists of milk and ghee.[278] The *Shandilya Upanishad* states the same, and links ghee and milk consumption to protection from burning sensations. In other words ghee and milk protect the alimentary canal from *agni* (fire), which is stoked in the process of Kundalini-rousing.[279] The *Shiva Samhita*, too, advises the consumption of milk and ghee,[280] and this was also espoused by the siddha Goraksha Natha.[281] That milk is especially helpful for advanced *pranayama* was confirmed by T. Krishnamacharya, who links it to his ability to stop his heartbeat during *Nadi Shodhana pranayama*.[282] Theos Bernard, too, learned from his teacher that *pranayama* could lead to the state of 'living on air', to which only milk was to be added.[283] Swami Rama says that ghee alleviates *vata*, cools *pitta* and rebuilds *kapha*, and for this reason is the ideal food for *pranayama*.[284] He also holds that ghee subdues vitiated *pitta*, making it a veritable miracle food.

Swami Ramdev considers milk, fruit and green vegetables the ideal food for *pranayama*,[285] and in another text he suggests taking

278. *Hatha Yoga Pradipika* II.14.
279. *Shandilya Upanishad* stanza 22
280. *Shiva Samhita* III.37
281. *Goraksha Shataka* stanza 53
282. A.G. Mohan, *Krishnamacharya: His Life and Teachings*, Shambala, Boston & London, 2010, p. 56
283. Theos Bernard, *Heaven Lies Within Us*, Charles Scribner's Sons, New York, 1939, p. 154
284. Swami Rama, *Path of Fire and Light*, vol. 1, Himalayan Institute Press, Honesdale, 1988, p. 12
285. Swami Ramdev, *Pranayama*, Divya Yog Mandir Trust, Hardwar, 2007, p. 18

green vegetables in large quantities.[286] Sahajananda, author of the
Hatha Yoga Manjari, recommends green food to avoid constipation.[287]
Shrikrishna, author of *Pranayama*, suggests living mainly on fruit and
vegetables.[288] In the *Jogapradipyaka*, Jayatarama recommends green
gram, a pulse, for rebalancing the *vayus* if they have become disturbed
by incorrect practice.[289] Food chosen by the yogic practitioner should
be high in pranic value,[290] and for this purpose it must be fresh and
untreated by preservatives and chemicals. Refining and packaging
foods makes them automatically tamasic, as they lose their *prana*
during processing and packaging.[291] In addition to giving most supermarket shelves a wide berth, you need to be aware that many vegetables
and fruits are radioactively treated and sprayed with chemicals such
as arsenic to preserve them. Although they may look good from the
outside, their pranic value has been significantly reduced. Radiation
treatment and chemicals are used to reduce the ability of bacteria
to break down foods. However our digestion process relies on very
similar bacteria to be efficient. If there are things in your fridge that
don't seem to go off, it is likely that they are completely denatured.
As a rule of thumb, what's not good enough for (exogenous) bacteria
in your fridge is also not helpful for the (endogenous) bacteria in
your alimentary canal. Without turning it into an obsession, eat as
much organic food as possible to avoid pesticides and fertilizers.
Fertilizers make vegetables and fruit grow large but they decrease
their nutritional value.

286. Swami Ramdev, *Pranayama Rahasya*, Divya Yog Mandir Trust, Hardwar, 2009, p. 84
287. *Hatha Yoga Manjari of Sahajananda* II.23
288. Shrikrishna, *Essence of Pranayama*, 2nd edn, Kaivalyadhama, Lonavla, 1996, p. 98
289. *Jogapradipyaka of Jayatarama* stanzas 800–806
290. Swami Niranjanananda, *Prana and Pranayama*, Yoga Publications Trust, Munger, 2009, p. 14
291. Swami Niranjanananda, *Prana and Pranayama*, Yoga Publications Trust, Munger, 2009, p. 211

CATEGORIES OF FOOD

I will enquire now into categories of food and the merit or demerit that they may confer on the yogi. Again, as I am not a nutritionist my advice only pertains to diet from a yogic perspective.

The most important rule in relation to diet probably is the one that says one person's food is another person's poison. Just because a particular category of food works for Indians does not necessarily mean that it will work for people of East Asian, Mediterranean or African descent. During evolution and history, humans have adapted to many foods that previously were unsuitable. However, many of today's yoga students come from diverse ethnic backgrounds that need to be taken into consideration. You need to ask yourself the question as to what your ancestors have adapted to. Your diet also needs to adapt to your personal situation, i.e. more protein for those who live a very physical life or are engaged in hard physical labour. For example, if you are of Caucasian or African descent and you perform a very intense multi-hour *asana* practice, you are likely to be in need of a higher protein intake than for example somebody of South Asian descent who puts more focus on a *pranayama* and meditation practice.

I will leave to one side any emotional discussion of which are the foods whose procurement involves violence and which foods are unethical. Dairy in India is considered non-violent on flimsy grounds, as its production is inevitably linked to the death of bull calves even if the milk cows are not slaughtered until their production recedes.

1. Dairy products are considered some of the most sattvic foods. Cheeses, in particular yellow cheeses, are considered too heavy and processed for yoga. They take too much energy to digest and their digestive process is too slow. Milk and ghee are considered yogic super foods. If you are dairy tolerant use plenty of them. However, milk can contain high levels of toxins, as it is further towards the end of the food chain. It is therefore important to use organic produce. It is now believed that dairy tolerance developed in the form of

a gene mutation in the Ural mountains about 5000 years ago and spread south and westwards from there. Individuals with this gene can digest dairy. Those without it have adverse reactions and may derive little consolation from the rave reviews milk gets in yogic scripture. The yogic tradition was carried by South Asian people. Since they developed agriculture very early on, they developed tolerance to dairy products. A yogi coming from an East Asian background, where no dairy culture developed, may have to look for suitable replacements.

2. Vegetables, tubers and legumes are also considered sattvic and have very high nutritional value. The also make the body alkaline and generally contain low levels of toxins. Vegetables are ideal for yoga, and you can eat as much of them as you like. I will not go into what particular vegetables, because again this depends on your ancestral background.

3. Fruit has many of the advantages of vegetables, with one disadvantage. They contain a lot of sugar. Eating too much fruit can disturb your sugar metabolism and lead to diabetes. As their energy and sugar content can easily be unlocked, it is wise to eat them in the morning or during the day, but not in the evening when little energy is required. Fruit generally contains low levels of toxins, as it is at the start of the food chain.

4. Seeds and nuts are very nutritious and contain high levels of protein and other nutrients, but some individuals are allergic to them. As long as they are stored properly they generally contain low levels of toxins.

5. Carbohydrates such as potatoes, wheat, rice and rye can be used by those who are tolerant to them. Many people are gluten intolerant. Carbohydrates are a cheap source of energy, are easily digested and generally do not contain high levels of toxins. However, they contain little in the way of nutrients, make the organism acidic and contribute to many modern diseases such as diabetes (high glycaemic index) and cancer (growth). As with milk, some experts argue that as a species we did not have enough time to adapt to agricultural

119

products such as simple carbohydrates. Many individuals are intolerant to simple carbohydrates but do not know it. If you do use simple carbohydrates then do not combine them with protein. Especially do not combine eggs, meat, dairy and fish on the one hand with bread, rice, potato, wheat etc. on the other. Proteins are broken down in the stomach in an acidic reaction and for this purpose stay in the stomach for quite some time. Simple carbohydrates are broken down in the small intestine in an alkaline reaction, and for this purpose travel very quickly through the stomach. If you mix both, the simple carbohydrates stay in the stomach too long and your body will become too acidic. You may combine both groups, the proteins and the simple carbohydrates, with vegetables or salad, which are complex carbohydrates. Most cases of obesity today are caused by a high-carbohydrate diet and not through a high-fat diet. Fat is a better and more natural source of energy, as the body accesses it over a longer time frame. It does not lead to large swings in energy availability as simple carbohydrates do.

6. Protein is used to build and repair muscle and other tissues, but it is hard to digest and may contain high levels of toxins. Foods that are rich in protein:

• Eggs are rejected by Indian vegetarians, using flimsy arguments like those that led them to accepting milk. Eggs contain the most highly available form of protein but may contain high levels of chemicals. If you use them buy organic.

• Soy is another good source of protein, but it is a phytoestrogen, and many Caucasians are intolerant to it due to lack of ancestral use. Beware of tofu and soy milk, which are unsuitable for many due to the highly industrial production method used. Fermented soy, i.e. tempeh, is much easier to digest.

• Red meats and poultry are heavy to digest and may contain high levels of chemicals. Although accepted by Buddhists, yogis reject them on the basis that you will eat the fear that the animal experiences when it is killed. The biochemical compounds, such as adrenalin, shed by the animal will make it more difficult for you to achieve spiritual states. Spiritual evolution is not just a waffly, abstract affair but is a biochemical process. By eating the body of a life form that is spiritually and intellectually less developed than you, you imbibe all of its neurotransmitters and they will have a tendency to bring about in your brain the same reactions as in the brain of the prey. Biochemically we are very, very similar to other mammals, and many hormones such as serotonin and adrenalin have almost the same function in us as in them.

In my first book on *asana* I explained that the body is the crystallized history of our past thoughts, emotions and actions. By devouring an animal you are in effect accumulating the entire history of its thoughts and emotions, which have crystallized as its body. You will then recycle them in your life. More than anything else, vegetarianism is therefore an act of inner hygiene. By importing the past of the animal into your tissues, meat-eating makes it less likely to attain and sustain spiritually exalted states, although it does of course not make it impossible.

Yoga, however, is a system that slowly and systematically increases the probability of experiencing spiritual liberation. For this reason all obstacles are progressively eliminated and all contributing factors are in the same manner put into place. No individual yogic method can cause spiritual liberation, but in their aggregate they make it more and more likely. The avoidance of mammalian meat is one of the actions that will stack the odds in your favour.

Meat is considered a category of food that makes the mind tamasic, as it is very hard to digest. It needs to be chewed for a very long time and even then its leftovers linger in the digestive tract, drawing *apana vayu* down. If you need to eat red meat and poultry, try to stick to organic varieties and to venison, as they contain lower amounts of toxins and chemicals than farmed animals. The main reasons for meat eating are health reasons. If your ancestors have not adapted to a meatless diet, you may find it difficult to switch quickly and extract enough nutrients from a vegetarian diet, and there is no point in becoming a sick and weak yogi. You will notice, however, that yogic methods like *Nauli* and *Kapalabhati* are very effective in increasing and purifying *agni*, so it may be possible to let go of meat later down the track. Additionally, *pranayama* is designed to extract more and more life force from air, so the advanced yogi needs less and less food.

• Fish contains important compounds such as omega 3 oils and is considered one of the best sources of protein. It is ruled out by yogic literature on similar grounds to the rejection of meat, although some Indian sages have accepted its use.[292] Another consideration is that farmed fish contains high levels of chemicals, and fish caught in the oceans are exposed to alarmingly increasing amounts of pollution, particularly mercury.

• Dairy products contain high levels of protein but many people are dairy intolerant. Additionally, the yogic texts are in favour of milk and ghee only, and not any other forms of dairy like cheeses and yoghurt. Since dairy is further up the food chain, it often contains high levels of toxins combined with antibiotics and other chemicals used in animal husbandry. If you use dairy, use organic produce whenever possible.

• Non-soy legumes such as the many types of beans and lentils contain high levels of protein, but several of them need to be combined to form a full protein. Since most people are tolerant to them and they do not contain a high level of toxins, they form an important source of protein for the yogi.

Summary: Apart from legumes, there is no easy and straightforward choice of protein: you will have to accept negative aspects with each choice you make. Those who are tolerant to milk can use it as an additional source of protein. Another important question, which I want only to allude to here, is whether some of the numbers relating to our daily required protein intakes are myths. Apart

292. Swami Nikhilananda (transl.), *The Gospel of Ramakrishna*, Ramakrishna Math, Madras, 1942, pp. 131, 199

from your lifestyle, your individual protein requirement is strongly influenced by what your ancestors have adapted to.

The question of whether yogis need to be vegetarian should not be answered merely on the basis of belief. Buddhist, Christian and Islamic mystics, most of whom ate some form of meat, have achieved mystical states similar to those experienced by Indian yogis, *siddhas* and *rishis*. The statistical occurrence of liberation appears to be higher in vegetarian Indian mystics than among any other group in the world. Yogic postures are today practised successfully by many non-vegetarians, but lengthy *kumbhakas* are thought to be safe only for vegetarians. Advanced *pranayama* forms the most straightforward approach to mystical experiences, but it comes at a price – vegetarianism. Swami Kuvalayananda suggests that the dictum of vegetarianism does not apply to the physical culturist, meaning somebody who practises *pranayama* only for its physical benefits. In this case *kumbhakas* should be limited to about 40 seconds each, which is enough to harvest the physical benefits.

Kumbhakas beyond 40 seconds are used to delete *karma* and conditioning, and eventually to raise Kundalini. None of these areas should be approached when eating meat. Kundalini-raising combined with meat-eating can be dangerous and painful. If you cannot let go of meat altogether, a wise approach would be to drop it for a time while you venture deeper into *pranayama*. The effect of *pranayama* may well enable you to abstain from meat for longer. If you are ready to let go of one category of meat, then abandon the eating of mammals first.

FURTHER NOTES ON WHAT NOT TO CONSUME

The *Hatha Tatva Kaumudi of Sundaradeva* suggests shunning sweets.[293] Cakes, chocolate, ice cream and other foods that contain sugar ideally are shunned by the yogi or taken in very small amounts. Sugars strongly influence the blood-sugar metabolism and can lead

293. *Hatha Tatva Kaumudi of Sundaradeva* XXXVI.66

to diabetes and other diseases. This also includes all other foods that have a high glycaemic index, such as white bread, baked beans and certain fruits.

The *Shiva Samhita* states that the yogi should abstain from acidic, astringent, pungent and bitter foods, also from salt and foods fried in oil.[294] The acid / alkaline balance has already been touched on and is a subject too vast to be treated here exhaustively. Acid / alkaline balance is for the yogi as important as the balance between the *doshas*. Many modern people are highly acidic and many chronic diseases occur as a result. Salt should be taken in moderation. It raises the blood pressure and damages the arteries. Frying food generally makes it cancerous. Eat as little fried food as possible and be aware of what you fry with. Certain oils when fried turn much more toxic than others. Coconut oil and ghee are very stable under increased temperatures, and hence become less toxic.

Jayatarama, author of *Jogapradipyaka*, warns that consumption of alcohol, tobacco, hemp and opium will result in painful hell for unending periods.[295] The warning appears grossly exaggerated, but the author means well. Of course people have managed to achieve great success even while consuming some of the above or even all of them. However it is again a question of stacking the odds against you. By using recreational drugs you will decrease the statistical probability of meaningfully and securely integrating spiritual exultation and bliss into your life.

This needs to be discussed without any emotional excitement. Alcohol simply mobilizes and expels *prana*. *Pranayama* tries to accumulate *prana* and increase the energy available for spiritual practice. Alcohol also makes your mind tamasic (torpid). Apart from that, it is an antiseptic that damages your brain and nervous system. Tobacco, hemp and opium are neuro-toxins that also make your mind tamasic, and they block the *nadis*, which you want to purify through *pranayama*. Danger from the smoking of any substance is

294. *Shiva Samhita* III.33
295. *Jogapradipyaka of Jayatarama* stanzas 372–380

increased when you practise *pranayama*. Through *kumbhaka* you may actually double the active surface area of your lungs. If you now smoke tobacco or marihuana, you increase the likelihood of lung cancer above that of a smoker who does not practise *pranayama*.

Shrikrishna, author of *Pranayama*, recommends staying away from spices and fried food, alcohol, tobacco, tea, coffee, cold drinks and, for advanced *pranayama* practitioners, also from meat, chicken, eggs and fish.[296] Spices are very rajasic and make your mind excited, agitated and fickle. Spices will make your mind jump about like a monkey that first drunk a bottle of whisky, then got stung by a scorpion and finally slipped and fell into a wasp's nest.

Coffee and tea are mobilizers and expellers of *prana* that do not go well with *pranayama*. Apart from that, coffee makes your mind very rajasic and disturbs your blood-sugar level. It mobilizes lots of energy suddenly, and after some time you crash and need another fix of some sort. Coffee also increases blood pressure and the heart rate, both of which *pranayama* seeks to reduce. It also makes the body very acidic. Coffee is therefore one of the most detrimental substances for the yogi.

Try also to avoid or reduce chemical cosmetics, chemical cleaning agents, chemical solvents and paints. Chemical medicines such as antibiotics, cortisone and some vaccines do have their place in life-threatening situations, but it must be asked whether the proclivity to constantly prescribe them helps others apart from the pharma-cological industry. A warning must also be given against combining *pranayama* with hallucinogenic drugs. When on hallucinogenic drugs, certain physiological safety mechanisms are suspended. You can easily damage your brain when combining them with *pranayama*. Opium and its derivatives such as morphine and heroin are suicidal for a spiritual practitioner. They cut off your spiritual antennae and reduce your world view to the survival perspective of the *Muladhara* (first *chakra*). Similarly dangerous are cocaine, crack cocaine, speed

296. Shrikrishna, *Essence of Pranayama*, 2nd edn, Kaivalyadhama, Lonavla, 1996, p. 98

and ecstasy, which prevent any development above the *Manipura* (third chakra). Coffee belongs in this group too; it is only much less potent than the others. It does not prevent development, but is unfavourable to it.

ASANA

Asana is the bedrock from which all other yogic techniques rise. Without *asana*, success in higher yogic techniques cannot be attained, much less can it be integrated. Success in *pranayama* is a realistic goal only if the body is beforehand baked in the fire of *asana* practice. Personally I found the Ashtanga Vinyasa sequences the ideal base from which to venture into *pranayama*, but it may not be the suitable form of practice for everybody. Whichever form of *asana* you practise and the more time and energy you invest in it, the faster you will progress in *pranayama* and the more advanced the *pranayama* exercises you can commence and successfully integrate. Until into his 90s T. Krishnamacharya practised *asana* twice a day to support his three-times-a-day *pranayama* practice.

The performance of *asana* is a prerequisite to *pranayama*, and *pranayama* has to be performed while being in *asana*, i.e. not while lounging, sitting in a chair or leaning against a wall.[297] The *Yoga Makaranda*, authored by T. Krishnamacharya, states that if *pranayama* is not practised with *asana* (and *yama* and *niyama*) little benefit is derived.[298] *Yama* and *niyama* I have described already in my book *Ashtanga Yoga: Practice and Philosophy*.[299] The *Yoga Rahasya*, handed down through T. Krishnamacharya, states that skill in *pranayama* cannot be acquired without practising postures and that meditation cannot be achieved without *pranayama*,[300] a statement that underlines the importance of *asana*. The same text says that after *asana* one must do *pranayama* and only after that *pratyahara* (sense withdrawal, the fifth limb) and only after that *dharana* (concentration, the sixth limb) is practised. According to the *Rahasya*, without this particular sequencing, no benefits can be obtained.[301]

297. The exception to the rule is *Ujjayi* without *kumbhaka*, which can be performed even when walking.
298. T. Krishnamacharya, *Yoga Makaranda*, rev. English edn, Media Garuda, Chennai, 2011, p. 55
299. Gregor Maehle, *Ashtanga Yoga: Practice and Philosophy*, New World Library, Novato, 2007, pp. 212–225
300. *Yoga Rahasya* I.45
301. *Yoga Rahasya* I.21

Patanjali, in his *Yoga Sutra*, describes not techniques as such but the results experienced once proper technique is performed. The sequence of *sutras* that describe *pranayama* starts with 'tasmin sati',[302] meaning 'being in this'. Being in this means being established in what has been described previously. The *sutras* on *pranayama* are preceded by the three *sutras* that describe the limb of *asana*. 'Being in this' means, then, commence *pranayama* after becoming established in *asana*.

The *Vasishta Samhita*, too, says that *asana* must be practised first, then *Nadi Shuddhi* (purification of the *nadis*), then *pranayama*.[303] This order is peculiar to sage Vasishta. Other *rishis* and *siddhas* considered *Nadi Shuddhi* to be the first exercise of *pranayama* rather than a separate exercise before it. In any case Vasishta says loud and clear that *asana* is first in line.

Rishi Vyasa says, in his commentary on the *Yoga Sutra*, that after having become victorious in an *asana* ('sati asana jaye') one now commences *pranayama*.[304] The *Hatha Yoga Pradipika*, too, states that *pranayama* is practised once empowerment in *asana* (*asana siddhi*) is obtained.[305] This is confirmed by the *Hatha Tatva Kaumudi of Sundaradeva*, which states that one who has mastered *asana* should practise *pranayama* and not otherwise.

Modern authorities and authors agree with these ancient injunctions. M.L. Gharote writes that only those who are stable in *asana* can achieve success in yoga.[306] Andre Van Lysebeth claims that *kumbhaka* is safe only when combined with *asana* practice and that any *kumbhaka* in excess of 40 seconds must be performed right after one's *asana* practice,[307] meaning not early in the morning before *asana* practice and not late in the afternoon many hours after one has concluded *asana*.

302. *Yoga Sutra* II.49
303. *Vasishta Samhita* I.84
304. *Yoga Sutra* II.49, Vyasa's commentary
305. *Hatha Yoga Pradipika* II.1
306. Dr M.L. Gharote, *Pranayama: The Science of Breath*, Lonavla Yoga Institute, Lonavla, 2003, p. 52
307. Andre van Lysebeth, *Die Grosse Kraft des Atems*, O.W. Barth, Bern, 1972, p. 98

WHAT EXACTLY ARE ASANA SIDDHI AND ASANA JAYA?

The above quotations drive home the point that a certain degree of mastery in *asana* has to be achieved prior to starting *pranayama*, although this still leaves out what exactly constitutes *pranayama*. Most of the quoted authorities understood *pranayama* as being serious spiritual *pranayama*, including long *kumbhaka*s, and not just simple therapeutic *pranayama*. We now need to inquire into what exactly this degree of mastery of *asana* is and what exactly constitutes *pranayama* in the context of those quotations. The degree of mastery has to be adapted to the difficulty of the *pranayama* one practises. T. Krishnamacharya, for example, taught simple *pranayama* to students who were too sick to practise *asana*, and noted *pranayama* teacher Swami Ramdev teaches introductory *pranayama* without much prior teaching in *asana*. It may be said that controlled breathing without *kumbhaka* or controlled breathing with *kumbhaka* up to 10 seconds may be executed without much in the way of safety precautions. In other words such simple practice does not constitute *pranayama* in the sense that the scriptures use the term: they often consider a 48-second *kumbhaka* as the entry level and, for that, *asana siddhi* (posture empowerment) or *asana jaya* (victory in posture) is required. Traditionally *asana jaya* is defined as the ability to do an *asana* for 3 hours at a stretch, and it is this very definition that was conveyed to me when I learned in India.

O.P. Tiwari, director of Kaivalyadhama, adds an important piece of information. He says that, once one has achieved *asana siddhi* in certain postures, one may commence *pranayama*.[308] In other words, *asana siddhi* is not a term that applies to the simultaneous mastery of all postures but only the postures that are applicable to *pranayama*. This was confirmed by T. Krishnamacharya, who used the term *asana siddhi* in the plural. He said that it was not possible to gain more than 24 *asana siddhi*s, nor was it necessary. Significantly, we find Rishi Vyasa's 'sati asana jaye' in the singular. He is not talking about general success in all *asana*s but success or victory in one of the important

308. O.P. Tiwari, *Kriyas and Pranayama*, DVD, Kaivalyadhama, Lonavla.

meditation postures. You can only practise *pranayama*, according to him, if you can sit extensively in one of the prescribed postures, and that excludes lying down, sitting in a chair, leaning against a wall or sitting simply cross-legged with the knees off the floor.

WHICH ASANAS ARE IMPORTANT AND NECESSARY?

About *asana*, Patanjali says that it needs to have the dual qualities of firmness and lightness.[309] In it, effort ceases and meditation on infinity occurs,[310] and one is beyond the assault of duality.[311] Here Patanjali puts the bar very high. Although he does not explicitly say so, there is only one posture that fits his description and that is *Padmasana* (lotus posture), once it is mastered. Sitting on a chair, for example, tends to make the mind dull and heavy as the gravitational force pulls us down, whereas in *Padmasana* the spine is perfectly aligned against gravity. This alignment lifts the spine and brain upwards, producing lightness. Importantly in *Padmasana*, the soles of the feet and palms are turned upwards, receiving energy from above, whereas while sitting in a chair there is an automatic discharge of energy out of the soles into the receptive Earth.

Padmasana, once it is mastered, also facilitates a natural alignment that is effortless. *Shavasana* (corpse posture) is also effortless, but of all postures it offers the largest area for gravitational down force. For this reason it induces heaviness whereas *Padmasana* induces lightness. Additionally, Patanjali's third condition asks for transcendence from duality, for example the duality between *rajas* (frenzy) and *tamas* (torpor). Again, *Shavasana* is the most torpid of all postures; therefore it presents an angle for the attack of the opposites. *Padmasana* is the only posture where the spine, through its miraculous alignment of the energy centres contained within it (*chakras*), automatically facilitates meditation on infinity and transcendence over duality. There are other postures, notably *Siddhasana* and *Swastikasana*, that

309. *Yoga Sutra* II.46
310. *Yoga Sutra* II.47
311. *Yoga Sutra* II.48

allow such alignment to a certain extent, but many traditional schools and teachers allowed *pranayama* to take place only in *Padmasana* for the above-mentioned reasons.

T. Krishnamacharya's perennial favourite, the *Yoga Rahasya*, states that of all postures *Shirshasana* (headstand) and *Padmasana* (lotus posture) are the important ones.[312] Headstand, of course, is not directly used to practise *pranayama*, but it achieves the steadying and reversing of *amrita* (nectar), which are essential for *pranayama*. The *siddha* Goraksha Natha taught that *pranayama* should be practised only in *Padmasana*.[313] Sage Gheranda also taught the use of *Padmasana*, but only with the right leg first in place and the left leg on top.[314]

Of the Vedic texts, the *Yoga Chudamani Upanishad* accepts only *Padmasana* for *pranayama*.[315] The ancient *Brhadyogi Yajnavalkya Smrti* also advises assuming *Padmasana* for the practice of *pranayama*.[316] The *Yoga Kundalini Upanishad* accepts both *Padmasana* and *Vajrasana*,[317] but gives *Padmasana* the preference.[318] The *Amrita Nada Upanishad* is somewhat more liberal, saying that *Padmasana*, *Svastikasana* or *Bhadrasana* will do as long as the practitioner can easily sit in it.[319]

The *Hatha Tatva Kaumudi* tightens the requirements by accepting only *Padmasana* for *pranayama*.[320] Bhavadeva Mishra, author of the *Yuktabhavadeva*, is somewhat less stringent in saying that *pranayama* was *preferably* executed in *Padmasana*.[321] Brahmananda, commentator on the *Hatha Yoga Pradipika*, prefers *Siddhasana* for the performance of *kumbhaka*.[322] *Siddhasana* is mentioned in many texts as the foremost of all yoga postures due to its propensity to induce *Mula Bandha* and

312. *Yoga Rahasya* I.103
313. *Goraksha Shataka* stanza 41
314. *Gheranda Samhita* II.8
315. *Yoga Chudamani Upanishad* stanza 106
316. *Brhadyogi Yajnavalkya Smrti* IX.186–190
317. *Yoga Kundalini Upanishad* I.2
318. *Yoga Kundalini Upanishad* I.22–23
319. *Amrita Nada Upanishad* 18–20
320. *Hatha Tatva Kaumudi of Sundaradeva* XXXVI.6
321. *Yuktabhavadeva of Bhavadeva Mishra*, lxvi
322. *Hatha Yoga Pradipika* II.9, Brahmananda's commentary

its suitability for rasing Kundalini. However, more often than not *Padmasana* is the preferred asana during *pranayama*.

According to van Lysebeth, of all postures it is *Padmasana* alone that guarantees correct spinal alignment, and it is this fact that makes it the posture of choice in most yogic scriptures. From my own *pranayama* practice I can confirm that *Padmasana* is the most efficient posture for it. However, I have to admit that I obtained *asana siddhi* in *Padmasana* not through mere *asana* practice itself. Even after a long phase of *asana* practice I still found *Padmasana* becoming uncomfortable after 10 to 15 minutes. This radically changed when I commenced *pranayama*. It might have been simply the fact that my mind was now focused on performing a task in *Padmasana* rather than simply waiting for signs of discomfort. After commencing *pranayama* in *Padmasana* I quickly managed to extend my time in *Padmasana* to 30 minutes and from there to 1 hour and eventually 3 hours, even if not in one sitting. Looking back now I would have been better off not to be so conservative but commence *pranayama* in *Padmasana* earlier. I would have been able to cover more ground rather than wait for some mythical stage of achievement in *asana* that will never come.

Another story illustrates the potency of *Padmasana*. At one point during *pranayama* in *Padmasana*, when adding external *kumbhakas* and Kundalini techniques I became so ecstatic that I literally lost any sense of time passing. I would come out of these sessions with my legs having gone completely numb. One day I must have folded my numb leg out of *Padmasana* in a very clumsy fashion because I acquired a micro-tear in the joint capsule of my left knee. For a period of 8 months after that I was unable to sit in *Padmasana* and had to be satisfied with *Siddhasana*. To my surprise my *kumbhaka* length decreased significantly and so did the total length of my *pranayama* sessions. Additionally, my capacity to concentrate diminished and so did my propensity for spiritual exultation. It was quite staggering to see what a difference it made to have simply lost my *Padmasana*. A modern Indian teacher that I hold in high esteem once told me 'You Westerners believe that mystical powers are obtainable by simply sitting in *Padmasana*.' Today I would reply that it is not just Westerners who believe that, but it's exactly what the *shastras* (scriptures) state. It comes at no surprise that most Hindu deities, Vedic *rishis* and tantric *siddhas* are depicted in *Padmasana*. It is a veritable laboratory for spiritual emancipation. But remember, it is not the laboratory that brings results. It is what you do in it, the actions you perform. These actions must be *pranayama* and meditation as described in the *shastras*. Mere sitting will not get you far.

I hope that I have created some curiosity and enthusiasm in you towards *Padmasana*. But please don't be as silly as I was, going up to the 3-hour level so fast. Your knees will thank you for it.

Let's look now at the requirements for postures in *pranayama*, and this will make clear why *Padmasana* excels. Any posture used for *pranayama* must fulfil the following requirements:

• Feet and hands must be turned away from the floor so that the ground cannot absorb *prana* being projected out of them. This rules out sitting on chairs, where the feet face downwards.

• Legs must not be lower than the *Muladhara* (base *chakra*) so that *prana* and blood flows are directed upwards. Again this rules out sitting on chairs and leaning against walls.

• The pelvis must be tilted forward quite strongly so that the spinal double s-curve is exaggerated and the spine assumes the shape of a cobra ready to strike. This is a prerequisite for the serpentine power to rise.

• To stimulate *mula bandha* the perineum must either press into the floor, which is achieved in *Padmasana* through the strong forward tilt of the pelvis, or be stimulated by the left heel, which is given in *Siddhasana*.

• Ideally, through forward tilt of the pelvis, the heels should press into the abdomen to stimulate *Uddiyana Bandha*. This is only the case in *Padmasana*.

• The posture must provide a firm base that can be held naturally for a long time. It must align the whole body effortlessly against gravitation, so that there is no slumping or slouching at all. Again, *Padmasana* reigns supreme here.

The posture that fits this brief best is *Padmasana*, with *Siddhasana* second and *Swastikasana* or *Virasana* acceptable if neither of the first two can be achieved.

The postures are here given in order of importance, *Padmasana* being the most important but most difficult. Learn the postures in the opposite order, starting with *Virasana* and slowly graduating towards *Padmasana*. Meditation *asana*s such as these are to be practised towards the end of one's general *asana* practice, when the body and particularly the hip joints are warmed up. If you do not know how to rotate and move your hip joints, you may injure your knees. Consult a yoga teacher to learn postures. I have described postures in my two previous books *Ashtanga Yoga: Practice and Philosophy* and *Ashtanga Yoga: The Intermediate Series*. Here I have described the meditation postures only in a basic fashion, as this is a book on *pranayama*. In these descriptions I am assuming that you have a general *asana* practice. You will need to have a certain foundation in *asana* to practise *pranayama*.

Padmasana

This is the best posture for *pranayama* because of the forward tilt of the pelvis and the spine being aligned like a cobra ready to strike – necessary for the serpent power to rise. Goraksha Natha, Gheranda and other authorities accept only the placing of the right leg first but T. Krishnamacharya recommends switching sides. If you can sit a few minutes in *Padmasana*, start practising for example your *Kapalabhati* in *Padmasana*. At some point you will be able to do a few rounds of your main *pranayama* practice in *Padmasana*. Do not suddenly extend the time spent in *Padmasana*. Add only a minute, or at most a few minutes, per week. The posture is extremely powerful and hour-long stints should be left to advanced practitioners of *pranayama*.

To enter the posture safely from a straight-legged position, flex the right knee joint completely by first drawing the right heel to the right buttock. The inability to touch the buttock with your heel would indicate that your quadriceps is too short to enter *Padmasana*

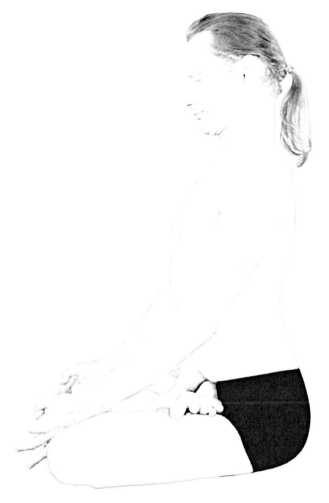

Padmasana, sometimes called Muktasana or Kamalasana

safely. In this case go to *Virasana* to lengthen your quadriceps or instead sit cross-legged. If you can touch your heel to your buttock, let the right knee fall out to the side, pointing and inverting the right foot. Now draw the right heel into the right groin to ensure that the

135

knee joint remains completely flexed in this abducted position. From here lift the right heel in towards the navel, bringing the knee closer to the centre-line. Keeping the heel in line with the navel, place the ball of the foot into the opposite groin.

Repeat these steps on the left, as if the right leg were still straight. First flex the knee joint completely until the underside of the thigh touches the back of the leg over its entire length. Drawing the knee far out to the left, first place the left ankle under the right ankle on the floor. From here lift the left foot over the right ankle in towards the navel, while drawing the left knee out to the side. Do not lift the left foot over the right knee, as this would mean opening the left knee joint, which would induce lateral movement into the knee during the transition. Keep the left knee joint as flexed as possible in the transition, allowing you to move the femur (thigh bone) and tibia (shin bone) as a unity with no gap in between.

Once the left leg is in position, move both heels towards each other so that they touch the navel area. Bring both knees close together so that the thighbones become almost parallel (depending on ratio of length between femur and tibia). Now inwardly rotate your femurs until the front edges of the tibias point downward and the soles and heels of the feet face upward. In this way the knee joints are completely closed and thereby protected. Do not sit in *Padmasana* while retaining the initial lateral rotation of the femurs used to enter the posture. The key to mastering *Padmasana* is being able to rotate your femurs internally while being in the posture. This is difficult to learn by merely sitting in *Padmasana* itself without being warmed up. An ideal tool for learning this is the femur rotation pattern of the Primary Series as described in my book *Ashtanga Yoga: Practice and Philosophy*.

Siddhasana

Siddhasana means 'posture of the adepts'. It is so called because it is used to raise Kundalini. In this posture the curves of the spine are not as accentuated as in *Padmasana*, and hence it is slightly inferior

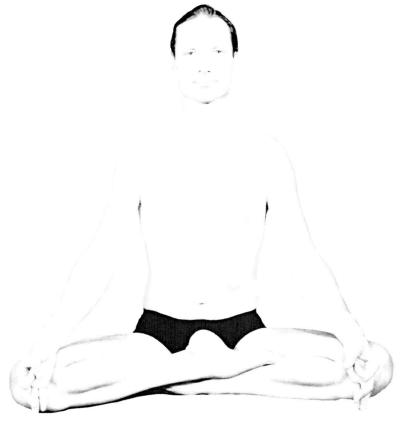

Siddhasana, sometimes called Vajrasana

for *pranayama*. However, with the left heel in the perineum, *Siddhasana* is the posture of choice to ignite *Mula Bandha*. Goraksha Natha and other authorities state that the left heel must be placed first to stimulate *Muladhara Chakra*. In this regard the posture is a mirror image of *Padmasana*, for which the classical authorities stipulate placement of the right leg first.

The characteristics of *Siddhasana* are very different from those of *Padmasana*. Whereas in *Padmasana* we bring the knees as close together as possible, in *Siddhasana* we take them apart as wide as possible. In the beginning you may choose to sit on a pad such as a folded blanket and decrease its height as you gain proficiency. The pad will assist you in tilting the pelvis forward more.

From a sitting, straight-legged position (*Dandasana*), bend the left leg and place the heel against the perineum, the location of *Muladhara Chakra*, between anus and genitals. Now bend the right leg and place the right ankle on top of the left one so that the right heel presses against the pubic bone. The organ of generation is now located between the left and right heels. Now insert the toes of the right foot between the calf and thigh of the left leg. Using both hands, move the calf and thigh of the right leg apart, reach through and pull the toes of the left foot up so that they are inserted between the calf and thigh of the right leg. Pay close attention to how this changes the location of the heel and what it does to the rotation of the left femur. It is only through this final action that the heel of the left foot comes into the right contact with the perineum between anus and genitals. This is the position necessary for Kundalini-raising.

There is an easier variation of this posture for beginners, called *Ardha* (half) *Siddhasana*. Here, instead of stacking the heels on top of each other, they are placed in front of each other, with both feet on the floor. Use this posture only as a warm-up, and graduate to *Siddhasana* when possible.

Svastikasana

Unfortunately, in modern times the swastika was popularised around the world by the German Nazis. But they got it all wrong. Su-asti-ka means 'symbol of goodness'. It symbolizes the life-giving forces of the sun and the divine order on planet Earth represented by the world axis, Mount Kailasha in Tibet, the throne of Lord Shiva. Prior to global warming, pilgrims approaching

Mount Kailasha could still see a giant swastika in the ice dome of Kailasha. Even today, when seen from space the four giant rivers Indus, Yamuna, Ganges and Brahmaputra can be seen forming a swastika when descending from the plain around Mount Kailasha,

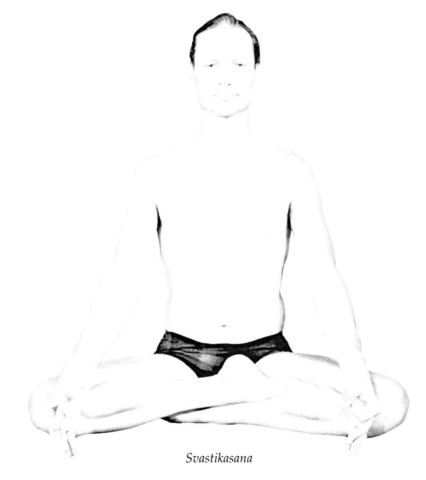

Svastikasana

bringing water to over a billion people. This is a reminder of the life-giving meaning of the swastika, far from the delusion of modern political movements.

In *Svastikasana* the legs and feet are arranged in the formation of a swastika. The knees are here wider than in *Padmasana* but closer than in *Siddhasana*.

139

Svastikasana is considered inferior to *Padmasana* and *Siddhasana*, and there is no preference as to which leg is placed first. Feel free to exchange sides. From a sitting, straight-legged position (*Dandasana*), bend the left leg and place its heel into the right groin. Then bend the right leg and place the right heel into the left groin. Now insert the toes of the right foot between the calf and thigh of the left leg. Using both hands, now move the calf and thigh of the right leg apart, reach through and pull the toes of the left foot up so that they are inserted between the calf and thigh of the right leg.

The posture is similar to *Siddhasana* but less ambitious. The heels are not on top of each other but laterally displaced. This makes tilting of the pelvis easier, but there is no stimulation of *Mula Bandha*.

Virasana

Virasana means 'hero's posture'. It is the way in which ancient warriors used to sit. An excellent introductory posture, it should be a regular part of one's practice before all other postures in this category (i.e. meditation postures) are attempted. Through daily *Virasana* practice the quadriceps are elongated and all other meditation postures are mastered easily. It is good to sit in Virasana every morning for 10 minutes before your general asana practice. First prop yourself up on folded blankets high enough for you to not feel any pain in your knees. As your thighs warm up and stretch slowly, decrease the height of the pad on which you are sitting until eventually, possibly after years, you sit flat on the floor. This is the ideal preparation for *Padmasana*.

Once you have come down to the floor, change to one of the other postures. If you can sit in *Virasana*, use it to do your *pranayama* practice until you can sit straight on the floor without padding. Then switch to *Ardha Siddhasana* or *Svastikasana*, followed by *Siddhasana* and eventually *Padmasana*.

Virasana is far superior to sitting in a chair, even if you have to prop yourself up quite high. The soles of the feet are turned upward and there is a natural upward flow of *prana*, whereas when sitting in a chair gravitation will always pull *prana* down.

In *Virasana* it is important that your thighs are parallel and not

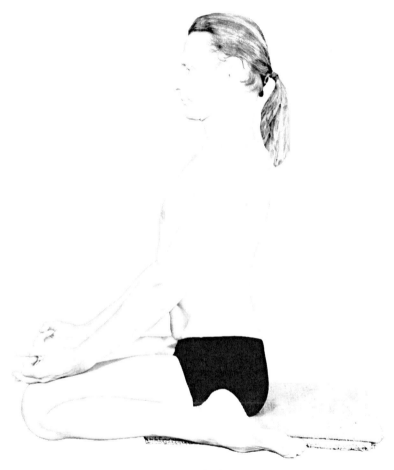

Virasana, sometimes called Bhadrasana or Vajrasana

turned out. The feet have to point straight back and never out to the side in the way children frequently sit. This is a sure way to ruin your knees. Soles and heels have to point straight up and the toes out to the back. Bring the feet wider than your hips and place a folded blanket between your feet. This way, by slowly reducing the height of the blanket, you will eventually sit between your feet.

Maintain the forward tilt of the pelvis as much as possible. This is more difficult in this posture than in the other meditation postures. Because of this weak spot, you will eventually slouch in *Virasana* and that's why you want to eventually graduate to the others. It is only in *Padmasana* that you can sit effortlessly for 3 hours with your spine assuming the characteristic of a cobra ready to strike.

Please note that the *asana* names in scripture are not set in concrete. There was no tradition that preserved the exactness of *asana* names, in the way that there was, for example, for traditions that precisely preserved the *Vedas*, *Upanishads*, *Yoga Sutras* and *Brahma Sutras*. Different schools in India may use different names for the same *asana*. For example different schools used the name *Vajrasana* for *Padmasana*, *Siddhasana* or even *Virasana*. *Asana* names were not considered to be that important.

IMPORTANCE OF INVERSIONS

An important adjunct to *Pranayama* is *Viparita Karani Mudra*, translated as inverted-action-seal. *Viparita Karani* means to invert the body daily for a significant time. It is a principle, not the name of a posture. There is no posture going by the name *Viparita Karanyasana*. You may invert the body in a modified shoulder stand, shoulder stand or headstand, with efficiency rising in exactly that order. Some schools accept only headstand (*Shirshasana*) as *Viparita Karani* because it is the most efficient and powerful form of it. The rationale of *Viparita Karani* lies in the importance of the centre of the cranial cavity. This area above the soft palate that includes the thalamus, hypothalamus, pineal and pituitary glands, all centred around the larger area of the third ventricle, is in yoga called the lunar *prana* centre, or simply the moon. It is thought to exude *amrita*, the nectar of immortality, but note that *amrita* is nothing but another name for *prana*. In the navel area is thought to be located the solar centre of *prana*, or simply the sun, which also represents gastric fire. In our normal body position, *amrita* gravitates downward and is burnt by the sun. When the body is inverted daily for an extended period, *amrita* becomes stored/ arrested. This can be taken to the extent of *amrita siddhi* when the *amrita* is permanently stored and does not fall any more into the fire. This state is very important for the development of *pranayama* and the higher limbs, as it automatically keeps the senses focused inwardly.

In order to work towards this state, you need to first slow down your breath during inversions as much as possible. T. Krishnamacharya's idea of headstand was to take only 2 breaths per minute. Slow your breath down gradually, not suddenly. In inversions the blood pressure initially rises only to drop off again after a few minutes. If you have high blood pressure, you need to take steps to reduce your blood pressure before working on inversions. Once you have achieved a very slow breath rate in your inversions, start to add breaths, perhaps one every few days. Be sensitive and stop adding on before you experience adverse symptoms. If you do experience symptoms such as headache, irritability, neck pain, ear pain, ringing in your ears, pressure or a fuzzy feeling in your head, do not extend your time any further until you have consolidated. In some cases you may need to reduce the time spent in inversions. Get the advice of a qualified teacher.

The question of how fast you can extend time spent in inversions is determined by your age and general condition. If you are young, athletic and in pristine health you may add on quite fast, whereas an older person with certain chronic health problems might have to do it very, very slowly. Some teachers are of the opinion that those over 50 should not embark on taking on extended inversions.

GENERAL ASANA PRACTICE

Your general *asana* practice outside of the classic meditation postures and the inversions is also very important for *pranayama*. Generally speaking, the more advanced your *asana* practice is the quicker you will improve in *pranayama*. An advanced *asana* practitioner with a 2-hour daily practice will be able to progress quickly in *pranayama*, but will have to go through the process of *pranayama* nevertheless, as its benefits cannot be obtained through *asana* practice, however advanced it may be.

A yogi with a less advanced *asana* practice will progress more slowly in *pranayama* but will progress nevertheless. It is essential to practise *asana* and *pranayama* daily; otherwise the gains created through *pranayama* cannot be secured but will dissipate. As with most information in this book, this rule is slanted towards *pranayama* as a spiritual discipline and not towards simple therapeutic *pranayama*, for which it does not apply. Some yogis have talked about pranic pressure that is built up through practice and simply escapes like fluid out of an open valve when practice is interrupted.

Yogic scriptures that talk about mastery of *asana* as a prerequisite for *pranayama* are referring to an intense form of *pranayama*. For example the *Hatha Yoga Pradipika* and *Gheranda Samhita* call a 48-second *kumbhaka* an inferior *kumbhaka*. This is because these texts addressed only a small elite of students who were prepared to throw at yoga everything they had and were ready to practise for most of the day. Both texts recommend practising 4 to 5 hours a day. To follow this advice and start one's *pranayama* practice with a 48-second *kumbhaka* is a possibility for those who have a very advanced *asana* practice, whereas for everybody else it would be sheer madness. Nevertheless, even for those who are very advanced in leg-behind-head postures, backbends, arm balances and extreme hip rotations, it is still not a good idea to put on such a load from the outset. It is much better to choose a comfortable ratio and then extend slowly while becoming proficient.

One should never, never get stressed, anxious or strained in one's *pranayama* practice. This will set off a sympathetic reflex (i.e. activate the sympathetic nervous system) and, once this pattern is established, it is hard to undo it. It is then very unlikely that you will experience mystical states, which are triggered generally through the parasympathetic nervous system. Similarly, if you experience your practice as stressful or laborious, it is less likely that you will continue it. I have talked to several advanced *asana* practitioners who did not, or found it very hard to, continue their *pranayama* practice, simply because they started with breath counts that were too difficult. It also has to be remembered that if your mind gets tamasic (torpid) or rajasic (frantic) during practice your count may simply be too long.

Many contemporary teachers set *pranayama*'s entry requirements in respect to *asana* practice at a very low level. This is due to the fact that *pranayama* has undergone a radical change. It is now used in yoga therapy and for health purposes, and prescribed for people who have a very low *asana* capability. When two teachers talk about *pranayama* they do not necessarily talk about the same thing. Those who say that one needs no or almost no *asana* requirement are talking about a very, very non-demanding form of *pranayama* that would not even be recognized as such by someone who teaches it for accessing mystical states.

If you use *pranayama* for health reasons, keep it very simple, and in this case it might consist only of simple breathing exercises. If you use *pranayama* as described in traditional yogic texts and in this book for attaining mystical states, then you need a sincere, daily *asana* practice. If you are looking to *kumbhakas* of 48 seconds and beyond, you need a daily *asana* practice of at least 60–90 minutes. If there are ways to cut one's *asana* practice in half or do away with it altogether, and yet sustain a top-shelf *pranayama* practice, this author has not yet found them.

BANDHAS

Serious *pranayama* should not be practised without prior knowledge of the *bandhas*. Modern practitioners often fail in *pranayama* and discontinue their practice because, in most cases, they commence it without a proper working knowledge of the *bandhas*. *Bandhas* are neuromuscular locks that prevent the *vayu* from going astray in *kumbhaka*. *Kumbhakas* in excess of 10 seconds should not be practised without *bandhas*. Breath retentions of less than 10 seconds may occur due to surprise, happiness, fear etc., but as such they do not really constitute *pranayama*. We could say that a proper *pranayama kumbhaka* starts at above 10 seconds. Deep and controlled slow breathing can be performed without the *bandhas*, but it becomes more efficient by applying some of them.

Let's have a look at the evidence. The *Yoga Rahasya* states that *pranayama* without application of the three *bandhas* does not confer benefits[323] and that without the *bandhas pranayama* is useless and may give rise to disease.[324] Contrarily, if done with all three *bandhas*, *pranayama* will destroy the causes of all diseases, according to its author, Nathamuni.[325]

This text, handed down through T. Krishnamacharya, also continues to emphasize the importance of the *bandhas* in its descriptions of individual *pranayamas*. According to the *Rahasya*, *Nadi Shodhana*, the most important *pranayama* method, can live up to its standing only when accompanied by all three *bandhas*. The *Hatha Ratnavali* states that applying all of them makes *prana* enter the central energy channel (*sushumna*),[326] a claim that is also to be found in the *Hatha Yoga Pradipika*.[327] The great Shankaracharya also said that, through the practice of the three *bandhas*, Kundalini arises and enters the

---

323. *Yoga Rahasya* I.61
324. *Yoga Rahasya* I.95
325. *Yoga Rahasya* II.50
326. *Hatha Ratnavali of Shrinivasayogi* II.8
327. *Hatha Yoga Pradipika* II.46.

sushumna.[328] He added that, through mastery of the *bandhas, Kevala Kumbhaka* (the culmination of *pranayama*) is achieved.[329] The *Yoga Kundalini Upanishad* declares that, by applying *Mula Bandha* during *kumbhaka, apana vayu* rises through the *chakras* and pierces the *granthis* (energetic and karmic blockages).[330] The same text says that the three *bandhas* should always be applied when *kumbhaka* is about to be performed.[331] The *Shandilya Upanishad*, too, proclaims that during *kumbhaka* the *bandhas* need to be applied to draw *prana* into *sushumna.*[332] The *Yuktabhavadeva of Bhavadeva Mishra* is supportive in declaring that all *pranayamas* are to be accompanied by the three *bandhas.*[333] The *Kumbhaka Paddhati of Raghuvira* goes as far as talking of 'shat anga kumbhaka', meaning the six limbs of breath retention.[334] These are named as inhalation, retention, exhalation and the three *bandhas.* The *Hatha Tatva Kaumudi of Sundaradeva* also proclaims that *prana* is moved into *sushumna* by *kumbhaka* with *bandhas*, and specifies which combination of *bandhas* needs to be applied during which respiratory phase.[335]

Among modern authors, Swami Ramdev, too, asserts that *pranayama* without *bandhas* is incomplete and that the *bandhas* are extremely helpful in mastering it.[336] The researcher Shrikrishna declares that in *kumbhaka* the three *bandhas* should always be applied and, additionally, *Mula* and *Uddiyana Bandhas* during inhalation and exhalation.[337] He also proclaims that, without applying the three *bandhas* during *pranayama*, detrimental results may manifest.[338] This is likely to be the main reason for the reduced attraction of *pranayama* to modern

328. *Yoga Taravali of Shankaracharya* stanza 6
329. *Yoga Taravali of Shankaracharya* stanzas 8–9
330. *Yoga Kundalini Upanishad* I.64–86
331. *Yoga Kundalini Upanishad* I.40
332. *Shandilya Upanishad* stanzas 26–30
333. *Yuktabhavadeva of Bhavadeva Mishra* lxviii
334. *Kumbhaka Paddhati of Raghuvira* 186–187
335. *Hatha Tatva Kaumudi of Sundaradeva* XXXIX.87
336. Swami Ramdev, *Pranayama*, Divya Yog Mandir Trust, Hardwar, 2007, p. 21
337. Shrikrishna, *Essence of Pranayama*, 2nd edn, Kaivalyadhama, Lonavla, 1996, p. 81
338. Shrikrishna, *Essence of Pranayama*, 2nd edn, Kaivalyadhama, Lonavla, 1996, p. 119

students. If you start *pranayama*, and particularly *kumbhaka*, without proficiency in *bandha*, adverse effects may set in. By studying the following instructions, and having one's progress checked by a teacher knowledgeable in *bandha*, success in *pranayama* will be achieved safely.

DIFFERENCE BETWEEN KUMBHAKA DURING BANDHA / MUDRA AND DURING PRANAYAMA

The *bandha*s are part of a larger group of yogic techniques called *mudra*s, energy seals. The *bandha*s have in common with many other *mudra*s their use during *kumbhaka* in diverting *prana* into a desired direction. To learn some of the *bandha*s properly we need to use *kumbhaka*. However, the *kumbhaka* here does not constitute *kumbhaka* proper in the sense of *pranayama*, because there is no count. When *kumbhaka* is practised in *pranayama*, we may decide to do 20 *kumbhaka*s of a length of 64 seconds preceded by a 16-second inhalation and followed by a 32-second exhalation. To perform the *kumbhaka*s safely, we would add the *bandha*s as an ancillary technique.

When we are learning the *bandha*s or practising any other *mudra*s, we do not count the *kumbhaka*s. The instruction will always be 'hold to capacity and focus on the quality of execution of the *bandha*'. You may repeat the exercise several times, but without any predetermined number of rounds. Practise the *bandha*s, particularly *Jalandhara Bandha*, until you have mastered them, and only then insert them into counted *kumbhaka*s. Once you start counted *kumbhaka*s, you will need to have acquired competence in *bandha*s so that you can focus on other aspects of your *pranayama*, such as count, *mantra*, visualization of *chakra*, sun, moon and meditation deity.

Jalandhara Bandha

Swami Kuvalayananda explains that the term *Jalandhara* comes from jalan (the brain) and *dhara* (upward pull).[339] Through the forward bending of the head, the *bandha* creates a pull on the spinal cord. Even more so than during internal *kumbhaka*, this is the case during external *kumbhaka*.

It is essential that *asana* practitioners acquire an understanding of *Mula* and *Uddiyana Bandha* before venturing into *asana* practice, as it is more difficult to cultivate the *bandha*s once one is used to faulty *bandha*-less *asana* practice. The same is true for *Jalandhara Bandha* in regard to *pranayama*. It is by far the most important *bandha* for *pranayama* and, while one may be able to ignore the other two *bandha*s in the beginning to some extent, *Jalandhara* is the essence of internal *kumbhaka*.

Its name comes from the stimulation it applies to the brain and spinal cord when placing the chin down on the chest in *kumbhaka*. One must first learn *Jalandhara Bandha* and only then commence internal (*antara*) *kumbhaka*. External *kumbhaka* with *Jalandhara Bandha* is a more advanced form of practice, which should be learnt later on.

BENEFITS OF JALANDHARA BANDHA

The *Hatha Yoga Pradipika* proclaims that, at the end of one's inhalation and before *kumbhaka* commences, one must apply *Jalandhara Bandha*,[340] a statement that is repeated in the *Yuktabhavadeva*[341] and the *Hatha Tatva Kaumudi*,[342] among other texts. The ancient *Brhadyogi Yajnavalkya Smrti* mentions *Jalandhara Bandha* together with a host of *Yoga Upanishads*.[343] The *Dhyana Bindu Upanishad* expounds that when *Jalandhara Bandha* is performed, *amrita* (nectar of immortality) does not fall into the gastric fire (*agni*), where it is usually burned, and

339. *Yoga Mimamsa* II.3
340. *Hatha Yoga Pradipika* II.45.
341. *Yuktabhavadeva of Bhavadeva Mishra* lxviii
342. *Hatha Tatva Kaumudi of Sundaradeva* XXXIX.87
343. *Brhadyogi Yajnavalkya Smrti* IX.186–190

hence a long life is gained.[344] The same claim is made by the *Shiva Samhita*, which adds that through *Jalandhara Bandha* the yogi absorbs the nectar, which otherwise is destroyed.[345] The *Yoga Rahasya* proclaims that *Jalandhara* impedes the downward flow of *amrita*, hence prolonging life.[346] It also states that *Jalandhara* maintains virility[347] and, by controlling the vital airs (*vayus*), overcomes many diseases.[348] The *Hatha Yoga Pradipika*[349] and the *Yoga Kundalini Upanishad*[350] both agree that *Jalandhara Bandha* moves *prana* into the central energy channel (*sushumna*). The two *nadis* should be stopped firmly by contracting the throat.

Among modern authorities, Swami Kuvalayananda affirmed that under no circumstances should *kumbhaka* be practised without *Jalandhara Bandha*. T. Krishnamacharya taught that *Jalandhara Bandha* awakens Kundalini, but for this purpose the chin must be positioned way under the collarbones.[351]

Most responsible authorities stated that, if (internal) *kumbhaka* is performed for longer than 10 seconds, *Jalandhara* is compulsory. Swami Ramdev teaches[352] that *Jalandhara Bandha* directs *prana* into the *sushumna* (central energy channel), awakens the *Vishuddha* (throat) *Chakra* and alleviates throat ailments like thyroid malfunction and tonsillitis.

JALANDHARA KEEPS PRANA FROM ENTERING THE HEAD
AND PREVENTS HEADACHE AND EAR PAIN

The *Yoga Kundalini Upanishad* informs us that *Jalandhara Bandha* prevents the air compressed in *kumbhaka* from entering the head,[353] a fact that can easily be verified by established practitioners when,

344. *Dhyana Bindu Upanishad* stanzas 78–79
345. *Shiva Samhita* IV.38–39
346. *Yoga Rahasya* I.72
347. *Yoga Rahasya* I.80
348. *Yoga Rahasya* I.81
349. *Hatha Yoga Pradipika* III.72
350. *Yoga Kundalini Upanishad* I.52
351. T. Krishnamacharya, *Yoga Makaranda*, rev. English edn, Media Garuda, Chennai, 2011, p. 105
352. Swami Ramdev, *Pranayama*, Divya Yog Mandir Trust, Hardwar, 2007, p. 21
353. *Yoga Kundalini Upanishad* stanza 51

upon releasing *Jalandhara* during internal *kumbhaka*, blood pressure in the head suddenly rises and one experiences ringing in the ears. *Jalandhara* also protects the ears, as the rising air during *kumbhaka* would otherwise enter the inner ear through the Eustachian tubes and cause ear pain and, in extreme cases, damage. Yogeshwaranand Paramahamsa similarly opines that internal *kumbhaka* without *Jalandhara Bandha* should not be held for long, as *prana* may force itself into the brain, leading to fainting.[354] A faulty *Jalandhara Bandha* will usually announce itself first through headaches resulting from *pranayama*. This signal should be heeded before more damage results.

TECHNIQUE

Assume a yogic meditation position, ideally *Padmasana*. Only in *Padmasana* does *Jalandhara Bandha* apply the maximum stretch and thus stimulation to the brain and spinal cord. Although this is also experienced to some extent in *Siddhasana* and the other meditation positions, it is only experienced to the maximum in *Padmasana*. There are two traditions in India in regard to *Jalandhara Bandha*. In the somewhat more lenient tradition, the chin is simply placed into the jugular notch and, according to that teaching, *Jalandhara Bandha* and any *pranayama* sessions should be precluded by *Viparita Karani Mudra*. *Viparita Karani Mudra* is then interpreted as a somewhat watered down version of *Sarvangasana*, in which the angle of the torso does not have to be vertical to the floor.

CHIN ON CHEST

The other tradition is somewhat stricter in its requirements. T. Krishnamacharya taught in this tradition,[355] which has the chin placed way down on the sternum (breast bone). According to this teaching, *Viparita Karani Mudra* does not refer to a particular body position but simply means to invert the body for a very long time until

354. Yogeshwaranand Paramahamsa, *First Steps to Higher Yoga*, Yoga Niketan Trust, New Delhi, 2001, p. 359
355. T. Krishnamacharya, *Yoga Makaranda*, rev. English edn, Media Garuda, Chennai, 2011, p. 105

amrita is steadied and thus *pratyahara* achieved. The two postures used for *Viparita Karani* are *Shirshasana* and *Sarvangasana*. Paramount in both is alignment, i.e. the body has to be absolutely vertical to the floor in either of them. According to this tradition, *Sarvangasana* and *Halasana* need to be practised prior to practising *pranayama*, because these postures teach the right position for *Jalandhara Bandha*, which is not to place the chin into the jugular notch but down on the sternum at exactly the place where it is located in *Sarvangasana*. Please note that placing *Jalandhara Bandha* is defined as placing the chin on the chest also in the Shiva Samhita[356] and Gheranda Samhita.[357] As it is generally not advised to go straight into *Sarvangasana* without preparation or warm-up, the necessity for practising *Sarvangasana* before *Jalandhara Bandha* and *pranayama* requires you first to perform your general *asana* practice, then inversions such as *Sarvangasana*, followed by *pranayama* practice with *Jalandhara Bandha*.

Having prepared the neck by means of *Sarvangasana* for *Jalandhara Bandha*, we inhale deeply and lift the chest high. The lifting of the chest will allow us to inhale more deeply as the thorax expands more, but it will also decrease the range of movement that we have for bending the neck down. Lifting the chest high decreases any strain on the neck, which is especially important for novices. The powerfully expanded chest created through the lift will eventually enable us to stay in *kumbhaka* for longer.

LOCKING THE THROAT

The next important step in establishing *Jalandhara Bandha* is to lock the throat through swallowing. Be sure to understand that simply placing the chin on the chest does not constitute *Jalandhara Bandha*; it only means that now you have assumed '*Jalandhara Bandha* position'. This fact is perilously left out in the teaching of many modern schools, and without it *Jalandhara Bandha* remains impotent and *kumbhaka* is dangerous. *Jalandhara Bandha* is defined as contraction of

356. *Shiva Samhita* IV.38
357. *Gheranda Samhita* III.10

152

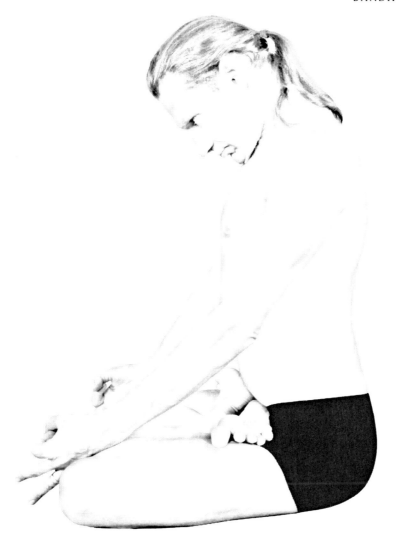

Jalandhara Bandha during internal kumbhaka

the throat in the *Hatha Ratnavali,*[358] *Shiva Samhita,*[359] *Gheranda Samhita,*[360] *Hatha Yoga Pradipika*[361] and *Yoga Kundalini Upanishad.*[362] How

358. *Hatha Ratnavali of Shrinivasayogi* II.8
359. *Shiva Samhita* IV.38
360. *Gheranda Samhita* III.10
361. *Hatha Yoga Pradipika* III.71
362. *Yoga Kundalini Upanishad* I.51

anybody can teach it as simply placing the chin down is beyond my understanding, as it means that *vayu* can enter the head and cause damage.

To activate *Jalandhara Bandha* means to swallow as if one is swallowing saliva and, once the throat muscles grip, to maintain that grip for the remainder of the breath retention. The test of whether *Jalandhara Bandha* is on properly is to try to breathe in or out. If you cannot breathe, even if trying, then and only then is *Jalandhara* correct. Apply this test the first few hundred times you perform the *bandha*.

Even if you have mastered it, re-check yourself regularly, particularly if you experience adverse symptoms such as pressure in the head, irritability or headaches. If you can breathe despite the fact that you have your chin in position, you are not applying *Jalandhara Bandha*! If need be, swallow several times until the throat is locked so that no air can pass into the head.

Contract the throat and place the chin low down on the sternum. The lower down you place it, the more stimulation the brain and the spinal cord will receive. However, especially in the beginning, proceed with care and don't strain the neck, as it may lead to headaches.

Now hold *kumbhaka* to capacity and not more. The fact that we hold *kumbhaka* only to capacity, but do not hold a *kumbhaka* of predetermined length (i.e. *matra*), means that we are not yet performing *pranayama* but only exercising the *bandha* in the *mudra* stage. Once you have reached your capacity to retain the breath, lift your head, release your throat and exhale gently – but exactly in this order and no other. Never release your throat first and then lift your head, as the *prana* may still enter the head. The air should not burst out, but come out in an even stream for the entire length of the exhalation. If you have to let the air out in bursts or gasp for the inhalation, you have exceeded your capacity. The bursting out and gasping constitute a loss of *prana* rather than a gain. In other words you have created demerit instead of merit.

154

It is important always to accept and honour one's limitations in *pranayama*. If not, lung tissue can be damaged, which in cases of ruthless practice can lead to emphysema. Ranjit Sen Gupta believes that a proper *Jalandhara Bandha* is a safety precaution against emphysema.[363] In any case it is important not to inhale so deeply that the lungs are overstretched. Nobody else can tell you how much you have to inhale. Be sensitive.

JALANDHARA BANDHA DURING EXTERNAL (BAHYA) KUMBHAKA

There is agreement about the fact that *Jalandhara Bandha* has to be applied during internal *kumbhaka* to prevent the rise of air and *prana* into the head. Opinions differ, however, where external (*bahya*) *kumbhaka* is concerned. The *Yoga Rahasya* insists on *Jalandhara Bandha* during external *kumbhaka*.[364] Other authorities mention *Jalandhara Bandha* only in the context of internal *kumbhaka*. The reason why *Jalandhara Bandha* during external *kumbhaka* is more difficult is that you have to bend your head down much lower to reach the chest, as the chest in external *kumbhaka* is deflated and dropped.

The main reason for *Jalandhara Bandha* – protecting the brain from the pressure of the fully inflated chest – does not apply to external *kumbhaka*, as the air pressure is very low after a full exhalation. Nevertheless, *Jalandhara Bandha* during external *kumbhaka* is very beneficial due to the intense stimulation it applies to the brain via the spinal cord. It is a powerful Kundalini technique, but much more difficult than *Jalandhara Bandha* during internal (*antara*) *kumbhaka*.

Jalandhara Bandha during *antara kumbhaka* must be thoroughly mastered before this more advanced version of the *bandha* is tackled. When building up to *Jalandhara Bandha* during external *kumbhaka*, prepare by increasing your time spent in *Sarvangasana* and *Halasana*. Also, always practise your external *kumbhaka*s after your *asana* practice, as only in this case will your neck be adequately prepared for

363. Ranjit Sen Gupta, *Pranayama: A Conscious Way of Breathing*, New Age Books, Delhi, 2000, p. 61
364. *Yoga Rahasya* I.62

the additional workload. When practising *Jalandhara Bandha* during external *kumbhaka*, lift your chest as high as you can and draw your

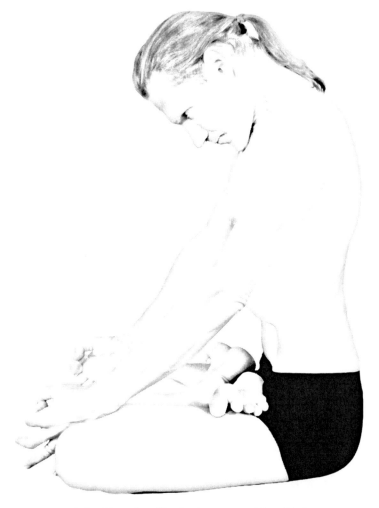

Jalandhara Bandha during external kumbhaka

shoulders forward so that the sternum and clavicles move forward and upwards to meet the chin.

This amounts to 'hunching of the shoulders around the ears', which is usually sneered at in all *asanas*. The only other posture where this is allowed is *Sarvangasana* (shoulder stand), which interestingly enough is the posture that induces the correct *Jalandhara Bandha* position.

Additionally, extensive internal *kumbhaka*s with *Jalandhara Bandha* must be mastered before serious external *kumbhaka*s with count are tackled. Apart from the Kundalini pull on the spinal cord, another strong reason why teachers like T. Krishnamacharya insist on *Jalandhara Bandha* during external *kumbhaka* is its influence on the nervous system and blood circulation.

JALANDHARA BANDHA AND THE PARASYMPATHETIC NERVOUS SYSTEM
By bending the head down low and contracting the throat, pressure is exerted on the carotid sinuses. This activates the parasympathetic nervous system, lowers the blood pressure and drops the heart rate. The general purpose of the carotid sinuses is to detect rising blood pressure in the carotid arteries, which if unchecked could damage the delicate blood vessels in the brain and eventually lead to a stroke. When the blood pressure in the carotid arteries rises, for whatever reason, they will expand and thus put pressure on the carotid sinuses. The sinuses are now stimulated and, as a safety mechanism, they activate the parasympathetic nervous system to both drop the blood pressure back down and slow the heart rate. *Jalandhara Bandha* uses this very mechanism to improve and increase *kumbhaka*. The parasympathetic nervous system enables you to relax into the *kumbhaka*s, and lowering the heart rate and dropping the blood pressure lead to a decrease in oxygen consumption of the organism. Hence, through *Jalandhara Bandha* the length of *kumbhaka* can be increased, resulting in many benefits such as deeper meditation and eventually the deletion of negative conditioning. Not only that, but success in *kumbhaka* and *pranayama* is reliant on success in *Jalandhara Bandha*. Its importance cannot be overemphasized.

Uddiyana Bandha

Uddiyana means flying up. The *Dhyana Bindu Upanishad* expounds that it is so called because it drives *prana* upwards into the central energy channel.[365]

DEFINITION

During inhalation, only the lower abdominal wall is contracted to drive part of the inhalation up into the thorax and prevent the abdomen from distending. During internal *kumbhaka* the entire abdominal wall is isometrically contracted to increase intra-abdominal pressure and drive *apana vayu* (vital down-current) up.[366] During exhalation the entire abdominal wall is isotonically contracted to drive air out without *apana vayu* turning down. During external *kumbhaka* the abdominal contents are sucked into the thoracic cavity to raise *apana vayu*. Technically speaking this is not a *bandha*, as there is no muscular contraction involved, but energetically it achieves what *bandhas* do – the diversion of *prana* and *vayu* into another direction. To make clear the stark difference between this method and the other three phases of *Uddiyana Bandha*, I call it *Bahya Uddiyana*.

Thus there are four different forms of *Uddiyana Bandha* / *Bahya Uddiyana*, applying to the four respiratory phases: inhalation, internal *kumbhaka*, exhalation and external *kumbhaka*. At any point of the breathing cycle one or another from of *Uddiyana Bandha* / *Bahya Uddiyana* applies.

CONTRAINDICATIONS FOR UDDIYANA BANDHA

Do not practise *Uddiyana Bandha* on a full stomach or during pregnancy. Apart from inhalation-*Uddiyana Bandha*, the other three versions are unsuitable to varying degrees for anyone suffering from peptic ulcers.

365. *Dhyana Bindu Upanishad* stanza 75
366. Muscle length does not change during contraction, static contraction.

158

ADDITIONAL CONTRAINDICATIONS FOR BAHYA (EXTERNAL) UDDIYANA

Additionally to the above, the more extreme form of *Bahya Uddiyana* should not be done during menstruation. However, if practised outside of menstruation, *Bahya Uddiyana* particularly has the potency to cure menstrual disorders, especially if they have resulted from a prolapsed uterus. Do not practise *Bahya Uddiyana* with a weak heart, heart disease or high blood pressure.

WHY UDDIYANA BANDHA?

There are numerous references to the miraculous effects of *Uddiyana Bandha*. The *Yoga Rahasya* states that it moves *prana* into *sushumna*,[367] that it cleans *chakras* and *nadis*[368] and that it helps with *apana*-related diseases such as menstrual disorders.[369] The *Hatha Ratnavali* declares that *Uddiyana Bandha* confines *prana* to *sushumna* and makes it rise therein.[370] The *Gheranda Samhita* proclaims *Uddiyana Bandha* to be a lion against the elephant death – due to its royal status, the lion was thought to be able to subdue even the elephant. It also claims that it is capable of conferring spontaneous liberation.[371] The *Goraksha Shataka* goes as far as stating that *Uddiyana Bandha* conquers death.[372]

INHALATION-UDDIYANA BANDHA

A complete yogic breathing cycle consists of filling the breath into the torso as if one would fill a receptacle with water, i.e. from the bottom up. The yogi inhales first into the abdomen, then into the thorax and finally into the upper lobes of the lungs, the clavicular area. Hence a yogic inhalation establishes a wave that initiates at the pubic bone and terminates at the manubrium of the sternum (upper end of the breast bone).

367. *Yoga Rahasya* I.65
368. *Yoga Rahasya* I.67
369. *Yoga Rahasya* I.69
370. *Hatha Ratnavali of Shrinivasayogi* II.53
371. *Gheranda Samhita* III.8–9
372. *Goraksha Shataka* stanza 77

Try the following experiment: Breathe in while keeping the abdominal wall completely relaxed. You will find that the belly expands more and more but the breath never reaches the thorax and clavicular area. This is a denatured and devitalizing way of inhaling. Now keep the lower abdominal wall firm and controlled, and inhale again. You will notice that now you will be able to draw the breath as high up as you choose. It is important that you do not contract the entire abdominal wall but only the part below the navel. Since the abdominal muscles interdigitate with the diaphragm, contracting the upper part of the abdominal wall will also lead to arresting the diaphragm. This would then make us chest-breathe exclusively – a form of breathing that is as denaturized and devitalizing as exclusive abdominal breathing.

We need to fully involve the entire torso in the breathing cycle to become a complete and integrated human being. The way to do so is to keep the lower abdominal wall controlled, slightly engaging the lower transverse abdominis muscle with the effect of drawing the abdominal contents gently in against the spine. The diaphragm is then free to descend downwards, increasing intra-abdominal pressure and massaging and compressing the abdominal organs. This will also lead to a slight protrusion of the abdominal wall above, but not below, the navel. The slight protrusion above the navel is feedback from the body that the diaphragm is moving freely up and down. You need to watch out for this sign.

The limited expansion of the upper abdomen will now lead to the excess volume of the inhalation expanding the thorax. It is very important for the health of the heart that the thorax is kept vibrant and pulsating. Exclusive abdominal breathing with a completely relaxed abdominal wall makes the thorax rigid, which is detrimental to *prana* supply to the heart. After the thorax is fully expanded, the controlled lower abdominal wall will then additionally drive the remainder of the inhalation all the way into the upper lobes of the lungs. It is very important for the upper lobes of the lungs to get properly ventilated, and only a few of us draw enough air into this area. Additionally, drawing the breath all the way into the upper lobes makes the wave of the breath reach this uppermost part of the thoracic spine. The proper function of the uppermost thoracic vertebrae will in turn guarantee that the nerves exiting along this area can properly supply their respective areas, mainly the arms, hands, wrists and shoulders. Any problems in this area are often related to a weak, inactive abdominal wall.

Readers of my previous books will have noted that it is this form of *Uddiyana Bandha*, which I will now call inhalation-*Uddiyana Bandha*, that is used during the entire *Ujjayi* breathing cycle in Ashtanga Vinyasa Yoga. Andre Van Lysebeth, the first Westerner to visit K. Pattabhi Jois, noted the teacher's emphasis on a controlled abdominal wall during *pranayama*,[373] and Van Lysebeth's book contains pictures depicting Jois supervising this form of *Uddiyana Bandha* in an advanced *pranayama* student.

We generally encounter the controlled abdominal wall in yogic texts when talk is of *Uddiyana Mudra*. This form of the *bandha* can be kept on for hours.

INTERNAL (KUMBHAKA) UDDIYANA BANDHA

We look next at the form of *Uddiyana Bandha* that is applied during internal *kumbhaka*. The *Hatha Ratnavali* says *Uddiyana Bandha* should be initiated after inhalation and before (internal) *kumbhaka* begins. The *Hatha Tatva Kaumudi* proclaims that by practice of *Jalandhara Bandha* and *Uddiyana Bandha* during (internal) *kumbhaka*, *prana* can be moved into *sushumna*. The *Kumbhaka Paddhati* recommends the initiation of *Uddiyana Bandha* after inhalation and before *kumbhaka* begins, and the *Gheranda Samhita* says the same.

We encounter here a form of *Uddiyana Bandha* different to the one already discussed. The *Uddiyana Bandha* performed during internal *kumbhaka* consists of the vigorous contraction of the abdominal muscles not only below but also above the navel.[374] Its purpose is

373. Andre van Lysebeth, *Die Grosse Kraft des Atems*, O.W. Barth, Bern, 1972, p. 138
374. *Hatha Ratnavali of Shrinivasayogi* II.55

to increase the pneumatic and pranic pressure in the torso to such an extent that *prana* enters *sushumna* and rises therein, and *apana vayu* is forced up. For this to happen, the yogi needs to have already obtained mastery in *Jalandhara Bandha* and *Mula Bandha*; otherwise *prana* will escape from the torso altogether. This constitutes a more advanced form of *Uddiyana Bandha*, and one should only worry about it after inhalation- and exhalation-*Uddiyana Bandha*s are learned.

One should not attempt internal *kumbhaka* of more than about 10 seconds without proficiency in *Jalandhara Bandha*. Initial sessions of internal *kumbhaka* must be devoted to checking again and again that *Jalandhara Bandha* is applied properly, so that *prana* does not force itself into the head and air into the ears and cause damage. Once *Jalandhara Bandha* is mastered, awareness in internal *kumbhaka* has to be diverted towards mastery of *Mula Bandha*, although *kumbhaka* can be performed without this *bandha* and not cause harm. But it is only after gaining mastery of both that the third *bandha*, *Uddiyana Bandha*, can be applied during internal *kumbhaka*. It will make the holding of the other two *bandha*s initially more taxing; it will also increase pressure on the lung tissue, which the novice needs to avoid. Lung tissue needs to be made strong by slowly increasing length and intensity of *kumbhaka*. This is the same principle as applies to muscles and tendons in *asana*, and in fact it applies to most things in life. The intensification of *kumbhaka* is the last thing a beginner should look for.

Apart from aiding the entry and rising of *prana* in *sushumna*, according to M.L. Gharote application of *Uddiyana Bandha* during internal *kumbhaka* also slows down the heartbeat by triggering the pressoreceptors in the abdominal viscera.[375] It has this effect in common with *Jalandhara* and *Mula Bandha*. All three *bandha*s (*bandhatraya*) work together to slow down the heart, deepen meditation, reduce the oxygen consumption of the body and hence prolong *kumbhaka*.

375. Dr M.L. Gharote, *Pranayama: The Science of Breath*, Lonavla Yoga Institute, Lonavla, 2003, p. 25

EXHALATION-UDDIYANA BANDHA

The *Yoga Kundali Upanishad* proclaims that *Uddiyana Bandha* should be performed at the end of internal *kumbhaka* and at the beginning of the exhalation.[376] The same is recommended in the *Yuktabhavadeva*,[377] the *Hatha Tatva Kaumudi* and the *Hatha Yoga Pradipika*.[378] When these texts talk about *Uddiyana Bandha* they are referring to what I call exhalation-*Uddiyana Bandha*. This form or phase of *Uddiyana Bandha* is similar to the internal *kumbhaka Uddiyana Bandha* in the regard that it uses the entire abdominal wall, i.e. the parts above and below the navel. But it is different in its effect and level of difficulty. Pulling the entire abdominal wall back in and towards the spine enables one to exhale fully and not leave a cubic centimetre of one's respiratory volume (i.e. vital capacity) behind. This way the maximum amount of CO_2 is exhaled and space for the new inhalation is created. This method creates the potential for a new larger inhalation and thus a longer subsequent *kumbhaka*. But there is another important effect. The instinctive action to create a complete exhalation would be to completely collapse the ribcage, but if you do that you will notice a distinct drop and let-down of energy (descending *apana vayu*) at the end of the exhalation, with the thoracic spine flexing (becoming more kyphotic) and the head tending to droop forward. Exhalation-*Uddiyana Bandha* enables one to keep one's spirit lifted and keeps the spine and head upright by supplying a necessary burst of energy. This way it enables the yogi to extend the exhalation as long as is needed.

Mastery of *pranayama* is not achieved during inhalation or *kumbhaka*. It is achieved during the exhalation. During serious *pranayama* the exhalation is to be made double the length of the inhalation and half the length of internal *kumbhaka*. The most frequently quoted *pranayama* count is 16 seconds for inhalation, 64 seconds for *kumbhaka* and 32 seconds for the exhalation. There would be some people who could

376. *Yoga Kundalini Upanishad* stanzas 47–48
377. *Yuktabhavadeva of Bhavadeva Mishra* lxviii
378. *Hatha Yoga Pradipika* II.45

hold their breath for 64 seconds if they sucked the air in within a few seconds, then held it and after that exhaled with an open mouth in a few seconds. But that is not the point of *pranayama*. The point is to be able, after a 64-second *kumbhaka*, to distribute one's exhalation gracefully over another 32 seconds, not rush at the end and not run out of exhalable air either.

This is much, much more difficult than the preceding 64-second *kumbhaka*. But it is here that the magic of *pranayama* happens. While *prana* is extracted from the environmental air in internal *kumbhaka*, the distribution of *prana* to the various areas of the body takes place during a smooth, long, even exhalation. And it is also generally during the exhalation that Kundalini eventually rises. But all of these things are possible only when exhalation-*Uddiyana Bandha* is mastered, which consists of drawing both the upper and lower abdominal walls in towards the spine. This must not, of course, be applied too rapidly, as otherwise the air would burst out of the nostrils. A smooth, even and long exhalation is required in *pranayama*. The application of external *Uddiyana Bandha* is a fine art that is learned in daily practice over a significant time frame.

In the hierarchy of the three forms of *Uddiyana Bandha*, the inhalation-*Uddiyana Bandha* needs to be learned first, because without it there is no complete yogic breathing cycle. Next in line, the exhalation-*Uddiyana Bandha* needs to be learned. It provides stamina in *pranayama* but requires constant remembrance. Only after that comes the internal (*kumbhaka*) *Uddiyana Bandha*. One should tackle it only once firmly established in *pranayama*.

EXTERNAL (KUMBHAKA) UDDIYANA / BAHYA UDDIYANA

There are two very different exercises described in yogic literature with almost the same name. One is often called simply *Uddiyana* and the other *Uddiyana Bandha*. Both are used to drive the vital down-current (*apana vayu*) up. Although they are similar in name they are very different in their application. *Uddiyana Bandha* is a muscular contraction that pushes the abdominal contents in and up. It can only have an effect when there is air in the lungs and when the abdominal muscles can push against something. Therefore it is used only during inhalation, internal *kumbhaka* and *exhalation.*

When the lungs are empty, instead of the *bandha* a vacuum is used to suck the abdominal contents up into the thoracic cavity. This also raises *apana vayu*, but the physiological mechanism is entirely different. *Uddiyana* takes place after a complete exhalation. During external *kumbhaka* the breath is arrested, the throat locked and a faked inhalation is performed during which the diaphragm rises. The abdominal muscles are completely relaxed and the abdominal contents are sucked into the thoracic cavity, a process that is supported by the latissimus dorsi and trapezius. M.V. Bhole, MD, argues in a journal article in *Yoga Mimamsa* that this is not really a *bandha*.[379] Strictly speaking this is correct, as it does not involve contraction of the muscle group central to the *bandha*, here the abdominals. For example in *Jalandhara Bandha* the throat is contracted and creates a barrier. The same applies in *Mula Bandha*, due to the controlled pelvic diaphragm. *Uddiyana Bandha* in its narrower sense is thus only a true *bandha* when the abdominal wall is controlled. Readers often mistake the significance of why the technique is sometimes named *Uddiyana Bandha* and at other times *Uddiyana*. Adding to that confusion, some rather recent schools of yoga are entirely ignorant of the fact that, apart from *Uddiyana*, there exists an *Uddiyana Bandha*, which is not only entirely different in nature but the true *bandha*. Compounding that confusion even more, Theos Bernard, following his teacher's nomenclature, named *Uddiyana* the dynamic flapping of the abdominal wall, which is sometimes called *Agnisara* or *Vahnisara Dhauti* and which in this present text is called *Nauli* stage 1. This is an entirely different exercise, and Swami Kuvalayananda taught that *Agnisara* does not even contain *Uddiyana* (i.e. no faked inhalation).

To differentiate *Uddiyana Bandha*, which is a muscular contraction that occurs during inhalation, internal *kumbhaka* and exhalation, I have named the passive *Uddiyana*, which only occurs during external

379. *Yoga Mimamsa* XV.2

(*bahya*) *kumbhaka, Bahya Uddiyana* throughout this book. In doing so I have followed a tradition that to my knowledge was initiated by Shrinivasayogi, the author of the *Hatha Ratnavali*.[380] This text was probably set down during the 17th century, and its author was well aware of the need to disambiguate *Uddiyana* from *Uddiyana Bandha*.

The *Yoga Rahasya* states that, after exhalation, external (*bahya*)

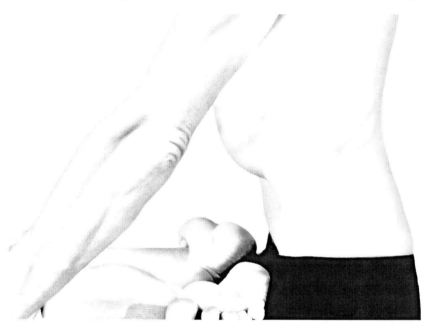

Bahya Uddiyana, sitting

kumbhaka should be performed with a strong *Uddiyana* and *Jalandhara Bandha*.[381] *Bahya Uddiyana* is said to alleviate abdominal-organ malfunctions such as diabetes and purify the *Manipura Chakra*. Apart from its application during external *kumbhaka*, it is also used in *Nauli kriya* and in *mudras* such as *Tadaga Mudra, Yoga Mudra* and *Mahamudra*. It is a passive exercise in the regard that its effect is not brought about by contracting the abdominal muscles but by creating upward suction through a faked inhalation after the throat is locked. Whereas the

380. *Hatha Ratnavali of Shrinivasayogi* II.56
381. *Yoga Rahasya* I.62

166

previous three active versions of *Uddiyana Bandha* tend to activate the parasympathetic nervous system, slow down the heart and reduce blood pressure, this passive *Bahya Uddiyana* tends to stimulate the sympathetic nervous system and speed up the heartbeat. This it does mainly through the suction that it applies to the adrenal glands. It can thus be used to create a balance between the sympathetic and parasympathetic nervous systems, but its function also explains why external *kumbhaka* is more difficult than internal *kumbhaka*. The heart tends to accelerate and consume more oxygen while the lungs are completely empty. This might be another reason why T. Krishnamacharya put so much emphasis on the difficult task of performing *Jalandhara Bandha* during external *kumbhaka* with *Bahya Uddiyana*. *Jalandhara* then tends to neutralize the sympathetic effect of *Bahya Uddiyana*.

While the other *bandhas* increase pressure in the abdominal organs, *Bahya Uddiyana* rapidly decreases intra-abdominal pressure from the normal. By applying both types sequentially while going from internal to external *kumbhaka* and back, the organs are massaged. Old stagnant fluid is sucked and squeezed out of the organs, and then fresh blood is pumped back into them. Elimination of toxins is greatly enhanced and the vitality of the organs is increased. The same is to be said for lung tissue.

In *pranayama*, *Bahya Uddiyana* is an advanced exercise that can only be tackled once the previous versions of *Uddiyana Bandha* have been learned. Especially if combined with *Jalandhara Bandha*, *Bahya Uddiyana* exerts a powerful suction on the brain and the cerebrospinal fluid. *Bahya Uddiyana* must be learned slowly during *Nauli*, *Tadaga Mudra* and *Yoga Mudra*. The beginner should initially perform not more than 2 or 3 repetitions per day and then slowly increase the rate over weeks and months.

Due to the intense pressure exchange, *Bahya Uddiyana*, like *Nauli*, should not be practised by women during a time when they wish to conceive, during menstruation or during pregnancy. However, at all other times it is very beneficial for the female reproductive system.

Like *Nauli*, it can aid in repositioning a prolapsed uterus. *Bahya Uddiyana* and *Nauli* can function as a form of natural contraceptive if used together with certain yoga postures.

Mula Bandha

Mula Bandha means root lock, referring to the pelvic floor as the root of the spine and nervous system.

WHY MULA BANDHA?

The *Dhyana Bindu Upanishad* proclaims that the old become young again when performing *Mula Bandha*.[382] The *Gheranda Samhita* agrees that *Mula Bandha* destroys all weakness and infirmity,[383] a claim that is supported by the *Shiva Samhita*.[384] Weakness and ageing are, according to yoga, due to a loss of life force, and this loss is partially due to the downward flow of life force. *Mula Bandha* preserves life force and makes it flow upwards.

The *Yoga Kundalini Upanishad* calls *Mula Bandha* the forcing up of the vital downward current *apana vayu*. It states that directing *apana vayu* upwards, together with igniting internal fire, will make the serpent Kundalini enter its hole, the central energy channel.[385] The same mechanism is explained in the *Hatha Yoga Pradipika*.[386] It is to be noted that *apana* must be raised to the 'region of fire', i.e. the *Manipura* (navel) *Chakra*, where it meets *agni*, which is to be stoked by wind (*vayu*). Together they have the power to ignite Kundalini. *Mula Bandha* is also used to awaken *Muladhara Chakra*.

TECHNIQUE

Mula Bandha initially is the pressing of the perineum with the left heel (in *Siddhasana*) and its subsequent contraction.[387] It is ideally

382. *Dhyana Bindu Upanishad* stanzas 74–75
383. *Gheranda Samhita* III.12–14
384. *Shiva Samhita* IV.41
385. *Yoga Kundalini Upanishad* I.40–46
386. *Hatha Yoga Pradipika* III.60–64
387. *Goraksha Shataka* stanza 81

168

learned in *Siddhasana* because the left heel will apply stimulation to the pelvic floor. This can, however, be replicated in *Padmasana* by tilting the pelvis forward enough to bring the perineum in contact with the floor. *Mula Bandha* may be experienced and practised in any yoga posture, but the two mentioned above are ideal. When proficiency is gained, the *apana vayu* will turn upwards.

In the beginning, *Mula Bandha* may be brought on by contracting the anus or the urethra as if one wanted to stop urination. However, to be precise, *Mula Bandha* is located right in the middle between the anus and genitals, at the centre of the pubococcygeus muscle. To some extend the contraction of the pubococcygeus will activate the entire pelvic diaphragm. In this context imagine the inhalation reaching all the way down to the pelvic floor, hooking into the pelvic floor and drawing it upwards. When wanting to focus on *Mula Bandha*'s connection to the exhalation, feel the exhalation dropping down and, as it turns into the inhalation, feel the breath rebounding off the pelvic diaphragm as if off a trampoline.[388]

Mula Bandha stimulates the filum terminale and cauda equina, which are anchored at the coccyx. Through that, *Mula Bandha* stimulates the entire brain and particularly the parasympathetic nervous system. It slows down the heart, lowers the blood pressure and decreases the respiratory rate. T. Krishnamacharya stated that *Mula Bandha* was instrumental in gaining his ability to stop his heartbeat.

WHEN

Ideally *Mula Bandha* is always applied during *kumbhaka*, as it activates the parasympathetic nervous system, making *kumbhaka* easier. *Mula Bandha* should also be held during inhalation and exhalation. Apart from that, *Mula Bandha* should also be applied when practising any *asana*, apart from *Shavasana* and during any Kundalini-raising exercise. During *kumbhaka*, however, *Mula Bandha* is second in importance to *Jalandhara Bandha*. Divert intellectual bandwidth towards *Mula Bandha* only when you are sure that *Jalandhara* is perfectly turned on.

388. Metaphor courtesy of Richard Freeman

WHEN NOT

The yogic scriptures recommend holding *Mula Bandha* all the time. However, this applies only to a very advanced practitioner who has completed his/her duties towards society and raises Kundalini. A person who still performs all normal functions in society and tries to hold *Mula Bandha* all the time may experience constipation. Food intake needs to be adapted if *Mula Bandha* is held all the time. Menstruation is also powered by *apana*, and turning *apana* up by means of *Mula Bandha* may interfere with the natural menstruation process. *Apana* is also responsible for the delivery of the foetus. During pregnancy *Mula Bandha* may have to be decreased, depending on the condition of the individual. For example, a female with a very advanced *asana* practice and an athletic *Mula Bandha* may benefit from releasing it, certainly towards the end of her pregnancy. If a strong practice of *Mula Bandha* is continued until the end of pregnancy, it may make giving birth more difficult. On the other hand, females with a generally low muscle tone and weak pelvic floor may benefit from practising *Mula Bandha* for longer.

TRIBANDHA OR BANDHATRAYA

These are terms used for the simultaneous application of all three *bandhas* in external or internal *kumbhaka* with miraculous effects. *Mula Bandha* drives *apana vayu* upwards; *Jalandhara Bandha* sends *prana vayu* downwards where it fans *agni*. The fanned *agni / apana* compound is then moved up into *sushumna* by means of *Uddiyana Bandha*.

Jihva Bandha

Jihva Bandha means tongue lock. It is the folding of the tongue backwards, placing its underneath side up against the hard and soft palate and pushing it as far back as possible towards the naso-pharyngeal cavity.

The *Hatha Tatva Kaumudi* promulgates that when the tongue is fixed against the palate behind the uvula, *prana* will enter *sushumna*

170

and one hears *nada*. *Nada* means inner sound, and it is regarded as the most straightforward method to enter *samadhi*. However, the stanza in the *Hatha Tatva Kaumudi* does not really pertain to *Jihva Bandha*. The tongue in *Jihva Bandha* cannot be moved beyond the uvula, being stopped by the tendon on the tongue's inferior surface, called the frenum.

The technique mentioned by the *Kaumudi* is really *Khechari Mudra*, which requires the frenum to be cut so that the tongue can be swallowed. The term *Khechari Mudra* should not be used to refer to *Jihva Bandha*. *Jihva Bandha* is the basic ingredient of *Nabho Mudra*, which refers to the milking of the uvula by means of the tongue, which releases *amrita* (nectar). *Khechari Mudra* is an advanced version of *Nabho Mudra*.

Khechari Mudra is reputed to greatly reduce respiratory speed, thus enabling much longer *kumbhaka*s. It makes *prana* steady and thus steadies the mind. These effects are also provided by *Jihva Bandha*, albeit to a lesser extent. One of the mechanisms through which the subconscious (*vasana*) can express and manifest itself is through subtle movements of the tongue and eyes. If the yogi arrests these movements, the subconscious loses its grip and *kumbhaka* and meditation can deepen. One of the main reasons for applying *Jihva Bandha* is that it steadies the subconscious by removing one of its expressions. In that way it is related to *drishti* (focal point) and its advanced form *Shambhavi Mudra*, where the attention is fixed at the third eye for a long time.

Jihva Bandha is thus an important adjunct for *pranayama* and all forms of meditation. Some yogic schools claim it can be used to replace *Jalandhara* in *kumbhaka*. This is not the case in my experience. It is better to add it to *Jalandhara Bandha*. This view is also supported by the Jyotsna commentary on the *Hatha Yoga Pradipika*.[389] Following this suggestion, one first applies *Jihva Bandha* and then, while maintaining it, enters *Jalandhara Bandha*. Alternatively, *Jihva Bandha* may be applied during the entire breathing cycle. Be aware of tension

389. *Hatha Yoga Pradipika with Commentary Jyotsna*, Adyar Library, Madras, 1972, p. 30

building up in your head. If you contract a headache release *Jihva Bandha*. Phase it into your practice slowly.

Jihva Bandha is a helpful ancillary of *pranayama* practice, but it is an extensive subject that is beyond the scope of this book.

KRIYAS

I am using the term *kriya* to refer to the gross purification processes that are called *shatkarmas* (six actions) in some texts and *ashta karmas* (eight actions) in others. In reality there are more than 40 *kriyas*, when the subdivisions are taken into consideration.

The *Hatha Yoga Pradipika* in chapter 2 first describes the main *pranayama* technique *Nadi Shodhana* (*nadi* purification) and then suggests the *kriyas* to those whose *nadis* are so clogged that *Nadi Shodhana* alone is not sufficient. Only after that does the *Pradipika* describe all the other various forms of *pranayama*. In other words the *Pradipika* suggests that some yogis may be in a condition good enough for the *kriyas* not to be required. However, Balakrishna, one of the commentators on the *Hatha Yoga Pradipika*, says that *asanas* and *kriyas* are both recommended as preparations to *pranayama*, as no single practice can eliminate all impurities.[390] The *Hatha Yoga Pradipika* does, though, insist on the performance of the *kriyas* before *pranayama* if fat and phlegm are present in the student's body, as these clog the *nadis*.[391] This view is also held by the *Yuktabhavadeva of Bhavadeva Mishra*.[392] Additionally, the 10-chapter edition of the *Hatha Yoga Pradipika* suggests, as an order of practices, first establishment in *asana*, then the purification of the *nadis* through *kriyas* and only then the practice of *pranayama*.[393]

The *Gheranda Samhita* states that purification can happen either through *Nadi Shodhana* with *mantra* or through the *kriyas* (purification processes).[394] In any case, a teacher of yoga should know the *kriyas* in order to be able to teach them, even if she will not teach all the *kriyas* to all students. The *Hatha Tatva Kaumudi* gives us a different view of the importance of the *kriyas*. It proclaims that the gross body gets purified through the *kriyas* whereas the subtle (energetic) body

390. *Hatha Yoga Pradipika* (10 chapters) II.24–25, Balakrishna's commentary
391. *Hatha Yoga Pradipika* II.21
392. *Yuktabhavadeva of Bhavadeva Mishra* lxxii
393. *Hathapradipika* (10 chapters) III.1
394. *Gheranda Samhita* V.36–37

is purified through *pranayama*, but its author, Sundaradeva, nevertheless admits that the *kriya*s are secondary to *pranayama*.[395]

The *Hatha Ratnavali*, authored by Shrinivasayogi, gives us some very important additional details. Firstly, he agrees that before *pranayama* the body must be purified through the *kriya*s [as asana alone is not sufficient to prepare for *pranayama*].[396] He then goes on to explain that the *kriya*s purify the 6 *chakra*s.[397] Shrinivasayogi states that *Nauli* purifies the *Manipura Chakra*, *Dhauti* purifies the *Anahata Chakra*, *Neti* purifies the *Ajna Chakra* and so on. This amounts to ascribing to the *kriya*s the ability to purify the subtle body too. Jayatarama, the author of *Jogapradipyaka*, makes the *kriya*s compulsory by stating that they and *pranayama* are both necessary as preparation for *samadhi*.[398]

Let us turn to the views of modern authorities. O.P. Tiwari, director of Kaivalyadhama, says that meditation is not possible if the *nadi*s are blocked, and if this is the case one may hypnotize oneself into the assumption that one is making progress in meditation whereas it is not the case.[399] He accepts, however, that cleaning of the *nadi*s can be brought about by such different tools as *kriya*, devotion to the Divine and *pranayama*. Swami Niranjanananda, successor of Swami Satyananda, holds that the effects of *asana* and *pranayama* increase profoundly if, through practice of the *kriya*s, toxins are expelled beforehand.[400] He adds that adverse effects may be encountered in *pranayama* if the *kriya*s have not been practised previously.

If problems are encountered in *pranayama* or Kundalini-raising, practitioners often make yoga responsible. This is similar to making the science of architecture responsible if a house collapses although the true cause was insufficient foundations and weak walls. If the yogi practises prudently and is grounded in *asana, kriya* and devotion, no adverse effects of *pranayama* will be observed.

395. Hatha Tatva Kaumudi of Sundaradeva VIII.18
396. *Hatha Ratnavali of Shrinivasayogi* I.60
397. *Hatha Ratnavali of Shrinivasayogi* I.61
398. *Jogapradipyaka of Jayatarama* stanzas 825–838
399. O.P. Tiwari, *Kriyas and Pranayama*, DVD, Kaivalyadhama, Lonavla.
400. Swami Niranjanananda, *Prana and Pranayama*, Yoga Publications Trust, Munger, 2009, p. 210

M.L. Gharote suggests that, without the background of the *kriyas*, *pranayama* is not likely to succeed.[401] He also explains that in our modern times, due to artificial ways of living, we are more likely to have unbalanced *doshas* (bodily humours), and due to that the *kriyas* have become even more important than in the olden days.[402] It is not the case that the *kriyas* are an obscure medieval practice. There would be few yogis in today's world who could afford not to do them (save those who have a very advanced *asana* practice). Chemical pollution of food, water and air, radiation, electricity, microwaves, cell-phones and radio activity, today make it much more necessary to practise the purification processes to expel some of the many toxins that confront us. The *kriyas* have assumed much greater importance in the modern, industrial, urban society.

T. Krishnamacharya proclaimed in *Yoga Makaranda* that both the *asanas* and the six *kriyas* need to be mastered to eliminate the negative influences of the three humours of the body (*vata*, *pitta* and *kapha*).[403] He also declared, however, that the *kriyas* are not necessary if somebody has achieved a high level of *asana* and *pranayama* practice.[404] However, such a standard of practice is rare these days. Krishnamacharya also held that some of the *kriyas* are rather part of Ayurveda and need to be part of treatment plans addressing individuals. The kriyas, which are part of Ayurveda, are the various versions of Dhauti, Basti and Gaja Karani. The two most important *kriyas*, however, *Nauli* and Kapalabhati, are not contained in Ayurveda, and it is these two processes that are very important for modern *pranayama* practitioners. Additionally the processes of *Neti* are described here due to air pollution in modern cities. The Kriya Trataka is an important *pratyahara* and *dharana* exercise, but it does not fall within the scope of this book. *Basti* (the yogic enema) is an extremely important adjunct to Kundalini-

---

401. Dr M.L. Gharote, *Pranayama: The Science of Breath*, Lonavla Yoga Institute, Lonavla, 2003, p. 53
402. Dr M.L. Gharote, *Yogic Techniques*, Lonavla Yoga Institute, Lonavla, 2006,p. 56
403. T. Krishnamacharya, *Yoga Makaranda*, rev. English edn, Media Garuda, 2011, p. 93.
404. A.G. Mohan, *Krishnamacharya: His Life and Teachings*, Shambala, Boston & London, 2010, p. 63

raising, but again, since it is not the subject of this book, I hope to cover it at a later stage.

Generally, performance of the chosen *kriyas* early in the morning before *asana* and *pranayama* is suggested, this being especially the case for *Nauli*. *Kapalabhati* should be performed right before one's *pranayama* practice. *Trataka* and *Neti* can be performed at any time of the day.

In my own practice I have found the *kriyas Nauli* and *Kapalabhati* extremely powerful, and I cannot imagine succeeding in higher yoga without practising them daily. *Neti* is extremely important in the beginning, to go beyond the 'blocked-nostril phase'. It may be discarded once this aim is achievn mned.

Nauli

Nauli is the churning of the abdominal muscles. The abdominal recti are isolated and then a wavelike motion is initiated, which first churns from the right to the left and then from the left to the right.[405] A vacuum is created in the intestines and abdomen, which helps to massage the abdominal organs, makes the heart, lungs and abdominal organs strong, returns them to health and expels any accumulated toxins.

The *Hatha Yoga Pradipika* says about *Nauli* that it removes dyspepsia, increases appetite and improves digestion. According to the *Pradipika*, *Nauli* is like the Goddess of Creation in that it creates happiness and destroys all disorders of the body.[406] But the benefits of *Nauli* are not only physical. The *Hatha Yoga Manjari* states that *Nauli* helps to turn the *chakras* upwards.[407] The *chakras* are always facing the Kundalini. In a person who has not awakened Kundalini, the *chakras*, thought of as lotus flowers, hang with their heads down facing the Kundalini in the *Muladhara* (base *chakra*). *Nauli* is an important exercise in raising Kundalini; hence Sahajananda, the author of the *Hatha Yoga Manjari*, remarks that it assists in turning up the lotuses.

405. starting, however, by isolating the rectus abdominis on the left, which is why it is called *Vama* (left) *Nauli*
406. *Hatha Yoga Pradipika* II.34
407. *Hatha Yoga Manjari of Sahajananda* II.48

The *Hatha Ratnavali* states that *Nauli* is also one of the main actions that bring about purification of the important *Manipura Chakra*,[408] the other being, as stated in the *Yoga Rahasya*, external *kumbhaka* with *Bahya* (external) *Uddiyana*. For the *pranayama* practitioner, one of the greatest benefits of practising *Nauli* is that it confers mastery over *Bahya* (external) *Uddiyana*. Without this version of *Uddiyana Bandha*, external *kumbhaka* cannot be effectively practised.

WHEN AND WHEN NOT NAULI?

According to Swami Kuvalayananda, Nauli can be done from puberty onwards but not before. It should not be practised in case of hyper-acidity and not for six weeks after giving birth. Additionally, it should not be done during pregnancy and menstruation, or if suffering from high blood pressure, heart problems, ulcers, hernia or glaucoma. Due to the intense pressure exchange, *Nauli* should not be practised during a time when women wish to conceive; however, it is very beneficial for the female reproductive system at times other than menstruation, conception and pregnancy.

Acharya Bhagwan Dev tells us that women suffering from menstrual problems will get swift improvement through *Nauli*.[409] It also helps with fanning the digestive fire, burning fat around the waist, *removing* sluggishness of the liver and alleviating constipation. If you are suffering from an aggravated *pitta* condition, do less *Nauli*, particularly stage 1. However, *Nauli* is part of the parcel of techniques that are used to purify *pitta*/*agni*. In case of vitiated *pitta*, slowly increase *Nauli* together with making diet changes and embracing devotion to the Divine and other yogic techniques under supervision of an experienced practitioner.

I teach Nauli in four stages. Nauli's first stage in yogic literature is variously called *Agnisara* (fanning of digestive fire) or *Uddiyana*. I regard the label *Uddiyana* as particularly confusing since, even without this present technique, *Uddiyana Bandha* has already four distinct

408. *Hatha Ratnavali of Shrinivasayogi* I.63
409. Acharya Bhagwan Dev, *Pranayama, Kundalini & Hatha Yoga*, Diamond Books, New Delhi, 2008, p. 18

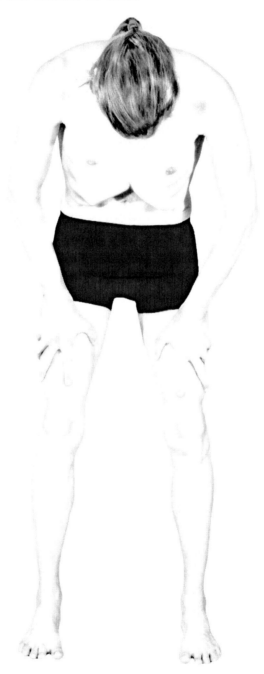

Nauli stage 1, standing

phases and need not be made more complex. Since this present technique forms a necessary prelude to the more advanced stages of *Nauli*, I will simply call it *Nauli* stage 1.

NAULI STAGE 1

The action should be performed on an empty stomach and after evacuation of the bowels. The early morning is ideal – before other yoga practices such as *asana* and *pranayama*. Although advanced Kundalini-raising *Nauli* is later to be done in *Padmasana* or a similar meditation posture, it is most easily learned while standing. Place your feet hip-width apart and your hands on your thighs just above the knees. Now stoop forward and look at your abdomen. It is helpful to bare your abdomen so that you see and understand the effect of your actions.

Now exhale fully, and at the end of the exhalation use the contraction of your abdominals to expel the last bit of air. Now lock and contract your throat and completely relax your abdominal muscles. Keeping the throat firmly contracted, perform a faked inhalation. This means you act as if you are inhaling but can't since your throat is locked. There is a limited expansion of the ribcage through the intercostal muscles. Additionally, lift the ribcage upwards to the head. The effect of these combined actions is that the vacuum in the lungs will suck the lungs up towards the clavicles. This raises and stretches the diaphragm (an act in itself very important and beneficial for the diaphragm), which now sucks the contents of the abdominal cavity into the thoracic cavity with all the pressure- changing effects this has for the abdominal organs. You will understand now that you need to be of average health (not of poor health) and without major disorders of the abdominal and thoracic organs to perform this intense action.

You have now arrived in external (*bahya*) *kumbhaka* (breath retention) with full *Uddiyana Bandha*, also referred to as *Bahya* (external) *Uddiyana*. If this is your first encounter with *bahya kumbhaka* or even with *kumbhaka* at all, then do not hold it longer than 10 seconds and get accustomed to this part of Stage 1 *Nauli* before you go further. If you are already practising external breath retention (*bahya kumbhaka*) and external *Uddiyana* (*Bahya Uddiyana*) you will find their performance greatly improved by *Nauli*.

If you are comfortable with and accustomed to external *kumbhakas*, suddenly release the intercostal muscles, latissimus dorsi and lower trapezius, and let go of the upward suction of the lungs. Your diaphragm will suddenly drop and the abdominal organs return to their original position. The action is performed without engaging the abdominal muscles, but only through creating and releasing suction with the thorax and the lungs. Once the abdominal organs have returned to their place of origin, you have completed one stroke of stage 1 *Nauli*. You may repeat the exercise up to 10 times in fast succession during the one breath retention, which will create a flapping, vertical wave-like motion of your abdominal wall. You have now completed 1 round of 10 strokes of stage 1 *Nauli*. Release your throat, inhale gently and come up to standing. If you find it hard to inhale due to the negative pressure in your lungs, exhale the last bit of air in your lungs forcefully and then only inhale gently. Over the next few days you may slowly increase the number of rounds from 1 to 3, taking a few breaths in between and coming up to standing if necessary. You may also slowly increase the number of strokes per round from 10 to 15 and eventually to 20, reaching a total of 60 strokes in 1 round. During that process make sure that you do not sacrifice amplitude of the strokes for increased frequency. Make sure that each individual stroke is vigorous, as otherwise the exercise becomes impotent.

A fast increase of strokes and rounds is not recommended during summer, particularly during a heatwave. Increase strokes more slowly if you live in a hot place of if you are used to spicy food with lots of chilli etc. You may also choose to decrease the amount of spices you use.

Do not go beyond this level of practice unless an experienced yogi supervises you. There are suggestions in literature that the practice might be extended to beyond 1000 strokes.[410] The reasoning behind such extreme forms of practice is that it may raise *agni* to such an extent that it can expel the *dosha*s, help in raising Kundalini and empower the intellect. The *Hatha Tatva Kaumudi* states that *pitta* in its pure form, that is when it is not impeded, ignites the fire of intelligence. It then causes rousing of Kundalini and expels the *dosha*s.[411] Without doubt we can call this quote one of the great secrets of yoga.

How, one may ask, can *pitta*, which is often the cause of disease, kindle the fire of wisdom and expel the *dosha*s? The mind is made up of three components, i.e. *tamas* (torpidity), *rajas* (frenzy) and *sattva* (fire of light and wisdom). These three qualities (*gunas*) of nature (*prakrti*) manifest themselves in the body as *kapha* (created by *tamas* – torpidity), *vata* (created by *rajas* – frenzy) and finally *pitta*, which is a product of *sattva*. However, while the connection in case of the other two can easily be understood, this is not so with *sattva* and *pitta*, apart from the fact that they are both related to the light and fire of the sun. *Pitta* is present in the body in vitiated or impeded form, and as such forms an obstacle. If vitiated *pitta* is aggravated/ increased it may cause inflammation, gastritis, stomach ulcers, hyper-acidity and liver problems. It is in such a case anything but the kindler of the fire of wisdom. If *pitta* is vitiated you can raise it only slightly and slowly, while purifying it at the same time. However, once *pitta* is purified it becomes a powerful ally in the spiritual quest, and yogis will use the stages of *Nauli*, combined with long sessions of *Surya Bhedana* and *Bhastrika pranayama*s, to raise Kundalini. If *pitta/agni* is vitiated, such a practice would damage or even destroy the body. An example of the destructive power of *agni* is the self-immolation at will of Sati, avatar of the Godmother and wife of Lord Shiva, when insulted by her father, Daksha.

Agni becomes impaired, for example, by a toxic diet, such as one containing meats, alcohol, coffee, etc., but the main cause of vitiation of *pitta* is the mind. Ideally the mind works like a laser, which is a form

---

410. Theos Bernard, *Heaven Lies Within Us*, Charles Scribner's Sons, New York, 1939, p. 21
411. *Hatha Tatva Kaumudi of Sundaradeva* XXXVI.55

of concentrated fire. A laser-like mind is said to be predominantly or almost exclusively sattvic. *Sattva* is the mental cause of the physical effect *pitta*. If toxic thoughts and emotions overtake the mind, they express themselves on the physical plane through impaired *pitta*, which turns against the body and destroys it. The mind, after all, is the root cause of disease. If the mind is purified through sequential application of the eight limbs, then practices like high-frequency *Nauli* can slowly be integrated into one's life, but only under the supervision of an expert.

Exercise *Nauli* stage 1 until you can easily practise 60 strokes over 3 rounds. Allow several weeks for this stage to develop. Once you are firmly established here, go on to stage 2, but continue to perform your 60 strokes daily as a preparation for the other stages.

Nauli stage 2 starts in the same way as stage 1. Stand in the same position, exhale, lock your throat and perform a faked inhalation so that the contents of the abdominal cavity are being sucked up into the thorax. Without reducing the suction thus created, press down with latissimus dorsi, trapezius and the lower part of the diaphragm, and also press on your knees with your arms. Now engage the two sides of the rectus abdominis and push it out while you continue to lift the thorax upwards. (If you have difficulty isolating the rectus, perform *Navasana* or a sit-up position and touch your belly. The muscles that are now bulging and keeping your legs from dropping down to the floor are the abdominal recti.)

You will now see that the two sides of rectus abdominis stand out while the more lateral parts of the frontal abdominal wall, where the obliques abdominis muscles are located, is being sucked inwards. This is due to the fact that by pushing out the recti a vacuum is created behind them. It is this vacuum that we will use in *Nauli* for therapeutic purposes. It is also used in *Basti*, the yogic enema.

Initially do one *kumbhaka* only and slowly build up to 3 rounds, bringing you to a total of six external *kumbhaka*s. This stage of *Nauli*

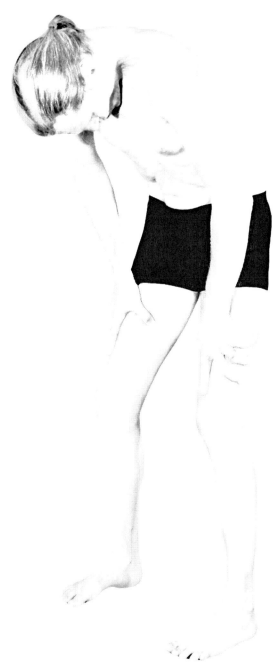

Nauli stage 2, Madhyama

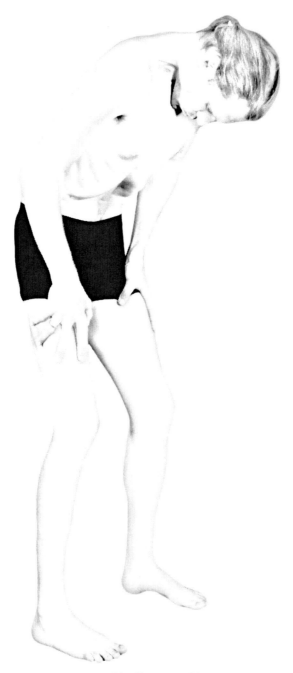

Nauli stage 3, Vama

is called *Madhyama,* because the abdominal muscles are pushed out in the middle.

NAULI STAGE 3, VAMA AND DAKSHINA

Once you have practised stages 1 and 2 for a while and are comfortable with them, move to stage 3. Stage 3 initially starts like stage 2. While standing, bend forward and perform external *kumbhaka* with *Bahya Uddiyana Bandha* (external *Uddiyana*). Keeping the abdominal contents sucked upwards, push out the abdominal recti in the middle (*Madhyama*) as in stage 2. Now lean to the left and push down with your left arm on the left knee, while you relax your right arm. You may exaggerate in the beginning by lifting the right hand off the right knee. This action relaxes the right side of the rectus abdominis, and you will now notice that the right side retreats and is sucked back into the abdomen, while only the left side protrudes. This is called *Vama Nauli,* i.e. *Nauli* on the left side. Hold it for the length of your *kumbhaka* and keep pushing the left side of your rectus out, bearing down on your left knee only. Now relax your throat, inhale gently and come up to standing.

Now reverse left for right and perform the exercise on the right. First perform external *kumbhaka* with *Madhyama Nauli.* Then relax the rectus on the left and continue to push out the rectus on the right by leaning into the right arm, pressing down on the right knee. Again, hold it for the duration of the external *kumbhaka.* Once accustomed to the exercise, take your time to isolate the two sides of the muscle by repeating the exercise once or twice. You may now discontinue *Nauli* stage 2 *Madhyama,* as you always enter *Vama* and *Dakshina Nauli* through *Madhyama.* In the early stages what is important is not how many repetitions you can do but the intensity and precision of your isolation.

NAULI STAGE 4, ROLLING, FULL VERSION

Stage 4 is the *Nauli* proper. Once it is learned, stages 2 and 3, which are for didactic purposes only, are to be discontinued. However, stage 1 is to be continued.

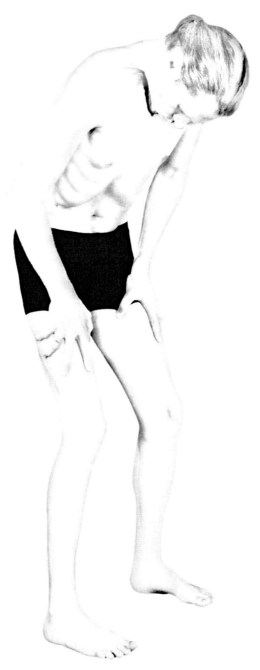

Nauli stage 2, Dakshina

Bending forward, perform external *kumbhaka* with *Bahya* (external) *Uddiyana*. Now push out the rectus abdominis in the middle, performing *Madhyama Nauli*. Next, take the pressure off the right arm and perform *Vama Nauli*, pushing out the rectus on the left. After you have clearly isolated the rectus on the left, take the weight off both arms, relax the rectus completely and suck the abdominal contents back into the thoracic cavity performing full *Bahya* (external) *Uddiyana*. Hold this for a second and then press down on the right arm and push out the rectus on the right (*Dakshina Nauli*). This is the first time that you access *Dakshina Nauli* straight from external *Uddiyana* and not from *Madhyama Nauli*. It may take a few rounds to get used to that. Then go on from *Dakshina Nauli* to *Madhyama Nauli*, which constitutes one churning. Take a breath and then repeat the exercise in the same order: *Bahya Uddiyana, Madhyama, Vama, Uddiyana, Dakshina* and *Madhyama*. What is essential is that you keep properly isolating each position and not concerning yourself with how fast you can do it.

Now repeat the exercise in reverse order. First perform *Bahya* (external) *Uddiyana*, then push out through the middle (*Madhyama*), from here go over to the right (*Dakshina*), suck back in with *Bahya Uddiyana* and go over to the left (*Vama*) and back to the middle (*Madhyama*). Come up, take a few breaths and then do a second *kumbhaka*, again churning to the right. Repeat this daily for a while, if necessary for a few weeks, until you have full control of all stages.

Once you can isolate all the positions, start to perform two churnings in one *kumbhaka*. This means that you hold each of the four positions for less time and have less time to isolate each one. For this purpose we are running the churnings into each other rather than starting each round anew. The order to the left is: *Kumbhaka, Bahya Uddiyana*, push out *Madhyama*, then *Vama*, then back to *Bahya Uddiyana*, then *Dakshina*, then *Madhyama*, from here straight over to *Vama* and back to *Uddiyana*, out on the right, *Dakshina*, back into the middle, *Madhyama*. Then take a few breaths and take another *kumbhaka's* worth of rolling to the left, performing as many churnings as you are comfortable with without losing the precision of the isolation.

Then do two *kumbhakas'* worth of rolling to the right, the order being *Kumbhaka, Bahya Uddiyana, Madhyama, Dakshina, Bahya Uddiyana, Vama, Madhyama, Dakshina, Bahya Uddiyana,* etc. As you slowly get more proficient and faster with the exercise, you will notice a wave-like motion going across your abdomen. However, make sure that you do not achieve this effect by losing precision.

After some time you may increase the number of *kumbhakas* to three in each direction. As you get more proficient you will be able to do more churnings per *kumbhaka*. Together with the three *kumbhakas* of stage 1, this makes a total of nine external *kumbhakas*. Do not go beyond this point without the supervision of a teacher. Even with a teacher, do not go beyond 5 rounds each (total 15 external *kumbhakas*) without making the lifestyle changes suggested above.

You will find that *Nauli* greatly improves your general health and digestion. It will also improve your grasp on *Bahya Uddiyana* and external *kumbhaka,* and will have a very beneficial impact on other aspects of your *asana* and *pranayama* practice.

Kapalabhati

For the *pranayama* practitioner, *Kapalabhati* (meaning 'shining skull') is the most important *kriya*. It should be mastered before any *pranayama* is commenced (unless it is very, very basic *pranayama*) and it should preclude any immediate individual *pranayama* session (unless the practitioner is very advanced). The majority of yogic scriptures treat *Kapalabhati* as a *kriya,* but some treat is as a *pranayama* technique itself. As a rule of thumb, if the *Kapalabhati* is taught without breath retention, then it is a *kriya,* and if it is performed with *kumbhaka* then it falls into the *pranayama* category.

DISAMBIGUATION OF KAPALABHATI FROM BHASTRIKA
Some yogic traditions do not clearly differentiate *Kapalabhati* from *Bhastrika*. Some call *Bhastrika* a *Kapalabhati,* with an active inhalation or *Kapalabhati* a milder form of *Bhastrika*. Some other schools define

Bhastrika as *Kapalabhati* with *kumbhaka*. However, the majority of yogic schools treat *Kapalabhati* (in Shyam Sunder Goswami's words) as abdominal short-quick breathing[412] and *Bhastrika* as thoracic short-quick breathing.[413] Following this school of thought, the present text describes the two exercises as two completely different methods. The disambiguation between *Bhastrika* and *Kapalabhati* and the views of the various schools are discussed in more detail in the chapter on *Bhastrika*.

THE BENEFITS OF KAPALABHATI

The *Hatha Yoga Pradipika* states that *Kapalabhati* dries up all the disorders stemming from excess of phlegm (*kapha*), which cause obesity, and through that drying-up leads to easy success in *pranayama*.[414] We also learn that it arrests the approach of old age and awakens the *chakra*s, reduces abdominal fat, massages, rebalances, purifies and awakens the brain, improves the functioning of the abdominal organs, cleanses lungs, improves respiratory functioning and may also be helpful for emphysema and asthma sufferers – if practised at times other than during an attack. It is also good for bronchitis and tuberculosis. *Kapalabhati* enriches the blood with oxygen and eliminates CO_2, thus making the blood alkaline. Apart from that it is thought to be helpful in curing obesity, acidity, flatulence, constipation, diabetes, blood sugar imbalance and depression. According to Swami Ramdev, 30 minutes of *Kapalabhati* per day practised over 2 sessions of 15 minutes is helpful in treating cancer.[415] He also considers it helpful for removing and avoiding blockages in blood vessels,[416] and curing prostate problems, stating that it is more helpful than all *asana*s combined.[417] For this purpose it should be practised vigorously so that all tissues vibrate. As the brain pulsates with the respiratory

412. Shyam Sunder Goswami, *Laya Yoga*, Inner Traditions, Rochester, 1999, p. 323
413. Shyam Sunder Goswami, *Laya Yoga*, Inner Traditions, Rochester, 1999, p. 307
414. *Hatha Yoga Pradipika* II.35–36
415. Swami Ramdev, *Pranayama*, Divya Yog Mandir Trust, Hardwar, 2007, p. 36
416. Swami Ramdev, *Pranayama Rahasya*, Divya Yog Mandir Trust, Hardwar, 2009, p. 49
417. Swami Ramdev, *Pranayama Rahasya*, Divya Yog Mandir Trust, Hardwar, 2009, p. 91

rate, *Kapalabhati* makes the brain vibrate at a very high frequency, purifying it. When practised for very long periods, *Kapalabhati* can lead to *Kevala Kumbhaka*. Swami Kuvalayananda explained that the increasing oxygen levels in the blood during *Kapalabhati* result in decreasing stimulation of the brain's respiratory centre.[418] The respiratory centre then does not initiate the next breath, which leads to the yogi being able to stay in *kumbhaka*. Additionally *Kapalabhati*, if practised properly low down in the abdomen, greatly improves *Mula Bandha*, which is very important for the *pranayama* practitioner. A veritable treasure chest is *Kapalabhati*, which is why all yogis should practise it.

WHEN TO PRACTISE KAPALABHATI

As with all *pranayama* techniques and most *kriya*s, one needs to wait at least four hours after a meal to practise *Kapalabhati*, which is why early in the morning is the best time. It cannot be practised late at night as it charges with energy, and sleeping afterwards may be impossible. It is generally advisable to practise *Kapalabhati* before any other *pranayama* techniques, as it is an ideal preparation for all *pranayama*s. *Kapalabhati* is to be mastered before *Bhastrika* is attempted. *Kapalabhati* purifies the lungs by removing congestion. It also opens up the alveoli through the rapid breathing and pumps up the organism with *prana* and oxygen. Additionally, it awakens the mind and refreshes the body. For these reasons it should always be practised between one's *asana* and *pranayama* practices, particularly when fatigued from *asana*. *Pranayama* cannot be practised when tired or when the mind is torpid (tamasic) – or frantic (rajasic) for that matter.

CONTRAINDICATIONS

Kapalabhati should not be practised during menstruation, but alternate nostril breathing without *kumbhaka* and *Mula Bandha* may be continued at that time. It also should not be done with high

418. *Yoga Mimamsa* IV.2

190

blood pressure, uterus or retina problems or nosebleed. Additionally it must be avoided in cases of heart disease, pneumonia, bronchitis, hernia and pregnancy, and when encountering dizziness. With an aggravated *pitta* condition, do not practise *Kapalabhati* for more than 2 minutes. Similarly, in summer its practice should be reduced. The reasoning behind this restriction will become apparent when looking at the similarity between *Kapalabhati* and *Nauli* stage 1. *Kapalabhati* is nothing but a *Nauli* stage 1 without *kumbhaka*. Through its vigorous flapping of the abdominal wall, it will, like *Nauli* stage 1, fan *agni* (digestive fire). That is why the safety precautions that apply to *Nauli* also apply here.

Practitioners commonly start coughing during *Kapalabhati*. Cough and then continue the practice. This is a normal way of releasing *kapha*. *Kapalabhati* may also bring on bronchospasms in asthmatics. In this case the practice should be discontinued and taken up in a gentler form on the next day, as it is very beneficial for asthma. Asthmatics need to practise more slowly, less vigorously and for shorter periods. By slowly increasing the intensity of the practice over a longer time frame, great improvement can be achieved.

TECHNIQUE

Practise *Kapalabhati* seated in a yogic meditation posture, ideally *Padmasana* or *Siddhasana*. For spiritual purposes the practice is done intensely for a long period to make all tissues pulsate. For such dynamic practice, *Padmasana* is a must. In *Kapalabhati* you will only move the abdomen, but the thorax is not kept relaxed but lifted by engaging the intercostal muscles, which produce inhalation. The thorax is then kept in a position as if completing the inhalation, meaning it is raised.

In a normal breathing cycle the inhalation is active and the exhalation is passive. *Kapalabhati* reverses this order. Here we make the exhalation active by forcefully driving the abdominal wall in against the spine. This action is performed by suddenly, forcefully contracting the abdominal muscles to drive the air out. It is essential to keep the shoulders and head steady. The shoulders should not bob up and down nor should the head move from side to side or backwards and forwards. Focus on each individual stroke of the abdominal muscles and make each stroke as vigorous as possible. For this purpose, in the early stages avoid speeding up. Speeding up leads to fast, shallow, superficial strokes, which have little effect. It is important to do the exercise slowly and methodically.

After you have expelled the air, inhale completely passively. When relaxing the abdominal muscles, the vacuum in the lungs will automatically suck in the air. The breath volume is increased by the fact that the thorax is kept lifted in the inhalation position. This will lead to the passive inhalation being three to four times as long as the active exhalation. It is this ratio that is defining for *Kapalabhati*. Whereas normal breathing has a ratio of approximately 1:2, with the exhalation almost double the length of the inhalation, during *Kapalabhati* the inhalation is up to four times as long as the exhalation; that is the ratio is 4:1.

The most common mistake made by novices is that they make the inhalation active too, and thus too fast. Apart from keeping the thorax lifted, you must completely relax after each vigorous abdominal stroke.

ADDITIONAL POINTS TO CONSIDER

Swami Kuvalayananda suggests visualizing the abdominal strokes hitting against the centre of Kundalini in the abdomen.[419] This action spiritually activates the nervous system.[420] The exercise cannot be performed properly without focusing on the lower abdomen, where the force of the strokes is the greatest. If one does not focus on the lower abdomen, one is likely to include the diaphragm, thorax or shoulders into the exercise. Make sure that you do not expel the air by using the diaphragm. The diaphragm must be kept relaxed. If in doubt, perform the exercise in front of a mirror. The ribcage should be frozen and not move. Movement should come from the abdominal

419. The original location of Kundalini is the *Svadhishthana* (own abode) *Chakra* in the abdomen, prior to it falling down to *Muladhara Chakra*.
420. *Yoga Mimamsa* IV.2

wall only. Movement of the lower ribs indicates activity of the diaphragm, which is another common mistake beginners make.

Kapalabhati tends to bring on *Mula Bandha* automatically. If *Mula Bandha* does not come on, you may be focusing too high in the abdomen. The brunt of the abdominal strokes and the mental focus need to be halfway down between navel and pubic bone. In other words *Kapalabhati* is a form of dynamic inhalation-*Uddiyana Bandha*.[421] Since the abdominal muscles, the domain of *Uddiyana Bandha*, and the pelvic muscles, the domain of *Mula Bandha*, are closely related, a strong, dynamic *Uddiyana Bandha* (i.e. *Kapalabhati*) will stimulate *Mula Bandha* into activity. Additionally, the vacuum that is created at the end of the active strokes not only sucks air passively into the lungs but also lifts the pelvic diaphragm, again stimulating *Mula Bandha*.

Keeping the thorax raised may lead to greater friction and pull on the bronchi. This may result in bronchospasm and coughing. If this is a constant problem for you, then you can reduce the inclination to cough by bending the head forward slightly. This can be taken as far as placing the head in the *Jalandhara Bandha* position (without contracting the throat) as suggested in *Yoga Rahasya*.[422]

STROKES PER MINUTE

Apart from using the diaphragm instead of the lower abdominals, the main common mistakes made in *Kapalabhati* are commencing the practice with too many strokes per minute and not keeping head and shoulders still. Another mistake is to make the inhalation fast and active, too, instead of slow and passive. You need to isolate each inhalation completely from each exhalation, as their nature is entirely different.

A standard breath (meaning a breathing cycle consisting of one inhalation and one exhalation) in *Kapalabhati* takes approximately 1 second with 1-fifth of that for the exhalation and 4-fifths of a second

421. This does not apply to the passive *Bahya Uddiyana*, which accompanies external *kumbhaka*. See more in the chapter on *Uddiyana Bandha*.
422. *Yoga Rahasya* I.101

for the passive inhalation. However, for a beginner it will be difficult to maintain vigour and force of the active exhalation and at the same time prevent this from spilling over into the inhalation. I recommend that a beginner practise as slowly as is necessary to maintain the salient features of this breathing method. This could mean that the technique is started with as few as 30 to 40 breaths per minute. This can increase significantly in advanced practitioners. In advanced *Kapalabhati* a yogi may raise the respiratory rate up to 120 strokes per minute. This is a very advanced form of practice, as at that speed it is difficult to maintain the different natures of inhalation and exhalation. For the beginner it is important to maintain the integrity, vigor and amplitude of each individual stroke rather increase their frequency.

NUMBER OF STROKES PER ROUND AND TOTAL NUMBER OF STROKES
Initially you will notice that you tire quickly. You may be able to perform only 15 to 20 strokes per round. Take a few normal breaths and then do a second round with an equal number of strokes. Over weeks of daily practice, slowly build this up to 60 and eventually over months and years to up to 120 per round. If you increase the frequency quickly you need to have breaks between rounds. If you increase the frequency more slowly you will be able to perform hundreds of strokes in one round without any breaks. This is beneficial when wanting to achieve meditative states. Swami Satyananda is known to have performed 5000 strokes of *Kapalabhati* in one stretch,[423] albeit at a low frequency.[424]

KUMBHAKA
Some teachers include *kumbhaka*s in *Kapalabhati* and some define *Kapalabhati* with *kumbhaka* as *Bhastrika*. You will find an exhaustive discussion of this subject in the chapter on *Bhastrika*. I recommend

423. Swami Niranjanananda, *Prana and Pranayama*, Yoga Publications Trust, Munger, 2009, p. 341
424. Swami Niranjanananda, *Prana and Pranayama*, Yoga Publications Trust, Munger, 2009, p. 273

using *Kapalabhati* as a *kriya* that is without *kumbhaka*. I suggest using it as a preparation for *Nadi Shodhana*. *Nadi Shodhana* is the most important *pranayama* technique, and you will find that you improve in it quickly if you perform several minutes of *Kapalabhati* right after your *asana* practice and right before *Nadi Shodhana*. This way you can use *Kapalabhati* to elongate your *kumbhaka*s in *Nadi Shodhana*.

KAPALABHATI AND HEAT

Kapalabhati is a heating technique. It increases *agni* and its vitiated form, *pitta*. If you practise *Kapalabhati* intensely in summer or in hot countries you may find that you aggravate *pitta*, which increases bodily heat, produces burning sensations and increases acidity. It can also decrease the quality of your sleep. In summer you may therefore have to decrease *Kapalabhati*, especially if you perform a second session in the afternoon. It is important to purify *agni* slowly rather than crank up its vitiated form, *pitta*. The purification of *agni* and the *nadi*s is the subject of almost all yogic techniques, such as *asana*, *kriya*, *pranayama*, *yama* and *niyama*, *mitahara* and *Ishvara pranidhana*.

You can also alleviate the symptoms of heat either by drinking milk after practice or by performing the cooling *pranayama*s, *Chandra Bhedana*, *Shitali* and *Sitkari*, which are described later.

Neti

There are two types of *Neti* – *Jala Neti*, in which water is used, and *Sutra Neti*, which utilizes a thread, traditionally dipped into beeswax.

SUTRA NETI

Sutra Neti is the one that is usually referred to in scriptures. According to the *Hatha Yoga Pradipika*, *Neti* consists of feeding a thread in through a nostril and out through the mouth.

Such a procedure is thought to purify the brain, remove disorders of the eyes and most other disorders of the cranial and cervical

425. *Hatha Yoga Pradipika* II.29–30

region,[425] and improve eyesight.[426] *Sutra Neti* is also believed to purify and open the *Ajna Chakra*, a fact that is stated both in the *Hatha Ratnavali*[427] and the *Hatha Yoga Manjari*.[428] M.L. Gharote informs us that the practice of *Neti* leads to a statistical improvement in cases of asthma.[429] A great advantage of *Sutra Neti* is that it also makes the membranes of the nose more resistant through the friction that it generates.

TECHNIQUE

When using a thread, make sure to start with the open nostril, i.e. the one through which the *svara* currently flows. Insert the thread into the open nostril, close the other nostril and then suck the thread through into the mouth by vigorously inhaling through the open nostril. More commonly used today than threads are rubber catheters or strings that are purposely made for *Neti* and obtainable through yoga suppliers. It is helpful to lubricate the string with ghee and feed it through the open nostril slowly. Once it reaches the back of the tongue, pull it out with two fingers and move it back and forth gently by pulling on both sides alternately. Once completed, repeat the procedure on the other nostril. Subjectively I have the impression that over time it enlarges the nasal passages or at least prevents them from swelling up. During *pranayama* the breath then becomes less audible and also less discernible when checked with a mirror placed at a certain distance. Some, but not all, schools use these methods to determine success in *pranayama*. The idea here is to reduce the distance to which breath and *prana* are projected out of the body.

JALA NETI

The second variety of *Neti* is *Jala Neti* and, while it is not lauded in yogic texts as much, it is far easier to perform and it has become increasingly important for yogis who practise *pranayama* in air-

426. *Hatha Ratnavali by Shrinivasayogi* I.42
427. *Hatha Ratnavali by Shrinivasayogi* I.64
428. *Hatha Yoga Manjari of Sahajananda* II.39
429. Dr M.L. Gharote, *Yogic Techniques*, Lonavla Yoga Institute, Lonavla, 2006, p. 66

polluted cities. The inside of the nose is speckled with thousands of minute hairs, which are directed outward against the incoming air. They are designed to comb pollutants and foreign bodies out of the air. The pollutants are then transported by the mucous membranes into the body and absorbed by the lymph system. The lymph system neutralizes them as much as possible, and they are then passed on to the blood circulation, eliminated via the liver and kidneys and then excreted. A much better method would be to let as few as possible of these toxins and chemicals enter the bloodstream, liver and kidneys. The workload of the body in relation to respiratory toxins and pollutants is then lightened significantly.

For this purpose the mucus membranes of the nose are rinsed and washed daily with a saline solution. This washes the toxins out of the body rather than letting them enter it. It is an important form of hygiene when living in an industrial city. *Jala Neti* also distinctly eases the workload on the heart when practising *pranayama*, as it tends to keep the nostrils obstruction free even if to a lesser degree than *Sutra Neti*. It is very frustrating when one tries to learn *pranayama* but is constantly confronted with blocked nostrils. This can be completely alleviated through *Jala Neti*. Additionally, it cures sinusitis and helps with other respiratory disorders such as the common cold and bacterial infections of the upper respiratory tract.

In regard to using water, please note that, although you do not swallow the water used for *Neti*, it is nevertheless entering a bodily orifice and will come in contact with mucous membranes. The water that you use needs to be of drinkable quality. In many communities tap water has become toxic through industrial pollution. The authorities often try to counteract that by adding certain compounds that are not fit for human consumption either. In many areas you will need to use either filtered water or bottled water.

TECHNIQUE
The easiest method is to use a purpose-made *Neti* pot, which can be obtained through yoga suppliers and local pharmacies. Fill it with

filtered water of body temperature. The water should not be cold or hot, otherwise the exercise becomes uncomfortable. Place approximately half a teaspoon of salt into the water, depending on the size of the pot, and dissolve it. The saline solution should be strong enough to purify the nose but not so strong as to provide an uncomfortable, stinging sensation, which would aggravate the mucus membranes. Now simply insert the spout of the *Neti* pot into one nostril, tilt the head to the side and gravity feed the water in through the top nostril and out of the bottom nostril. Don't tilt the head back, otherwise the water will enter your mouth. Then reverse the procedure for the other nostril. Finally, blow your nose several times vigorously to remove excess water. Do so with your head facing down and also out to each side to make sure that you remove all water from your sinuses.

The sensation of rinsing the nose with water is not unpleasant if the temperature of the water and the salinity are right. If you do not have a *Neti* pot you can also use a bowl or even your cupped hand. However, for this method you have to create suction, which requires a bit more skill. Lower your head and insert the lower nostril into the water. Close the upper nostril with your thumb. Suck the water into the nose and once your nose is full tilt your head over to the other side to let it run out. Repeat the process several times and then change sides. If you suck in too much water you can always let it run out of your mouth. Always keep your head bent forward and do not create too much suction, as otherwise you may end up with water in your trachea. I suggest doing *Jala Neti* daily until the problem of blocked nostrils is cured.

Techniques

LIBERATING THE BREATHING PATTERN THROUGH BREATH WAVES

If you go without preparation straight into applying traditional *pranayama* methods, you will take all breathing impediments that you have accumulated through past thoughts and actions into your *pranayama* practice, where they will manifest as obstacles. If obstacles are present, it will manifest in your *pranayama* practice as being uncomfortable: impatient, fidgety on the one hand or dull, lethargic and incapable of accessing spiritual states on the other. Both states are due to the presence of the *rajas* and *tamas gunas* respectively in your conditioning and mindset. Although you may iron all of that out by using traditional *pranayama* techniques, you will progress more quickly if you first work with some of the following methods. Their purpose is to re-initiate a natural breathing pattern that is often intercepted by mental activity.

Ideally, when practising *pranayama* we experience and apply something that I like to call the oceanic breath. The oceanic breath moves like a wave of *prana* through your entire organism and reaches every cell of your body. In the process, it absorbs your entire awareness and draws it away from thoughts and emotions of past and future. The inability to apply the oceanic breath spontaneously or, better, to hand yourself over to it and surrender, is determined by the density of your conditioning. Practically speaking this means that emotions and thoughts of fear, guilt, shame, pain, anger, etc. and their associated memories form energy blockages in your body, which prevent you from breathing into certain areas. This reduces or even prevents the ecstatic experience that breathing could be, and numbs us to the extent that experiencing spiritual states appears inaccessible. It may also manifest as experiencing states such as boredom, confusion or depression, which are unlikely during oceanic or complete yogic breathing. By liberating the breathing pattern beforehand, i.e. becoming able to breathe into every cell of the body, *pranayama* can become a deeply satisfying and revelatory experience from early on.

To liberate the breathing pattern fast and effectively and to experience the oceanic breath I suggest working with a set of exercises that I call breath waves. These breath waves will establish resonance frequencies in your body, which will break down energetic blockages that prevent you from breathing totally and feeling alive.

Reclining waves

The first set of these exercises requires you to lie down on your back. For some students it is easier to experience the breath when bending up the legs and placing the knees together. Lie on a soft surface such as a carpet or blanket for comfort. Now place one hand, say your left one, on your belly. After having exhaled, breathe exclusively into your belly so that your left hand is lifted up to the ceiling. For some people who are used to exclusive thoracic breathing this is difficult to achieve but it is extremely important that you persist until you have the experience that you can in fact breathe exclusively into your belly or, better said, distribute all of your breath into this area.

Exclusive chest breathing is related to holding on to pent-up emotions. The most effective way of dealing with emotions that surface during breathing is simply to acknowledge them for what they are, breathe them out and then let go of them. Emotions, especially the powerful ones like pain, fear, shame and guilt, tend to get bigger and more powerful when we don't look them straight in the eye. They grow bigger and bigger when we turn our back on them, and eventually they become so big that we get the feeling they may devour us, which is true in a metaphorical sense. Prefiguring a notion that gained currency only in the 20th century, the ancient *Bhagavad Gita* said that repression does not work and that we need to act according to our nature.[430]

430 *Bhagavad Gita* III.33

Instead of repressing negative charges like emotions and denying them, we need to turn around and look straight at them. Once acknowledged as a denied part of us, they will shrink to life size. It is usually the fear of the fear that is most fearful, and not the primary fear itself. Deep-seated emotions may need to be released and acknowledged before you go further in *pranayama*, and *asana* practice can be very helpful in that regard.

It is important to remember, when dealing with both emotions and thoughts, that you are not the emotion. You are the witness to the emotion. It cannot touch you as long as you don't identify with it. Just as a movie image cannot stick to the screen on which it appears, a thought or emotion cannot stick to the awareness to which it arises. Dis-identify with all mental images that occur during the breathing process and simply return to the breath. Releasing an emotion is different to acting it out. If you react to an emotion by acting it out you will increase its grip on you.

RECLINING TWO-STAGE UP-AND-DOWN BREATH WAVE
Place your right hand in the middle of your ribcage and draw the next inhalation exclusively into this area so that only your ribcage expands and your belly is completely static. When activating the ribcage and integrating it into the breathing cycle, make sure you let the breath rise only as far as the uppermost rib and not beyond. Ancient yogic texts warn of letting the *prana* rise into your head. Of course you cannot let actual air enter into your head, but, when you breathe too high up, the intracranial pressure rises, due to too much blood rushing into the brain. You would then get light-headed, but, more seriously, the oscillation of intracranial pressure is also detrimental to the blood vessels in your brain. Keep the air and pressure down in your chest and don't let it rise. Later on, in *kumbhaka*, we will use *Jalandhara Bandha* to prevent this, but if you find it difficult at this early point to isolate the chest from the head during inhaling, then simply do not breathe so high up into the upper lobes of your lungs.

202

Once you have inhaled, make sure that you exhale as consciously from this area as you inhaled, and expel all the air that is accessible to you. Similarly, as some are exclusive chest-breathers others are exclusive belly-breathers and, although this gets less attention in the media, it is as much as an impediment as exclusive chest breathing. It makes the ribcage rigid and the heart and lungs torpid. It also enlarges and weakens the abdominal organs and makes one addicted and a slave to one's emotions, which are stored in the abdomen. If you are incapable of fully using your ribcage in the breathing cycle, you are severely limiting your vitality.

For those not used to integrating the ribcage into their breathing, take some time to experience breathing into every area of your ribcage such as the back, where it touches the floor, the sides, the front and the clavicular area. Continue to breathe until you have the experience that you can fill every cubic centimetre of your ribcage with air and then empty it out as consciously as you filled it.

Once you have come to this state, place your right hand on your ribcage at the height of your heart and your left hand on your navel. Now distribute the first half of your inhalation into your belly so that your left hand rises. Then distribute the second half of your inhalation into your ribcage so that the right hand is lifted up towards the ceiling. Try to isolate both phases as clearly as possible.

On the first half of the exhalation, deflate only the ribcage so that only your right hand drops. With the second half of your exhalation, drop now your left hand by deflating the belly. With some practice you will learn which sets of muscles to use to achieve both of these ends. Keep breathing in this way, inhaling into the belly first and then inhaling into the chest. Then exhale from the chest first, and only then from the belly. Continue until you feel as if a two-stage wave travels upwards from the pelvis to the shoulders and then back down, reaching each area of your torso. Not only will this exercise help you to isolate the ribcage and belly from each other and access them individually, but by exhaling from the chest first you will prepare for an important *pranayama* technique called *Bhastrika*.

RECLINING TWO-STAGE DOUBLE-UP BREATH WAVE

This second exercise is identical to the first in regard to inhalation. Inhale into the belly first and with the second half of the inhalation fill the ribcage. However, with regard to the exhalation, this breath wave is the opposite. Because it takes more muscular effort to keep the ribcage fully inflated, the normal tendency is to exhale from the ribcage first. However, here we use our abdominal muscles to empty the belly first while keeping the ribcage inflated. Only once this is completed is the ribcage allowed to drop. Take some time to experience the difference of this exercise from the previous one by first letting your left hand on the belly drop and only then lower the hand on your heart. In order to do so you need to use a technique that was described earlier, called exhalation *Uddiyana Bandha*. This means that during the exhalation you contract the entire transverse abdominis muscle and draw it back against the spine. This way you can exhale from the belly yet keep the ribcage inflated.

This powerful breathing method should only be used when the body is static, such as lying down or sitting. When moving in and out of *asanas* a toned-down version of this technique, called inhalation-*Uddiyana Bandha*, must be used. During inhalation-*Uddiyana Bandha* only the lower part of the transverse abdominis, the part below the navel, is utilized.

Continue this exercise until you experience inhalation as a wave travelling up from the pelvis to the shoulders; as you exhale, in contrast to the previous exercise a second wave travels upwards from the pelvis to the shoulders, powered by the contraction of the abdominal muscles. This exercise forms the basis of another important breathing exercise called *Kapalabhati*, which is described under *kriyas*.

RECLINING THREE-STAGE UP-AND-DOWN WAVE

In this exercise we will divide the torso into three areas. The first extends from the pubic bone and pelvic floor up to the lower ribs. While lying on the floor, use your hands to feel the lowest ribs on the side of your torso. Feel how much further down the ribcage reaches here on the side and back than in the front of the chest. The lowest floating ribs form the lower boundary of the second area I propose we should breathe into. Now touch the lowest tip of the sternum (xiphoid process) on the anterior surface of your ribcage. This forms the upper boundary of this second or middle area, which is dissected by the diaphragm. The diaphragm is the large dome-shaped respiratory muscle that separates the thoracic from the abdominal cavity. It attaches to this point in the front and, since it slopes from here down to the lowest floating rib in the back, this middle area strictly speaking consists of thorax in the back and abdomen in the front.

The third and highest area consists solely of ribcage, extending from the lower tip of the sternum up to the collarbones. Strictly speaking it extends even higher than the collarbones, since the first and second rib and tips of the lungs reach up above the collarbones.

Lying on your back, place your left hand on the lower area of your belly. Keep in mind that the lower area this time is smaller than in the two-stage wave, which only isolated abdomen and thorax. Now let the distribution of breath into the lowest third of your torso lift your left hand up towards the ceiling and, exhaling, let it drop down towards the floor. Repeat this a few times until you have isolated this area clearly. Keeping your left hand in place, now position your right hand on the previously described middle area, consisting partially of thorax and partially of abdomen. Distribute the first half of your inhalation into the lower third of the torso, lifting the left hand, and only then the second part of the inhalation into the middle part, elevating your right hand. Exhaling, let the right hand drop first and only then the left hand, meaning you exhale from the middle area first, then from the lower part of the torso. Take a few breaths in this fashion until you have clearly isolated the two areas.

With that established, remove your left hand from your belly and place it on your upper thorax, between your heart and your jugular notch. Now distribute the first third of your inhalation into your lower belly, where your left hand was previously situated, then use the second third of your inhalation to fill the middle third of your trunk. When you have completed that, direct the final third of your inhalation into the upper third of your torso. Make sure that your breath reaches and ventilates the upper lobes of your lungs, which are often neglected, but do so without straining. Never fill your lungs to the extent that they feel like bursting. The feeling of bursting alerts you to the fact that the fragile septi, the separating walls between your alveoli, experience great strain. If you ignore this warning, you may end up actually bursting some of them, which may lead in the long run to emphysema.

When exhaling, empty first the area that you breathed into last, the uppermost third of your torso. To achieve this, focus on dropping your left hand down towards the floor. Once you have expelled the first third of air, exhale the second third now from the middle area of your trunk, dropping the right hand. Finally exhale the last third of breath from your belly. Continue this pattern until you have the experience of a wave travelling from your pubic bone to the jugular notch upon inhalation and back down upon exhalation. With some practice you will be able to create a resonance frequency by linking each breath wave up with the next one, thus enhancing its force or amplitude. Be aware what this does to your spine. You will feel a wave-like motion moving the vertebrae of your spine. It is very therapeutic to let this wave travel up and down your spine while reclining.

You will also be able to find energy blockages in your spine, i.e. fixated vertebrae etc. These areas are the ones where you will not be able to feel your breath moving your spine. Ideally you would feel the wave moving each vertebra individually. This takes time and practice, but it will make your spine more fluid and healthy. This three-stage reclining up-and-down wave is ideal for experiencing the oceanic breath and deep relaxation. Visualize a wave washing up onto the beach upon inhalation and back down into the sea upon exhalation.

206

You will feel now how, powered by the breath, a wave is going up and down the front of your torso. Feel how this influences your mind. It makes one serene and at the same time creates a detached observer within. Once you have established the wave, now work on equalizing wavelength and intensity. Wavelength refers to the time each breath takes and intensity refers to the amount of air inhaled and exhaled. Do this in as unobtrusive a fashion as possibly. Rather than ordering from above a 'correct' time, let each wave naturally take the shape of the previous one.

Once you have achieved this you will notice that a resonance frequency has established itself. And when you have made the shape and the length of the each breath wave equal, they link into each other and enhance each other. This is by itself a meditative experience, but the important thing to notice is its influence on the spine. The waves, previously felt at the front of the torso, move now to the spine, and you can feel them pulsating up and down this structure, previously imagined as rigid. This sensation helps with creating openness in the central energy channel (*sushumna*). It is also therapeutic for the functioning of the central nervous system, i.e. spinal cord and brain. The pulsating of the spine with the breath enhances the supply of cerebrospinal fluid to the brain and makes it literally pulsate with each breath.[431]

RECLINING THREE-STAGE DOUBLE-UP WAVE

This fourth exercise is an extension of the previous breath wave. Make sure you have become proficient in the reclining three-stage up-and-down wave before you tackle this exercise. The inhalation proceeds in exactly the same way as before: distribute a third of your inhalation into the belly, a third into the middle and the last third into the upper chest. With the exhalation, however, rather than let the wave wash back down from the jugular notch to the pubic bone, let the exhalation wave also begin at the pubic bone and travel upwards.

431. The brain does this to a certain extent in a healthy person, but this technique, like some other *pranayama* techniques, enhances the function.

This may sound counterintuitive, but it is this form of breathing that we will eventually utilize in slow-breathing pranayama techniques such as *Nadi Shodhana*, and *Surya* and *Chandra Bhedana*. The double-up wave will drive *prana* up the spine during exhalation. This is particularly important once you are integrating longer *kumbhaka*s into your practice. It is the upward movement during the exhalation that will then keep you on track.

The way to initiate the double up-wave is to engage the lower part of your transverse abdominis to drive the air out of the lower third of your torso. Then use your upper abdominals to expel the air from the middle part of your torso. And finally exhale from the upper part of the torso.

Continue this exercise until you have the feeling of one wave after another flowing from the base of your trunk up towards your collarbones. The appropriate visual image here is more akin to looking out on the ocean from far up and seeing one wave after another nearing the shore. Another interesting visual image in this context is to look at a snail from below as it travels across a pane of glass. You will see successive wave-like motions travelling across the lower surface of the snail in the same direction.

This wave will make more sense to you when you practise it upright, against the force of gravitation, as it will become obvious then that it counteracts gravitational force; but it is very helpful to imprint it already here in the reclining position.

RECLINING SIX-STAGE UP-AND-DOWN WAVE
Once you have imprinted the two forms of the reclining three-stage wave you can upgrade to the six-stage wave simply by subdividing into two parts each area of the torso that you learned to breathe into. We have then a lower abdominal area, an upper abdominal area, a lower mid-trunk area, an upper mid-trunk area, a lower thoracic area and an upper thoracic area. On the inhalation, let the waves travel from the pelvic floor to the jugular notch through these six distinctly separate areas. Upon exhalation let it travel back down

slowly from area to area, exhaling from the upper chest first and the lower belly last.

The great advantage of this is that you can slow down the wave, become more conscious which areas it touches, and increase its amplitude and thus its effect on the tissue it travels through, and also abandon yourself more to the oceanic character of the experience. By subdividing the wave more, the likelihood of experiencing its resonance frequency increases. Feel how the *prana* wave touches and heals every cell in your torso and every organ. If you have difficulty feeling this, use your imagination. Where *vrtti* (thought) goes, there goes *prana*. If you think that the wave touches and heals every organ it will tend to do so. If you identify any dead, dark and numb areas in your body, consciously direct breath into these areas, as they are the ones where you most need it.

Also here make sure that you do not let *prana* rise into the head, where it would lead to increased intracranial pressure. This wave is extremely useful for recharging with *prana* and it is very helpful for relaxation. It is beneficial to make this a regular exercise during *Shavasana* (corpse posture) at the end of your *asana* and *pranayama* practice.

RECLINING SIX-STAGE DOUBLE-UP WAVE

This wave starts again exactly like the previous one, but during the exhalation the direction is reversed. Exhalation commences in the lower abdomen and travels from there up the spine. Feel how this wave takes more effort but it also energizes. The main purpose of this wave is to imprint it here so that it is at your disposal once we move into the vertical plane and work against gravitation. Six-stage waves form the bedrock of meditation techniques, but more about that later.

The purpose of the reclining breath waves is to abandon yourself into the process of breathing without having to struggle against gravity. Continue to experiment with these waves until you have the experience that you are being moved by a powerful wave of breath and that this wave literally rolls through every cell of your body and breathes it. Once you are satisfied with this step, switch to the upright waves. They are initially more difficult to feel, as the imprinted holding patterns of your muscles will try to hold you in a way that does not require feeling the aliveness of the breath. However, once those waves are imprinted they are more powerful in carrying life force and breath up the spine to the brain.

Seated waves

After having learned to compartmentalize the torso and breathe into its various sections, we will now venture into the vertical plane. When lying down due to the impact of gravity on the supine body, the main thing we needed to learn was to breathe upwards to lift our hand up to the ceiling. It is different when sitting upright: the impact of gravitation is such that it supports us in distributing breath into the back, sides and front of the torso evenly; however, we need to become aware of this process. Apart from that, when sitting upright we need to make a more conscious effort to drive the air all the way up into the upper chest, as gravitation will limit breathing to the lower abdomen in individuals with a slouchy physique. The seated waves will make us experience the inner form of the various *pranayama* techniques.

UPRIGHT TWO-STAGE UP-AND-DOWN WAVE
As mentioned before, the two-stage up-and-down wave is the native breath wave for *Bhastrika*, thoracic bellowing. *Bhastrika* is an advanced high-volume, rapid-breathing *pranayama* that I describe extensively later in this text. It is important to learn this breath wave slowly and, after integrating it into *Bhastrika*, increase the speed only gradually. The reasons why many practitioners don't succeed in *Bhastrika* are that they do not study its native breath wave and they increase the speed (frequency) too quickly.

Sit upright in your preferred meditation posture with knees on the floor, palms and soles of the feet facing up and spine, head and neck in one straight line. As in the reclining two-stage wave, we will isolate the entire thorax from the complete abdomen. Take the first half of the inhalation into the abdomen. You need to keep the lower abdominal wall active (inhalation-*Uddiyana Bandha*) as otherwise all air will disappear into the abdomen and you will find it impossible to distribute any into the chest. Now draw the second half of the inhalation into the chest, expanding it into the front, back and sides and upwards. Make sure that you include the upper lobes of the lungs in the inhalation. When exhaling, let the chest drop first and, only when it is fully deflated, engage exhalation-*Uddiyana Bandha* to empty the abdomen completely. You will notice that this will happen quite automatically, as gravitation applied to the thorax will deflate it as if by itself. Using this wave you are able to take large-volume breaths very quickly; hence it is ideal for *Bhastrika*.

UPRIGHT TWO-STAGE DOUBLE-UP-WAVE
This wave is more counterintuitive than the previous one. As previously, sitting in your preferred meditation *asana*, distribute the first half of your inhalation into the belly and then the second half into the chest. Again, you will need to apply inhalation-*Uddiyana Bandha* to achieve this.

Once you have completed the inhalation, engage the entire abdominal wall (exhalation-*Uddiyana Bandha*) to drive all air out. Repeat this breath wave until you are established in it and can feel the difference to the previous one. Since we again isolate only two areas of the torso, this wave, like the previous one, can be used for rapid breathing. However, you will notice two important differences: Since we exhale from the abdomen first, the controlled abdominal wall will prevent the ribcage from dropping when we subsequently exhale from it. That means the exhalation is not as complete as in the previous wave, reducing the volume somewhat. Secondly, since we consciously exhale from the belly first, the life force in this wave is lifted, driven up, which makes the mind less tamasic (torpid) at the end of the exhalation. Double-up waves make you more alert than the up-and-down waves. This two-stage double-up wave forms the foundation for *Kapalabhati*, abdominal bellowing. Before practising *Kapalabhati*, however, study its description closely, as the breath wave is modified further for its purpose. In *Kapalabhati* we use mainly the lower abdomen (and not the entire abdominal wall) for exhalation. Additionally, the exhalation is fast and active whereas the inhalation is slow and passive.

UPRIGHT THREE-STAGE UP-AND-DOWN WAVE

Now we are ready to transfer the three-stage up-and-down wave into the vertical plane. Sit in your favourite meditation *asana*. Compartmentalize the torso in exactly the same way as during its reclining equivalent. Engaging inhalation-*Uddiyana Bandha*, fill first the lower abdomen with air. Then distribute the second half of your breath into the mid-torso. Finally draw the third part of your inhalation into the upper chest. Feel the amount of inhalation-*Uddiyana Bandha* needed to get the breath all the way up to the clavicles. Feel the benefit of liberating and ventilating the upper lobes of the lungs, which most individuals neglect for most of their lives.

For the exhalation we use the order that gravitation and *apana vayu* (vital down current) dictates to us. This means that we exhale first from the upper chest, then from the mid-torso and finally from the abdomen. During the inhalation this wave extends the torso and therefore lifts the head. During the exhalation this wave flexes the torso and thus moves your head forward and down. This wave therefore has the tendency to move you like a Bedouin on a camel, if you let it happen. This is the breath wave for the introductory deep breathing that can be used at the beginning and end of each *pranayama* session. It can also be used for relaxation and short meditations. If you use it for longer than a few minutes, it tends to make the mind too tamasic at the end of the exhalation. The exhalation is ruled by *apana vayu*, and this 'natural' wave tends to move our awareness up on the inhalation and down on the exhalation. It is therefore not suitable for higher yogic work such as serious *pranayama* and meditation. We are relying on turning *apana vayu* up to use it as one of the engines of Kundalini-raising, and that is exactly what the next wave is designed to do.

UPRIGHT THREE-STAGE DOUBLE-UP WAVE

We will now transfer the three-stage double-up wave into the vertical plane. Sit in your favourite meditation *asana*. As with the previous wave, engage inhalation-*Uddiyana Bandha* to fill first the lower abdomen, then the mid-torso and finally the upper chest. For the exhalation we go counter to the law of gravitation by driving *apana vayu* up. This means that we exhale first from the lower abdomen. Feel the amount of *Uddiyana Bandha* that is needed. Then exhale from the mid-torso and finally from the upper chest. In the beginning put some awareness towards the need to not overwork your diaphragm. The diaphragm has to work more in this method, as we are exhaling against gravity.

The three-stage double-up wave is good for energizing and learning to distribute breath. Do an experiment. Gently direct your attention towards *Bhrumadhya* (third eye). When exhaling upwards through using this wave, you will notice that *prana* is naturally flowing upwards towards the third eye. While the previous three-stage up-and-down wave surrenders to *apana vayu*, the three-stage double-up wave utilizes *apana gati*, the inner upward movement contained in the usually down-flowing exhalation. This is important for attaining and sustaining states during *pranayama* and meditation. By moving *prana* up, this wave tends to prevent the mind from becoming tamasic at the end of the exhalation. This three-stage double-up wave is the native breath wave for all slow-breathing *pranayama* techniques such as *Nadi Shodhana*, *Surya* and *Chandra Bhedana*, and Shitali.

SIX-FOLD WAVE UP-AND-DOWN WAVE

This wave forms the basic configuration for *chakra* breathing and purifying, with each wave top representing one of the six *chakra*s. Since the sixth *chakra* is located in the head, a safety precaution has to be built in so that the intracranial pressure does not rise. To achieve this we do not breathe through the entire torso but only through *sushumna*, which is a very thin stalk or hollow going through the spine. This sounds more difficult than it is. Since *prana* goes where *vrtti* goes, you only need to permanently focus on *sushumna* to achieve this.

SIX-FOLD DOUBLE-UP WAVE

This is the native breath wave for Kundalini-raising. One focuses on the *chakra*s during inhalation and exhalation but, instead of letting the *apana* move down, one raises it during the exhalation by focusing on the *chakra*s in an upward sequence, as is naturally done during the inhalation.

Six-stage meditation waves grow naturally out of the three-stage waves as meditation naturally grows out of *pranayama* and *pranayama* out of *asana*. These complex waves have many ancillary aspects such as *mantra*, *chakra*, *bandha* and *mudra*, which are beyond the scope of this book. I hope to be able to describe them in a later publication.

COMPLETE YOGIC
BREATHING CYCLE

IMPORTANCE OF COMPLETE BREATHING

The basic *pranayama* exercise on which all following techniques are based is the complete yogic breathing cycle. Rather than exclusive thoracic breathing or exclusive abdominal breathing, the complete yogic breathing cycle ventilates all areas of the torso. This enables us to breathe deeply, expel maximum amounts of carbon dioxide and toxins, take in maximum amounts of oxygen and distribute *prana* evenly throughout the entire organism. It also helps us to get rid of blockages that otherwise would impinge on our vitality. During the complete yogic breathing cycle we will utilize breath waves that, like a resonance frequency, pulsate up and down the spine and torso. Ideally it engulfs every cell of the body and makes it vibrate with vitality.

Once again, yogic breathing is different to exclusive abdominal breathing. Exclusive abdominal breathing weakens your abdominal muscles, which are important stabilizers of the spine. It also makes your abdominal organs distend, your belly protrude and your thorax become rigid; worst of all, it makes your mind tamasic (inert, dull, heavy). Of course it is the path of least resistance, as the abdominal wall offers less resistance to expansion than the thorax. But to exclude the thorax from the pulsating movement of the breath has a lot of detrimental results. It weakens the heart, the lungs and the abdominal organs, and also fixates the upper thoracic and cervical vertebrae, hence making neck, shoulder and wrist problems more likely.

Exclusive abdominal breathing has attracted a lot of positive attention. The reason for this is that it was heralded as a solution to the scourge of exclusive thoracic breathing (chest breathing). Exclusive chest breathing is of course very detrimental, as it makes the mind rajasic. Chest breathing is often done with the purpose of not feeling or accessing bottled-up emotions, which are stored in the abdomen. By not breathing into the abdomen, these emotions are not felt. Chest breathing triggers the sympathetic nervous system and gives one the feeling of being wired, much as if one had imbibed coffee.

Exclusive abdominal breathing, on the other hand, triggers a parasympathetic reflex and makes one relaxed. It may be useful in moments when only relaxation is wished for and nothing else. However, during *pranayama* and meditation it is not helpful, as it makes the mind too tamasic – dull and torpid. It keeps the *prana* low down in the abdomen, whereas the yogi seeks to transport *prana* up to the higher energy centres (*chakra*s). While it may be helpful at times to de-stress with exclusive abdominal breathing, it does not confer the energy and brightness of intellect that is necessary to perform spiritual work such as *pranayama* and meditation. The human being is a bridge from the animal to the Divine.

Bridges needs a certain level of inherent tension to span a chasm; otherwise they collapse. Many tasks in our life demand a certain amount of creative tension and a balance between the sympathetic and parasympathetic nervous systems, which exclusive abdominal breathing cannot provide. Integrated thoracico-diaphragmatic breathing delivers this balance. Additionally, it also leads us beyond the dichotomy of tamasic abdominal breathing and rajasic chest breathing, and makes the mind sattvic by creating a balance. For this purpose, however, the entire torso needs to participate in the breathing process. During the breathing cycle we will first become proficient in *rechaka* (exhalation), then *puraka* (inhalation), only after which *kumbhaka* (retention) is tackled. It is important that you experience and integrate all of the various exercises relating to inhalation and exhalation before thinking about *kumbhaka*.

COMPLETE YOGIC EXHALATION
We will start our exploration of the complete breathing cycle with the exhalation. When trying to breathe more deeply, students often try to inhale more, but the start of deep breathing is simply exhaling

216

completely. The yogic term for exhalation is *rechaka*, but *rechaka* doesn't just mean exhaling: it means exhaling completely. Any left-over used air that remains in the lungs without being exhaled decreases the emission rate of your CO_2 and other gaseous waste matter, and also decreases the potential for the next inhalation and thus rate of oxygen and *prana* intake. The first thing that we need to learn about yogic exhaling is that all air possible needs to be exhaled. For this to occur, the development of a powerful exhalation-*Uddiyana Bandha* is required. This means that the entire abdominal wall, and particularly the entirety of the transverse abdominis muscle, is used to drive out the air (remember to use this form of exhalation only when the body is static in a meditation *asana* and not during *vinyasa* practice).

Engaging the entire abdominal wall, gently but determinedly pull it back towards the navel. In an established practitioner this may feel as if the abdominal muscles touch the front of the spine. The advantage of exhaling in this fashion is that you remain very upright whereas, if your exhalation consisted mainly of deflating the thorax, your posture would become more stooped with an accompanying downward flow of life force.

Students sometimes ask how one can exhale from the abdomen first. Imagine for a moment that you hold in your hands a soft plastic water bottle full of water with its lid removed. Now place your hands around the upper half of the bottle and squeeze. Of course you will notice that water is being squeezed out. Now place your hands around the lower half of the bottle and squeeze again. You notice wherever you squeeze water will come out. The torso works in a similar fashion during exhalation. When I recommend exhaling from the abdomen first, I merely want to convey that the muscular effort, the act that drives air out, is initiated in the abdomen and not in the chest.

While there is comparatively little that can be done wrong during the inhalation (apart from inhaling too deeply and causing alveoli to burst, which could lead in the long term to emphysema) and during the *kumbhaka* phase (apart from not holding the *bandha*s properly or retaining the breath too long), it is the exhalation that clearly shows the level of proficiency or mastery in *pranayama*. For example Raghuvira, in his *Kumbhaka Paddhati*, says that by mastering *rechaka* (exhalation) one masters all aspects of *prana*.[432]

Once great proficiency in the art of exhalation is gained, it is used to distribute *prana* to the required areas – *prana* that has been taken in during the inhalation and absorbed during *kumbhaka*. The exhalation needs to be smooth and even, without acceleration in the beginning or end and subsequent gasping for air, because only then the fixation of *prana* will be effective. If we hold *kumbhaka* too long and then have to exhale fast and gasp for air, that round of *pranayama* is wasted and in fact has contributed to a depletion of *prana*. Hold *kumbhaka* only to such an extent that the subsequent exhalation can still be performed smoothly.

Exhalation needs always to take place through the nose and never through the mouth, as otherwise *prana* will be lost. To extend the exhalation reduces *rajas* (frenzy) in the mind, which is why exhaling for double the length of the inhalation will create relaxation. On the other hand extending the exhalation for too long can make the mind tamasic. Exhaling for double the length of the inhalation may be helpful for somebody who suffers from anxiety but counterproductive for someone suffering from depression. For this reason breathing with the proper prescribed ratios is important. A qualified teacher is required to recommend ratios suitable for the individual.

The exhalation also should not be extended by force but only within the capabilities of the individual practitioner on that particular day. According to M.L. Gharote, exhalations that are drawn out too much can lead to heart problems.[433] This cannot happen, however, if the yogi uses common sense and progresses slowly and methodically. As with most human endeavours, in *pranayama* the application of brute force rarely pays off.

432. *Kumbhaka Paddhati of Raghuvira* stanza 73
433. Dr M.L. Gharote, *Yogic Techniques*, Lonavla Yoga Institute, Lonavla, 2006, p. 110

COMPLETE YOGIC INHALATION

Puraka means complete yogic inhalation. By definition this is only possible if a complete yogic exhalation precedes the inhalation. If the exhalation leaves a litre or two of stagnant air in the lungs, the subsequent inhalation can never be complete. That is why many traditional *pranayama* teachers say that each *pranayama* technique must start with a complete exhalation.

Let's undertake an experiment here. After exhaling completely, relax your abdominal wall. Let any muscle tension dissipate out of it. Now breathe in. If the abdominal wall is completely relaxed you will find that (a) the belly begins to protrude like a large watermelon and (b) however hard you try, you cannot get any breath whatsoever into the ribcage. When you then exhale, you will also notice that the volume of the abdominal inhalation was surprisingly small. You can only take in a large volume when you fully inflate your thorax. Due to the fluids and organs that are already contained in the abdominal cavity, an abdominal inhalation cannot accommodate a large breath volume. Now begin your next inhalation with the firm purpose in mind to take in the largest amount of air. As you do so place your fingers against your lower abdomen and see what happens. In an attempt to fully inflate the relatively rigid thorax, the lower abdominal wall automatically contracts. After your thorax has fully inflated, note the large volume during your subsequent exhalation.

The conclusion of this experiment is that the controlled and engaged lower abdominal wall is the engine that powers a full, yogic inhalation. As stated above, I call this engine 'inhalation-*Uddiyana Bandha*' to differentiate it from other forms of *Uddiyana Bandha*, and it is this form that can also be used during movement such as a *vinyasa* practice. Keep clearly in mind the different forms of *Uddiyana Bandha* that we use in the complete yogic breathing cycle for exhalation and inhalation. During the exhalation the entire abdominal wall is used to drive the abdominal contents in against the spine, which will help in driving all air out of the lungs. How different from the inhalation: Here only the lower part of the transverse abdominis is used, so that the diaphragm may descend freely to create space for the inrushing air.

A note: It is detrimental to contract the upper part of the transverse abdominis during inhalation. Since the upper transverse abdominis interdigitates with the diaphragm, you will then tighten and harden it and prevent it from moving freely with a concomitant loss of vitality and vital capacity (Interestingly enough, western medicine calls the maximum amount of air inhaled after a maximum exhalation your vital capacity.)

To inhale completely you need to keep the lower abdominal wall firm but above the navel stay relaxed. For this purpose you need to isolate the lower half of the transverse abdominis muscle from the upper half. The transverse abdominis is the innermost (fourth) layer of the abdominal muscles, and its function is to draw the abdominal contents back against the spine. Practice will develop this ability, and it is helpful to check frequently with your fingers or visually whether you remain soft above the navel. If you do remain soft there, then the belly will protrude slightly above the navel but not below. This restriction below the navel will enable you to draw the second half of your inhalation into the lower part of the chest, which will now expand. Notice how this training also increases the strength of your lower abdominal muscles.

When inhaling, let the inhalation commence all the way down at the pubic bone and fill your entire torso with air, similarly to filling a pitcher with water. The idea is that water will automatically fill all volume available and not leave empty spaces. Similarly, imagine drinking air slowly and it penetrating all the remote areas of your torso, which you would never usually think about. Attempt to time your inhalation so that when your lungs are completely filled your visual image is that the water level has just submerged your collar-bones or has gone slightly higher. Never let air or its related pressure get any higher than the throat and enter your head.

How much air to inhale? The maximum amount that the average adult can inhale after a complete exhalation is said to be 4.8 litres in males and 3.1 litres in females. The average amount of air inhaled or exhaled per breath, the so-called tidal volume, is said to be 0.5 litres in both sexes. This means that theoretically we could increase the volume by 6 to 9 times for a deep inhalation. Practically speaking the situation in *pranayama* is much different, as we will not just make a few attempts to reach the maximum but repeat it over and over again and eventually also add *kumbhaka*. Of course we then need to be much more cautious and slowly increase the amount of air that we inhale. In other words, when inhaling during *pranayama* we never go to our absolute limit. In the beginning we may inhale close to 80% of our vital capacity and slowly over months let this grow to 90% and possibly eventually to 95% in an advanced practitioner, but hardly more. Of course you don't need to resort to a spirometer to measure these volumes; you can simply gauge it by the amount that you could inhale on top of what you have already inhaled if you had to. Once you have some practice with *pranayama* you can measure this simply by the amount of time you could continue to inhale relative to the time you have inhaled already. During *pranayama* we train ourselves to have a steady volume of inhalation and exhalation relative to time unit. This corresponds to a steady flow of *vrtti* (thought pattern).

As you continue to practise, you will exercise your lung tissue, make it more resistant and notably open alveoli in the upper lungs, which are full of mucus because you hardly ever use them. This process must be undertaken slowly. The lungs are more akin to joints and ligaments rather than muscles in the regard that they adapt to exercise rather slowly. Never inhale to the extent that you feel your lungs will burst, because if your mind conjures up this visual image that's what your alveoli are probably just doing. Inhalations that are too deep may cause lung damage. Even the wording 'filled to the brim' indicates that you probably have gone a bit too far. Take 10% off 'filled to the brim' and you will be okay.

Interestingly enough, if for a moment in your mind's eye you visualize yourself 'brimming' from your inhalation, the image indicates that if we inhale too much the mind will get rajasic (frantic). This is exactly what yogic tradition says. You could never imagine yourself 'brimming' from an exhalation. Correspondingly, yogic tradition says that excessive exhalation makes one tamasic (torpid). You have now acquired a yogic tool for self-medication. If you feel you are too torpid and need more energy, increase the length of the inhalation. If you feel that your mind is running amok and isn't giving you rest, then increase the length of the exhalation.

COMPLETE YOGIC BREATHING CYCLE

The complete yogic breathing cycle is the basic technique of *pranayama*. It consists of a complete exhalation combined with a complete inhalation or, according to some authorities, vice versa. A *pranayama* session consists of ongoing sequences of such breathing cycles. During the exhalation, all air available is exhaled purposefully but without force. During the inhalation the entire torso is filled from the bottom up like a pitcher being filled by water poured into it.

The cycle is the framework into which the breath wave required for the particular *pranayama* / meditation technique is placed. If the purpose of your breathing cycle is relaxation, use the three-stage up-and-down wave. Generally speaking, during rapid breathing *pranayamas* like *Kapalabhati* and *Bhastrika*, the complete yogic breathing cycle is combined with a two-stage wave, as rapid breathing makes it too difficult to isolate more than two areas of the torso. During slow-breathing *pranayamas* like *Nadi Shodhana* and *Surya Bhedana*, the three-stage double-up wave is utilized. Here we have more time to distribute our attention to more areas and make sure that all tissue gets ventilated. During extremely slow *pranayamas* like *Bhutashuddhi Pranayama* and *Shakti Chalana Pranayama*, and during meditation, six-stage waves are combined with the complete yogic breathing cycle.

During all of these waves the inhalation always follows the same format: it starts at the pelvic floor and ends at the base of the neck. Depending on the purpose of the technique, the phase of the practice session (i.e. beginning, middle or end) and the experience of the practitioner, the exhalation runs either downwards (up-and-down wave) or upwards (double-up wave).

UJJAYI

Jaya means victory. *Ujjayi* means victorious or conquering. It is so called because the technique allows us to become victorious in *pranayama*. *Pranayama* means extension or stretching of *prana*, and this is exactly what *Ujjayi* does. To stretch or extend the breath and *prana* we need to create some form of constriction to the breath to make its distribution into the various targeted areas easier. Constriction of breath can for example be created by closing one nostril, and if the other one should be flowing at that time (i.e. the *svara* goes through this nostril), then even by half-closing that open nostril. This way enough friction is created to stretch (*ayama*) the breath (*prana*) long. In some other techniques you may create constriction by inhaling through the rolled and protruding tongue (*Shitali*) or by opening the lips but keeping the teeth closed and inhaling through the crevices between the teeth and the tongue (*Sitkari*).

If one inhales through both nostrils, the technique used is *Ujjayi*, the victorious breath. In *Ujjayi* the epiglottis, the lid on the throat that prevents water or food from entering the bronchi when swallowing, is partially closed. This produces a gentle hissing or whispering sound. You can use this sound to distribute the breath and *prana* to whichever area in your body you want.

The sound is quite similar to that of a wave washing up on the shore and then washing back down again. Make sure that the sound is even, calming and gentle. If you strain, you will trigger the sympathetic nervous system and the method will not achieve its aim. The easiest way to get the idea of *Ujjayi* is to whisper and then close your mouth while you continue to whisper. When whispering we use the half-closed or 70% closed epiglottis to produce a sound that doesn't travel far, but during whispering the mouth is open so that we can form words. It is important that the vocal cords are not engaged, so that there is no humming component to the sound.

224

Close now your mouth but keep producing this whispering sound, with the effect that you now produce *Ujjayi*. The reason why we whisper is that the breath proclaims the great secret. But it will only work its magic if you do keep it secret. The *Ujjayi* sound should be audible mainly to you or, in a quiet room, to the people right next to you. If the sound is too loud you will strain, thereby activating the sympathetic nervous system, and fail in slowing down the heartbeat and lowering blood pressure, which are important components of *pranayama*.

Now, what is the secret that requires whispering? During *Ujjayi* we try to make the inhalation even with the exhalation and we try to make the sounds as similar as possible. But note that, even after all your efforts, each has its own distinct character. The inhalation has a more sibilant character, while the exhalation sounds more aspirate. The secret that the breath whispers consists of the sibilant *sah* on the inhalation and the aspirate *aham* on the exhalation. If we combine these two Sanskrit terms (using a set of tools called *sandhi*, i.e. junction), we arrive at *soham*, the great *mantra* of *prana / prakrti*. *Soham* is one of the so-called *mahavakya*s (great words) of the *Upanishads*. It means 'I am that'. It is by means of this *mantra* that prana breathes and enlivens us throughout our whole life from our first to our last breath. 'I am that' means that deep down we are not what we think we are. It means that we are not the so-called phenomenal self, that is the self that is caught up with phenomena such as body and mind. Instead, we are 'that'. 'That' is the pure awareness to which all the phenomena arise. It is that which still remains after body and mind have passed away. It is the immutable, infinite and eternal consciousness, the true self.

Ujjayi is the constant pronunciation of a *mantra* that proclaims we are not that which changes and decays but that which is permanent, immutable, infinite and immortal – pure awareness.

IMPORTANCE OF ASHTANGA VINYASA YOGIS GOING BEYOND UJJAYI

Although this book is addressed to all practitioners of yoga, not just to practitioners of Ashtanga Vinyasa Yoga, I will have to address them separately here. My two previous books described the Primary and Intermediate Series of *asana*s of Ashtanga Vinyasa Yoga. As an Ashtanga Vinyasa practitioner I need to understand that *pranayama* practice is not exhausted nor is it completed by applying the *Ujjayi* breath during my *asana* practice. In fact this is only the tip of the iceberg. *Ujjayi* is a very potent practice, and its inclusion in *asana* practice, like the inclusion of the *pratyahara* and *dharana* techniques of *drishti* and listening to the breath, not only makes *asana* practice far more effective but also turns it into a preparation exercise for *pranayama* and meditation. *Ujjayi* certainly helps one to learn to direct the breath, to stretch it long and distribute it evenly into all areas of the body. However, *Ujjayi* breathing is only *pranayama* in a preparatory sense. Many of the earlier definitions of *pranayama* will have made it clear that most *shastra*s define *pranayama* as a formal sitting practice involving a variety of counted *kumbhaka*s. Similarly, as *drishti* and focusing the mind on the breath during asana are not a replacement but preparation for formal sitting yogic meditation practice, so is *Ujjayi* during one's *asana* practice not a replacement for formal sitting *kumbhaka* practice but preparation for it. *Ujjayi* without *kumbhaka* cannot by itself bring about the balance of Ida and Pingala, which is obtained through *Nadi Shodhana pranayama*, nor can it bring about the complete cessation of fluctuations of *prana*, which is obtained through extensive breath retentions (*kumbhaka*).

Drishti and *Ujjayi* are introductions and preparations of higher yogic techniques so that, when the time comes for taking up a sitting practice, we are firmly established in the fundamentals of *pranayama* and meditation. When practising *Ujjayi* properly, that is gently, smoothly and free of ambition, the Ashtanga Vinyasa practitioner will have a good head start into *pranayama* and will quickly progress in essential techniques like alternate nostril breathing and *kumbhaka*.

SLOW DOWN BREATH

Sitting in your favourite meditation posture, extend the breath using the *Ujjayi* technique. You will find that *Ujjayi* is a vital tool in slowing down the breath. Apply the complete yogic breathing cycle, expelling all air on the exhalations and breathing in the maximum amount of air available without straining. Initially we use a 1:1 ratio, which means that we make the exhalations exactly as long as the inhalations. Since the inhaling represents *rajas* (frenzy) and the exhalation *tamas* (torpor), giving them both the same length provides energy and a dynamic balance. We will use the three-fold up-and-down wave for the first few breaths in our breathing session to arrive at and relax in the present moment before we switch to the wave that is native for each *pranayama* technique.

Upon inhalation you will find that producing the *Ujjayi* sound will make it easier to distribute the air in the lower, then the medium and finally the upper third of the trunk, and to exhale in the opposite order. Once established in this breathing method, we switch now to the three-fold up-and-down wave, which is native to *Ujjayi*. (This does not refer to *vinyasa* practice but only to formal, seated *pranayama* practice.) This means that we start the exhalation just above the pubic bone and let it ripple up like a wave towards the collarbones. Take a few rounds to establish this wave and feel how much it empowers your concentration and your ability to focus your mind on noble, spiritual ends. But this wave is of course work. The up-and-down wave is relaxing but in the end tends to leave Kundalini at the base of the spine. The mind is then just happy to eat, drink and be merry.

Once driving breath and *prana* up with the double-up wave has become a natural process, start counting your breaths. The easiest way to do this is to have either a clock or a metronome ticking in the background. Do not look at the clock but keep your eyes closed or fix them on a sacred image. Right from the outset we want to get accustomed to having the visual sense as a meditation aid rather than using it to look at a clock. Similarly, when you hear the clock or metronome ticking, please do not count in your mind but use your fingers for digital counting as previously described. This way you can pronounce a *mantra* instead of a number in your mind. You will find that your intellect will develop faster and more powerfully and your spiritual growth will accelerate much more than when using your mind to count numbers. It usually takes only 2 or 3 sessions to adapt to the novelty of digital counting, i.e. counting on the digits of your hand.

If for example you counted on your first inhalation to four, then make sure that on the exhalation you count to four as well. Every time you touch a digit with your thumb instead of saying in your mind '1', '2' etc., say 'OM, OM'. OM will be our default *mantra* if no other is specified. OM gave rise to the terms 'omnipotent', 'omnipresent' and 'omniscient' and also to the Hebrew *Amen* and Arabic *Amin*. In other words OM is a universal term symbolizing the Supreme Being.

While chanting your *mantra* once every second, determine the length of each breath. Let us suppose you start with 4 seconds/*matras* for both inhalation and exhalation. Once comfortable at this level, on the next day choose to extend your breath to 5 seconds/*matras* for each inhalation and exhalation. However, do this without any ambition. Never strain and never force yourself. For some people, extending the breath is easier than for others. Accept however long it takes for you.

Once you are comfortable with 5 *matras*, go to 6, 7 and so forth. Sometimes you will have to stay at a particular count for a few days or weeks; sometimes you can move on more quickly. You will probably find that it is quite easy to extend your count to 10 or even 15; then it becomes slower. With practice over weeks you can make each inhalation and exhalation longer than 20 and eventually 25 seconds. It is important to practise each day for the same amount of time and ideally also at the same time. If you notice any detrimental signs, back off and stay at your level until you can continue to progress. As you slow down your breath, you will notice more and more how your mind slows down and meditation is naturally induced.

The long-term goal is to slow down the breath to one respiratory cycle per minute or less; that is, assuming a 1:1 ratio, one takes 30 seconds for the inhalation and 30 seconds for the exhalation. At this point concentration develops powerfully. Apart from slowing down your mind, breathing as slowly as that will also make your mind sattvic, that is it will make it gravitate towards the sacred. For this reason it is also very beneficial to have a sacred object or image of the Divine in front of you during *pranayama*.

PRANAYAMA WITH SACRED IMAGE

The image must have meaning for you rather than for me. For this reason there is little point in my suggesting one for you. What is important is that the image harmonizes with your cultural background or your concept of the Divine. This is relatively straightforward for Hindus and Christians. For Muslims and Buddhists it requires some elaboration.

In Islam it is not permitted to make images of the Divine; it is considered idolatry. Some Sufi groups use the image of a heart with the word *Allah* in Arabic engraved on it. Alternatively you could use your favourite *Sura* or place a copy of the Holy Qu'ran in Arabic in front of you.

Buddhism is ambiguous in its relation to the Divine, and it inherited this stance from the system of thought that it originated from, the *Samkhya*. Similarly to *Samkhya*'s founder, Kapila, the Buddha also said that the Divine was outside the scope of the Buddhist teaching. Theravada Buddhists may therefore visualize the Buddha during *pranayama* or place his image before them. Mahayana Buddhists are advised to use an image of the Bodhisattva of their choice. Followers of the Vajrayana (Tibetan Buddhism) may use an image of the refuge tree, consisting of *Dharma* protectors *Lama*, *Dharma* and *Sangha*.

One of the suggestions repeated in many yogic texts in regard to *pranayama* is that it should be performed with a sattvic intellect, i.e. an intellect that gravitates towards the Divine/sacred. The easiest way to achieve this is to place your sacred image in front of you while you perform *pranayama*. If you then find your mind straying you just need to open your eyes to remind yourself of your purpose.

You may also practise *pranayama* with your eyes open and fixed on a particularly point on your Divine or sacred image. In yoga this technique is called external *Trataka*. Generally there is a rule that *pranayama* should be performed with eyes closed to avoid distraction. However to focus on the Divine is not a distraction. It is rather a higher form of focus than what happens for most people with eyes closed. You will also quickly come to a new form of communion with the form of the Divine that you meditate on (*ishtadevata*). For me this is the main reason why I practise *pranayama* daily. There may be many health benefits to *pranayama*. Stronger than those may be the advantages that it produces in developing mind and intellect. All of those are, however, overshadowed by the closeness to the Divine that ensues when one practises *Trataka* on the Divine, particularly during *kumbhaka*.

Slowing down the breath more and more, using a *mantra* such as *OM* to count your breath and meditating on the Divine while doing so, the many benefits of *pranayama* will soon become evident to you. Needless to say, if the use of *OM* does not harmonize with your faith then replace it with a sacred word that has meaning for you.

WHY SWITCH TO A 1:2 RATIO
As described earlier, the inhalation has a rajasic effect and the exhalation a tamasic effect. To clothe it in positive terms, when extending the exhalation relative to the inhalation, *rajas* in your mind will be reduced. This leads to relaxation, an activation of the parasympathetic nervous system. It also makes your mind calm, lowers your blood pressure and slows down the heartbeat. The last two facts in particular imply a reduced oxygen consumption by the body, which means that the 1:2 ratio is a preparation for *kumbhaka*. Generally we will introduce *kumbhaka* after the 1:2 ratio has been mastered. There are exceptions to this rule of course.

Since the exhalation reduces *rajas* (frenzy), it also has the tendency to increase *tamas* (torpidity). Hence, a 1:2 ratio should not be tackled if from the outset excess torpidity is already present in the student.

This would be the case if you feel very lethargic, dull, heavy, depressed or excessively introverted. If this is the case, stay on a 1:1 ratio for now and increase your practice of *Kapalabhati* and *Nauli*, which are described in the chapter on *kriya*. Once you have mastered those techniques, add *Bhastrika* (which strongly energizes) and *Surya Bhedana* (which extroverts), both of which are described later in this book.

WHEN TO SWITCH TO A 1:2 RATIO

If you practise *pranayama* unsupervised, I suggest that you continue the above method until you reach a count of 30 seconds for each inhalation and exhalation. That way you can be absolutely sure your organism is well prepared for everything to come. However, if you do practise with a teacher, she may suggest that you change your ratio earlier. Some teachers say that mastery of 1:1 is reached with a 20:20 count or a 24:24 count. None of these ratios was ever described in a fixed manner in the ancient yoga texts. Yogis never thought that rigidly fixing these ratios would bring success. What is important is that the ratios work for you. It is left to the teacher to make the right decision according to the individual circumstances of the student. It has not been thought that fixing these ratios is what makes the difference. Rather follow the general guidelines.

A similar fact holds for switching from one ratio to the other. There is no hard and fast rule as to how it is to be done. One method I learned in India was to keep your inhalation as it is while slowly extending the exhalation. Another method is to extend the exhalation while reducing the inhalation. Yet another approach is to reduce the length of the inhalation to half while maintaining the length of the exhalation. This may sound invasive at first, but it is the method with which I have had the best results, and so it is the one that I will describe here.

Suppose you have reached a comfortable count of 30:30 and want to switch to a 1:2 ratio. You do this simply by reducing the inhalation by half of the count, i.e. 15, and leaving the exhalation as it is. Your new count for the day is then 15:30. You will notice that this is very easy compared to your previous 30:30 ratio. From then on, increase the count according to the 1:2 ratio. On the next day you could increase to a 16:32 ratio and would possibly still find that easy going. If so, then increase the next day to 17:34 – you are likely to meet some resistance here. Once you find resistance such as running out of breath towards the end of the exhalation, stay at this count until you have completely adapted. If you have added on too quickly, you need of course to go back. Generally speaking you want to avoid that and increase your practice only once you are absolutely sure that you are ready for it. For most people it is more difficult to arrive at a 20:40 count than to practise a 30:30 count, although the total length for both is the same.

DURATION OF EACH PRACTICE SESSION
I recommend practising this method for no less than 10 minutes and a maximum of 30 minutes per day, but 20 minutes would probably be enough. I strongly suggest practising 2 to 6 minutes of *Kapalabhati* (depending on season and constitution) right before your *Ujjayi* breath-extension practice. The best time to fit it in is right after your *asana* practice, that is *asana*s first, then *Kapalabhati*, then *pranayama*. If you can't fit it in, then practise it at any other time, but before meals, not after. Once you have achieved a 20:40 count you are certainly ready to move on to the next technique, *Nadi Shuddhi*. However, your teacher may let you move on before that.

PURIFICATION OF NADIS

WHY PURIFICATION OF THE NADIS?

The *Hatha Yoga Pradipika* declares that control of *prana* is only possible once the impurities have been removed from the *nadis*.[434] It adds that directing *prana* into *sushumna* must similarly be preceded by purification of the *nadis*.[435] Additionally, the *Pradipika* ascribes to *nadi* purification success in yoga[436] and health.[437] The *Gheranda Samhita* declares that cleansing of the *nadis* must take place before *pranayama* proper,[438] because *prana* cannot flow through *nadis* clogged with dirt and so they would preclude the attainment of knowledge.[439]

Sage Vasishta agrees, stating that purification of the *nadis* needs to take place before *pranayama*.[440] He even goes as far as to say that practising the higher limbs of yoga, from *pranayama* onwards, is futile if the yogi doesn't purify the *nadis* beforehand,[441] and that this is particularly the case for meditation.[442]

The *Hatha Ratnavali* states that, once the *nadis* are purified through *pranayama*, *prana* easily enters *sushumna* and one goes beyond the mind.[443] The *Hatha Tatva Kaumudi* informs us that unless the *nadis* are purified higher yoga is not possible.[444] Sundaradeva assures us that, without purification of the *nadis*, long *kumbhakas* are not possible.[445] Shyam Sunder Goswami says that purification of the *nadis* brings *mantra* alive.[446] With clogged *nadis*, application of *mantra* and the

434. *Hatha Yoga Pradipika* II.5.
435. *Hatha Yoga Pradipika* II.41
436. *Hatha Yoga Pradipika* II.19
437. *Hatha Yoga Pradipika* II.20
438. *Gheranda Samhita* V.2 and V.33
439. *Gheranda Samhita* V.35
440. *Vasishta Samhita* I.81–82
441. *Vasishta Samhita* I.83
442. *Vasishta Samhita* B49 (page numbers are double in this book)
443. *Hatha Ratnavali of Shrinivasayogi* II.2–3
444. *Hatha Tatva Kaumudi of Sundaradeva* XXXVI.36
445. *Hatha Tatva Kaumudi of Sundaradeva* XI.18
446. Shyam Sunder Goswami, *Laya Yoga*, Inner Traditions, Rochester, 1999, p. 115

higher limbs is ineffective. The *Goraksha Shataka* affirms that the yogi becomes capable of controlling *prana* only once purification of the *nadis* has taken place.[447]

I want to complete this section by quoting once again from the *Hatha Tatva Kaumudi*, which says that whoever commences practice of *kumbhakas* without first purifying the *nadis* is an 'idiot'.[448] We should see a sense of humour in play here, but the message is nevertheless clear.

DISAMBIGUATION OF NADI SHUDDHI FROM NADI SHODHANA

Nadi purification can be translated into Sanskrit either by the term *Nadi Shuddhi* or by *Nadi Shodhana*. To my knowledge they are synonymous. However, the term *Nadi Shuddhi* is used by the Rishi Vasishta in his *Vasishta Samhita* to describe alternate nostril breathing without *kumbhaka*.[449] The term *Nadi Shodhana* has been used by the *siddha* Goraksha Natha in his *Goraksha Shataka* to describe his technique of alternate nostril breathing with *kumbhaka*. Apart from the presence or lack of *kumbhaka*, there are also other important differences between the techniques. It is obvious that Vasishta's technique is more fundamental and is to be learned before Goraksha Natha's method, which is more advanced. In order to make absolutely sure at any point to which method we are referring I will refer to one as Vasishta's *Nadi Shuddhi* and to the other as Goraksha's *Nadi Shodhana*. The *Shandilya Upanishad* declares that these two techniques, i.e. alternate nostril breathing without and then with internal *kumbhaka*, should be practised sequentially one after the other.[450] That is, practise the second method after the first is mastered.

The second series of *asanas* of Ashtanga Vinyasa Yoga, which I have previously described in my book *Ashtanga Yoga: The Intermediate Series*, is also known under the name *Nadi Shodhana*. All outer limbs

447. *Goraksha Shataka* stanza 101
448. *Hatha Tatva Kaumudi of Sundaradeva* XXXIV.5
449. The same method is also described by sage Yajnavalkya
in *Yoga Yajnavalkya* V.17–20
450. *Shandilya Upanishad* stanzas 16–18

(*bahirangas*) have as their aim more or less *nadi* purification. Generally speaking, gross purification takes place through *asana* and *kriya*, and subtle purification through the methods described in this book. For members of modern societies, with their pollution from chemical, electronic, electromagnetic, radioactive and other sources, it is strongly advised to use several types of *nadi* purification by combining *asana*, *kriya* and *pranayama*. Those who have followed the descriptions in my earlier books and practised *asana* will find that they progress in *pranayama* much faster than others who are relatively new to *asana*, or not adept in it, but they will benefit nevertheless. If you found many of the *asanas* described in my earlier books too difficult to master then you will benefit from this course even more. I recommend the course outlined in this book to all who want to progress swiftly with the practice of the higher limbs.

Vasishta's Nadi Shuddhi

BENEFITS

This technique removes *kapha* and impurities from the subtle energy channels (*nadis*). It also balances brain hemisphericity, the sympathetic and parasympathetic nervous systems, efferent and afferent nerve currents, anabolic and catabolic function, and lunar (relativistic) and solar (fundamentalist) mind. *Nadi Shuddhi* (without *kumbhaka*) is a good form of practice during pregnancy.

THE RISHI VASISHTA

I have named the technique after the Rishi Vasishta, as he promulgates it in his text *Vasishta Samhita*.[451] Although this is not the only scripture that teaches the technique, it possibly is the original one. *Nadi Shuddhi* also prominently features in the *Yoga Yajnavalkya*[452] and the *Darshana Upanishad*.[453] All of these texts are very important in regard to Vedic yoga.

451. *Vasishta Samhita* II.61–67
452. *Yoga Yajnavalkya* V.17–20
453. *Darshana Upanishad* V.5–10

Vasishta is the first of the *sapta rishis* (seven *rishis*) and he is a mind-born son of Lord Brahma. Vasishta was the court priest of King Dasharatha of *Ramayana* fame, but he was already ancient at that time. His most important treatise is the *Yoga Vasishta*, a 30,000-stanza dialogue in which he teaches the juvenile Prince Rama, the sixth Vishnu avatar, about the supreme reality. The *Puranas* (mythological texts) contain a vast number of passages referring to Vasishta. He is one of the Indian culture bearers.

OPENING THE NOSTRILS

When commencing alternate nostril breathing initially, many students find that one of their nostrils is quite blocked. The number one practice for overcoming this is *Jala Neti,* which is described in the chapter on *kriya.* Please practise *Neti* daily and you will find yourself rid of the problem within a relatively short time. During my childhood I had an accident in which my nose was completely smashed, after which my left nostril was almost permanently blocked. *Neti* got rid of the problem within 6 months. Notice that having blocked nostrils is a sign of imbalance, with its adverse health consequences. So please be tenacious in applying *Neti.*

You may also need to look into ways of changing the *svara* (nostril dominance) so that you can open the blocked nostril when commencing your practice session. Ways to change *svara* were introduced in the chapter 'Svara and Nadi Balance'.

SHANKA MUDRA

In order to open and close the respective nostrils we use a *hasta mudra* (hand seal) called *Shanka Mudra.*

Traditionally only the right hand is used for performing this *mudra.* The left hand in India is used for cleaning ones *derriere.* For this reason it is considered unclean and therefore not used while eating or touching one's face. Even touching others with one's left hand can be considered an insult. This may be the reason why this *mudra* is limited to the right hand. If you do have a shoulder imbalance

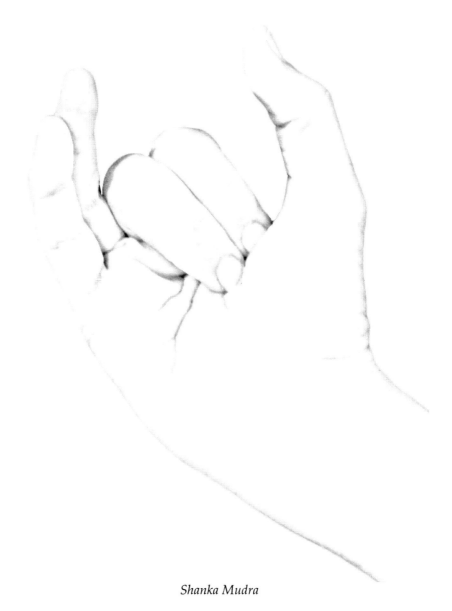

Shanka Mudra

caused by excess use of the right arm you may find it beneficial
to alternate.

Shanka Mudra is so called because in it the fingers form the shape
of a conch. The pointing and middle finger are folded and placed

on the mount of the thumb. The ring and little finger are placed together and are held opposite the thumb.

As already explained in *Ashtanga Yoga: Practice and Philosophy* the symbolism of the fingers is as follows:

Thumb	Brahman (infinite consciousness)
Pointing finger	atman (individual self)
Middle finger	buddhi (intellect)
Ring finger	manas (mind)
Little finger	kaya (body)

Shanka Mudra is used during an active purification process. The individual self and intellect are already in synchronicity with infinite consciousness and, in a gesture of obedience, are bowing to Brahman. The body and mind, however, need to be purified so that Brahman may be attained. Hence they are used here in interaction with the thumb, representing Brahman. Some schools teach an alternative version in which the first and second fingers are resting on the third eye.

When using *Shanka Mudra*, touch the nostril only to the extent that the nostril closes, not more. The septum should not be squeezed to the extent that it warps into one direction. The touch should be gentle. During alternate nostril breathing and when using *Shanka Mudra*, no *Ujjayi* sound is produced and the throat is kept completely unrestricted. Make sure that you keep spine and head upright. Do not turn the head to the left when your right thumb applies pressure to the right nostril. Also do not lift your right shoulder (assuming that you are using your right hand to manipulate your nostrils). Once in a while practise in front of a mirror (not too often, mirrors draw *prana* to the surface, the opposite of what you want to happen) or film yourself to ensure that head, shoulder and spine positions are correct. Additionally, see to it that both collarbones are on the same level and do not lift the collarbone on the right. Generally speaking, in the early days of *pranayama* it is easier to let the arm hang down so that your elbow touches the ribcage; otherwise you may tire quickly and build up tension. Later on, once you have adapted, you may lift the elbow further out to the side.

Obviously, as in all other *pranayamas*, we want to sit in a traditional meditation *asana*, which fulfils the following requirements:

- Head, neck and spine in a straight line
- Knees firmly on the floor and not hovering above it
- Both soles of the feet and palms of the hand turned upwards in a receptive position.

If in doubt please check the chapter on *asana*.

INHALE LEFT

Nadi Shuddhi and its more advanced cousin *Nadi Shodhana* always commence with an inhalation through the left nostril and finish with an exhalation through the same. This is a view that reverberates through all yoga *shastras* (scriptures). I will save you from tedious quotations of dozens of *shastras* and quote only one. The *Hatha Tatva Kaumudi* declares that the practitioner should always commence practice through Ida (the left nostril), because it produces *amrita* (nectar).[454] The same *shastra* also proclaims that *pranayama* is useless when commenced through the right nostril, as the right (*Surya*) creates heat and toxins.[455] I have earlier, in the chapter 'Svara and Nadi Balances', described the left nostril as nurturing and anabolic (building up tissue) whereas the right nostril is dissecting and catabolic (breaking down tissue). Naturally we need a balance between the two, but *Nadi Shuddhi* needs to start through the left to nurture the fledgling practitioner.

METHOD

As with all slow-breathing *pranayamas*, this one utilizes the three-stage double-up wave within the complete yogic breathing cycle. The *Vasishta Samhita* states that *Nadi Shuddhi* is alternate nostril

454. *Hatha Tatva Kaumudi of Sundaradeva* XLIV.47
455. *Hatha Tatva Kaumudi of Sundaradeva* XXXVII.4

breathing without *kumbhaka*.[456] As previously suggested, I recommend that you precede your *pranayama* firstly by your *asana* practice and secondly by a session of *Kapalabhati*. Since one of your nostrils will be more open than the other, I suggest that you reduce to half the count that you used lately in your *Ujjayi* breathing, described in the last chapter.

We will again start with a 1:1 ratio unless your teacher recommends otherwise. Generally speaking, as a safety precaution each new *pranayama* method is commenced in *sama* (even) *vrtti* mode. This means that all components have an equal length. Only then does one progress to *vishama* (uneven) *vrtti* mode, in which different lengths for the various components are used. This is only a general rule. The teacher can waive it if there are reasons for doing so. For example, say you have previously practised *Ujjayi* to a count of 30:30 or 20:40. Reducing this count to half means a new *Nadi Shuddhi* count of 15:15. You would now block your right nostril with your right thumb and take a 15-second inhalation through the left nostril. Now, without a break, open the right nostril and close the left one with the ring and little finger of your right hand. Exhale now through your right nostril for 15 seconds. Then reverse and inhale through the right nostril for 15 seconds. Close the right nostril with your thumb and open the left nostril by removing the ring and little fingers. Exhale now through the left nostril for 15 seconds. This constitutes 1 round. Immediately, without a break, continue into the next round by again inhaling through the left nostril for 15 seconds and so on.

I have recommended that during *Ujjayi* you pronounce the *mantra* OM or your *ishtamantra*[457] for each tick of the clock or metronome. This is different in *Nadi Shuddhi*. Here we pronounce the syllable of water (*vam*) during the lunar breathing cycle, and the *mantra* of fire

456. Swami Digambarji et al. (eds), *Vasishta Samhita (Yoga Kanda)*, Kaivalyadhama, Lonavla, 1984, p. 17
457. An *ishtamantra* is a *mantra* related to a specific *ishtadevata* such as OM Nama Shivaya for Lord Shiva.

(*ram*) during the solar cycle. The lunar cycle consists of an inhalation through the left nostril and an exhalation through the right nostril. During that time, pronounce the *bija akshara* (seed syllable) *Vam*. The solar cycle constitutes an inhalation through the right nostril and an exhalation through the left. During that time pronounce the *bija akshara Ram*.

The location into which we pronounce the *mantra* is also of importance. Intonate the syllable of water in the centre of the skull, the larger area of the third ventricle of the brain. This area in yogic parlance is called 'the moon', as it constitutes the lunar, life-giving, anabolic, nurturing reservoir of *prana* called *amrita*. While we pronounce *Vam* in this area, we visualize this centre as the disc of the full moon, shining like an ocean of liquid silver, with a cooling, nectar-like quality.

During the solar cycle we pronounce *Ram* in the circle of fire, i.e. the *Manipura Chakra*. The *Manipura* is called the circle of fire because it is the seat of *agni*, the element of fire. Each *chakra* is a representation of a particular element and it carries that element within itself. The *Manipura* (navel *chakra*) represents the element fire, in the body most notable as the digestive fire. Each *chakra* also has a seed syllable (*bija aksharas*) associated with it, which again represents the element. The *bija mantra* of the navel *chakra* is the syllable of fire, which is *Ram*. Strike the *mantra Ram* into the circle of fire, which you visualize at the navel or, precisely speaking, the point behind the navel where a projected horizontal line emanating from the navel would meet the spinal cord. This is the location of the *Manipura Chakra*.

This most effective method of purifying the *nadi*s combines alternate nostril breathing with *chakra* visualization and *mantra*. This method is so powerful that the *Darshana Upanishad* claims that, if practised in seclusion in nature, it will purify the *nadi*s in 3 to 4 days, but I wouldn't bet on that.[458] As stated earlier, *shastra*s do contain an element of *stuti* (exaggerated praise) to make sure that students practise the techniques with conviction.

458. *Darshana Upanishad* V.10

The *rishis* Vasishta and Yajnavalkya both state that, when practising 18 rounds per day (6 rounds at each of the 3 *sandhis*, i.e. morning, lunchtime and evening), you will purify the *nadis* in 3 to 4 months – or if not then in 3 to 4 years.[459] That's a bit more realistic, although quite vague. I prefer instructions to be given more precisely, but I can just imagine those two *rishis* sitting in a circle of students 6 or 8 thousand years ago and, after making this joke and noticing the helpless looks on their students' faces, bursting out into thunderous laughter. Indian teachers love to make such ambiguous statements: it's part of playing with the student. Luckily enough we do have methods to determine whether we have achieved the purpose of this method, as described below.

Pronounce the *mantras Vam* and *Ram* during their respective cycles, synchronized with the ticking of a clock or a metronome, and count the seconds with your thumb on the fingers of your left hand. This way you don't have to count in your mind and can utilize your mind for the *mantra* and the visualization. Practise for at least 10 to 15 minutes per day for the method to work, but you will progress faster with 20, 25 or 30 minutes. Starting from a 15:15 count, slowly build it up until you have again arrived at approximately a 30:30 count, extending each breathing cycle again to a minute. Try to avoid changing your count during a session. If you make up your mind to practise 24:24 then try to stick to that and don't go up and down with your count during a session. This presumes, of course, that you have chosen your count wisely and are capable of sticking to it. If you have repeatedly chosen a count that is too advanced for you, then you generally have to be more defensive, that is, do not be too ambitious. The main exception to the rule of sticking to your count comes about with the approach of summer. With the daily temperature increasing you might have to reduce the count, as otherwise your body may heat up too much.

Once you have reached a 30:30 count, again switch to the 1:2 ratio as described in the previous chapter and from there add on until

459. *Vasishta Samhita* II.67; *Yoga Yajnavalkya* V.17–20

you have reached a 20:40 count. It is important that you are comfortable at all times and never strain. *Pranayama* is not to be toyed with. It is a powerful tool to be respected. You may get away with pushing your way through *asana* practice but not through *pranayama*. The *shastras* state that, if practised prudently, *pranayama* will cure all diseases. However, if practised foolishly it will create diseases. On the other hand the *shastras* also state that avoiding *pranayama* creates the diseases. So practise *pranayama* we must, but it has to be technically precise.

You can go on to the next technique once you can comfortably, without straining, practise daily for around 15 minutes the 20:40 ratio with alternate nostril breathing, *mantra* and visualization. Alternatively, your teacher may let you move on faster, particularly if he notices about you the signs that Vasishta speaks about, which are lightness and effulgence of body and increased *agni*.

The next technique is a significant step up, so you will do well to be proficient at Vasishta's *Nadi Shuddhi*.

Ujjayi with kumbhakas

Ujjayi is not directly related to purifying the *nadi*s, but the technique is interpolated here as a safe and easy method to practise *kumbhaka* and then to integrate these *kumbhaka*s into the more advanced *Nadi Shodhana*. If you practise under the supervision of an experienced teacher she may take you straight past this technique and get you to integrate your *kumbhaka*s straight into *Nadi Shodhana*. Many teachers, however, prefer to separate the two so that you do not have to worry about alternate nostril breathing, *mantra*s and visualization while tackling the new task of *kumbhaka*. Either way, the aim is eventually to practise *kumbhaka* within alternate nostril breathing.

As it is too difficult to commence both types of *kumbhaka* at the same time, we need to choose one, practise it until some level of perfection is reached and then go on to the next. The decision as to which type of *kumbhaka* to learn first is not straightforward.

THE CASE FOR EXTERNAL KUMBHAKA

External *kumbhaka* is the one explicitly mentioned by Patanjali as clearing the mind.[460] It is also mentioned in the *Brhadyogi Yajnvalkya Smrti* and the *Yoga Rahasya*. The main advantages of external *kumbhaka* are:

- Combined with *Bahya Uddiyana*, external *kumbhaka* offers the most straightforward way to purify the *Svadhishthana* and *Manipura chakra*s.
- It leads to purification of the mind and attainment of Raja Yoga.
- T. Krishnamacharya taught that, in order to achieve a balance, internal *kumbhaka* needs to be counteracted by external *kumbhaka*. He taught internal *kumbhaka* as part of *Brmhana kriya* (expanding action) for those built lightly, and external *kumbhaka* as *Langhana kriya* (reducing action) for those of rotund built.[461] The rationale behind this is simple: internal *kumbhaka* increases your rate of absorbing *prana*, thus decreasing your dependence on food. If you do not decrease your food intake you may put on weight. External *kumbhaka* increases *agni* (part of which is digestive fire); hence your ability to burn food and fat rises. If you do not increase your food intake you will lose weight.

Reasons against starting with external kumbhaka

If practised without *Bahya* (external) *Uddiyana*, external *kumbhaka* is very apanic. This makes the mind tamasic and has little benefit.

If practised with *Bahya* (external) *Uddiyana*, which turns *apana* up, the problem is fully rectified and the *kumbhaka* now lives up to Patanjali's claim. However, when it includes *Bahya Uddiyana*, the technique is really quite advanced and not suitable as an introductory *kumbhaka*.

---

460. *Yoga Sutra* I.34
461. T. Krishnamacharya, *Yoga Makaranda*, rev. English edn, Media Garuda, Chennai, 2011, p. 79

THE CASE FOR INTERNAL KUMBHAKA

The majority of yoga *shastras* are silent about external *kumbhaka*, and if they do mention it they say it leads to Raja Yoga, meaning it is part of meditation yoga. What they do mention extensively is internal *kumbhaka*. Internal *kumbhaka* has several big advantages:

Since the lungs are full, we can continue to absorb oxygen during retention. This enables us to draw out *kumbhaka* much longer and use this time for advanced meditation techniques.

Internal *kumbhaka* is the one used to fixate *prana* in the various organs, and it therefore leads to health and life extension.

Since we can continue to absorb oxygen from the full lungs, internal *kumbhaka* is less frightening, enabling the student to come to terms with *kumbhaka* without fear.

Swami Niranjanananda taught that external *kumbhaka* was so out of reach for the novice that he demanded of his students that they first achieve a 20:80:40 count in internal *kumbhaka* before they even thought about external *kumbhaka*.[462] This places external *kumbhaka* and its massive benefits out of the reach of more than 98% of all practitioners.

Summarizing, I recommend the following approach:

Early on, start with a daily practice of *Nauli*. Over time *Nauli* will lead to mastery of external (*bahya*) *kumbhaka* and *Bahya Uddiyana*. Once you have a grip on both, start to integrate them into *Tadaga Mudra* after your shoulder stand and into *Yoga Mudra* at the end of your sitting postures. The ideal *pranayama* for integrating count into your external *kumbhaka*s is *Bhastrika*: due to the huge amounts of oxygen, you can hold even external *kumbhaka*s for quite a long time. Once you have familiarized yourself with counted external *kumbhaka*s, you may include them together with internal *kumbhaka*s into *Ujjayi* and *Nadi Shodhana*.

I suggest you start your counted *kumbhaka* practice here with

462. Swami Niranjanananda, *Prana and Pranayama*, Yoga Publications Trust, Munger, 2009, p. 224

internal k*umbhaka*s. This lowers the entry hurdle for beginners, as the idea of retaining the breath inside with full lungs is initially less alien than retaining it outside with empty lungs.

CONTRAINDICATIONS

The practice of *kumbhaka* is generally not advised during pregnancy or for anyone suffering from high blood pressure or heart disease. However, if these conditions exist in a mild form they can be improved through *pranayama*, under the supervision of a skilled yoga therapist. The same may be said about peptic ulcers.

Kumbhaka practice should never be combined with the use of psychedelic drugs. There are inhibitors in our nervous and endocrine systems that prevent us from tampering with our respiration and heart rate. Through years of skilful practice, the yogi learns to suspend some of these inhibitors and venture into areas not accessible to the untrained person. There are reasons why these areas are inaccessible to the untrained. However, these very same inhibitors may be suspended through some psychedelic drugs, and anything can happen if you practise *pranayama* under their influence.

KUMBHAKA WITH JALANDHARA BANDHA

As pointed out previously, every internal *kumbhaka* exceeding 10 seconds needs to be accompanied by *Jalandhara Bandha*. Please read the chapter on *Jalandhara Bandha* if you have not yet done so. When retaining the breath inside, *Jalandhara Bandha* exceeds by far in importance *Mula* and *Uddiyana bandha*s. Remember that it is not enough to just rest the chin on the jugular notch. That is only the *Jalandhara Bandha* position. A *bandha*, however, is a muscular contraction, not a position. To induce the *bandha* we swallow saliva and, when the throat muscles grip, maintain this grip and do not release it. Only then place the chin down on the chest and keep it there for the duration of the *kumbhaka*. The test of whether the *bandha* is on or not is to try to breathe. Only if no air gets through are you performing the *bandha* correctly.

246

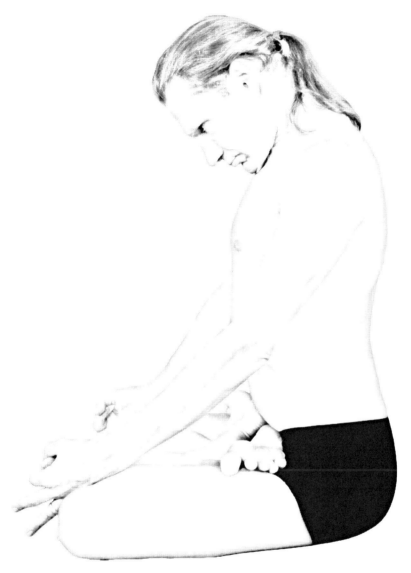

Internal kumbhaka with Jalandhara Bandha

Before placing your chin down, lift your chest as high as you can. This way you are less likely to strain your neck. A large amount of neck flexion is required to perform this *bandha* effectively. One of the reasons why *pranayama* ideally is done after *asana* practice is that

247

Sarvangasana (shoulder stand) prepares your neck for *Jalandhara Bandha*. When you come to the end of the *kumbhaka*, first lift your head, next release the grip of the throat muscles and then exhale slowly – not in any other order. If you release the grip first, then lift your head and then exhale, *prana* may still enter the head, which is to be avoided.

COUNT

Firstly, as we are integrating a new element into our count and are starting a new technique we will return to a *sama vrtti* count, in which all elements of the ratio are equal. Assuming that you were previously practising for example a 30:30 ratio in *Nadi Shuddhi*, we cut the inhalation into half to arrive at 15 seconds for the inhalation. Applying then the new 1:1:1 ratio, we arrive at 15 seconds for the inhalation, 15 seconds for the internal *kumbhaka* and 15 seconds for exhalation. It should not pose a problem, as the three phases combined add up to 45 seconds whereas your previous count totalled 60 seconds. If your previous count in *Nadi Shuddhi* was less than 30:30 or 20:40, reduce the new count accordingly.

Sit in your preferred meditation *asana* and, using the ticking of a clock or metronome, count digitally on your fingers, pronouncing *OM* or your *ishtamantra* once every second. Slightly contracting your glottis, produce an *Ujjayi* inhalation with a length of 15 seconds. Seeing that this is a slow-breathing *pranayama*, we are again placing the three-stage double-up wave into the complete yogic breathing cycle. Maintain the amount of inhalation-*Uddiyana Bandha* required to draw the inhalation all the way up into the upper lobes. Once having completed the inhalation, lift the chest high to reduce the necessary amount of neck flexion. Induce now the contraction of the throat by performing a swallowing movement and place the chin down low on your sternum where it would be when performing shoulder stand. Keep the throat firmly contracted and check whether any air can escape. If you do manage to breathe, repeat the swallowing until your throat is hermetically sealed and no *vayu* can enter the head.

248

Count again to 15 using your *mantra* and fingers. Once you have mastered *Jalandhara Bandha*, maintain *Mula Bandha* throughout the entire cycle. After 15 seconds, lift your head, release the grip of your throat and smoothly exhale with an even sound over the entire length of the exhalation. Use exhalation-*Uddiyana Bandha* to drive all air out, starting from just below the pubic bone.

This constitutes 1 round. Once you are proficient with this count, increase it, sticking to the 1:1:1 ratio. Once you have reached a breathing cycle length of 1 minute, i.e. 20:20:20, go on to *Nadi Shodhana*.

Once you have learned external *kumbhaka* and are comfortable with integrating it into *Ujjayi*, again reduce your previous *Ujjayi* ratio (20:20:20) to half, arriving at a 10:10:10 count. Adding external *kumbhaka*, you have a new count of 10:10:10:10, with the last number reflecting external *kumbhaka*.

Complete the first three respiratory phases as above but, after the completion of the *Ujjayi* exhalation, firmly contract the throat (initially without *Jalandhara Bandha*) and perform a faked inhalation. This means that you are lifting your ribs with your intercostal muscles but, as the throat is locked, no air can rush in. Instead, the ensuing vacuum will suck the diaphragm and with it the contents of the abdomen into the thoracic cavity. This *bandha* is called *Bahya Uddiyana*, and ideally the abdominal wall should touch the front of the spine. Thoroughly study the information on this *bandha* in the chapter on *bandha*s. At the end of your 10-second external *kumbhaka*, release the throat and gently perform the next *Ujjayi* inhalation. This constitutes 1 round.

Once you are accustomed to the count, slowly increase it, maintaining the 1:1:1:1 ratio. Once your breathing cycle exceeds 1 minute, you may take external *kumbhaka* across to *Nadi Shodhana* and integrate it there. You may also integrate *Jalandhara Bandha* into external *kumbhaka*. However, make sure that you lift the chest as high as possible, while keeping your arms straight and moving your shoulders forward to receive the descending chin. Since the chest is deflated, *Jalandhara* is here much more challenging.

Once you have achieved a certain proficiency, discontinue this practice and focus on *Nadi Shodhana*, which is the core *pranayama* technique. We used *Ujjayi* at this point only as a training platform for *kumbhaka*s.

If you have difficulty sleeping after performing *Ujjayi* in the evening, consider the following: Some Ashtanga Vinyasa practitioners form a connection between *Ujjayi* breathing and activation of the sympathetic nervous system. As soon as the *Ujjayi* sound starts, the body will trigger the sympathetic nervous system in an attempt to psych itself up for the intense *vinyasa* practice. This might be beneficial for *vinyasa* practice, but it requires the isolation of *Ujjayi* breathing from a more serious *kumbhaka* practice unless you break the link between *Ujjayi* and the sympathetic nervous system. Similarly, it may call for the practice of any *Ujjayi* being undertaken not too late in the evening. On the other hand the link between *Ujjayi* and the sympathetic nervous system can be utilized for staying alert in meditation as long as this does not happen too late in the evening.

Goraksha's Nadi Shodhana

INTRODUCTION TO GORAKSHA NATHA
The *siddha* Siddha Goraksha Natha was the illustrious founder of the Natha order. Or *is* the founder we should say, as he is considered to be an immortal. There were confirmed sightings spread over around 400 years dating from the 10th until around the 14th century. Since then he has made himself scarce. Many accounts of yogis performing miraculous deeds such as walking in thin air or over water, raising the dead or coming back from death, date back to the person of Goraksha Natha, or Goraknath as he is called in Hindi, Goraksha Natha being his name in Sanskrit.

Apart from Matsyendra Natha, his teacher, Goraksha Natha is the most famous of the *siddhas*. A *siddha* is a yoga master who has attained supernatural powers. Apart from performing numerous miracles, recruiting many disciples, and compiling several important yoga

250

shastras, Goraksha was also a great leader and organizer. He founded the Natha order, with many monasteries, and also created his own distinct *Shaiva* philosophy. Svatmarama, the author of the influential *Hatha Yoga Pradipika*, traces his own lineage back to the two *siddha*s and, upon close examination, we find the *Pradipika* nothing but an elaboration of the older texts authored by Goraksha Natha. It is fascinating to see how such a brief text as the *Goraksha Shataka* contains essentially everything that Hatha Yoga came to be 400 years later.

Some scholars claim that the teachings of the *Yoga Upanishads* are nothing but the methods of Matsyendra and Goraksha, which were eventually elevated to Vedic status by their includion in the *Upanishads*. They argue that this had been done because tantric Hatha Yoga had become so influential that it had to be included in the Vedic canon. Others believe that the teachings of the *Yoga Upanishads* and those of the *siddha*s are part of a much older tantric tradition and that Goraksha was nothing but its most important compiler and reformer. I hold this last position simply because I consider it unlikely that such a vast, complex and brilliant teaching as that of the *siddha*s could have been invented simply by one or two people in one lifetime, even if that life was 400 years long. The *shastras* themselves state that both Matsyendra Natha and Goraksha Natha received this teaching from Adhi Natha, the first and primordial *natha*, the Lord Shiva.

WHY NADI SHODHANA

Goraksha Natha declares that *Nadi Shodhana* frees one of all diseases. The *Yoga Rahasya*, handed down through T. Krishnamacharya, proclaims that *Nadi Shodhana* is the most important *pranayama*.[463] It also declares that, while other *pranayama*s have limited benefits, *Nadi Shodhana* has countless benefits.[464] In his *Yoga Makaranda* the *Acharya* (teacher) states that *Nadi Shodhana* purifies the *Ajna Chakra* (third

463. *Yoga Rahasya* I.103
464. *Yoga Rahasya* I.103

eye).[465] *Nadi Shodhana* is also accepted by the other yoga *shastras* as the prime *pranayama* and one of the prime elements of yoga. Since *Nadi Shodhana* creates a balance between the lunar (Ida) and solar (Pingala) *nadis*, it prepares the body to assimilate power (Shakti) and raise Kundalini. Once body and mind are purified, the ascent of power (*shakti chalana*) poses no problem.

INTERNAL KUMBHAKA

The difference between Vasishta's *Nadi Shuddhi* and Goraksha's *Nadi Shodhana* consists in the use of *kumbhaka*. While the inhalation has a rajasic impact and the exhalation is tamasic, *kumbhaka* has a sattvic influence. It stills the mind, and the underlying *sattva* begins to shine through. This can be understood in the following way: Thought (*vrtti*) is powered by *vata*, i.e. movement of *prana*. *Prana* is arrested in *kumbhaka*. Since *prana* is arrested in *kumbhaka*, there is no natural movement powering thought. Thought waves, which are expressions of our conditioning, warp our perception of the world to such an extent that we cannot perceive it as it truly is. They do this in a similar fashion to waves powered by the wind rippling the surface of a pond. The formerly still surface distorts reflections, which will be clearly discernible again if the surface of the pond returns to calmness. The surface-distorting force is *tamas* (torpidity) or *rajas* (frenzy), depending on which one is predominant. Yoga teaches that, if they are absent and the mind is devoid of thought waves, the object contemplated can be clearly reflected like the full moon in a forest lake during a windless, balmy summer night.

This capacity of the mind to not distort an object is only observable when the mind is completely still and this clarity of reflection-producing stillness is called the mind's *sattva* (intelligence). *Sattva* is automatically predominant in the mind during *kumbhaka*. Or should I say predominant with a certain qualification. Imagine a wind turbine propelled by a powerful gust of air: Once *kumbhaka* sets in,

465. T. Krishnamacharya, *Yoga Makaranda*, rev. English edn, Media Garuda, Chennai, 2011, p. 5

the impulse acting on the turbine is removed, but it will continue to rotate for a while due to the inertia of its mass. Similarly our mind will want to continue thinking due to the inertia of our conditioning, even though the impulse of the breath is removed. How long the propeller of the mind will continue to rotate is determined by the 'thickness' of the conditioning of the individual. This depends simply on the number of individual subconscious imprints (*samskaras*) supporting it.

During *kumbhaka* it is much easier to find the underlying stillness of the mind, but many practitioners fail to look for it. In *kumbhaka* the mind will go on only if it continues to be artificially driven by one's conditioning, and even the thickest of all conditionings will slowly use up its fuel. Look for and find in *kumbhaka* the underlying stillness of the mind.

Apart from the spiritual benefits just described, one of the important physical benefits of internal *kumbhaka* is that, under the pressure of the air held inside, the alveoli in the upper lobes of the lungs open and become ventilated. These neglected upper alveoli are breeding grounds for many respiratory diseases, but they also impinge on our general vitality by reducing our potential CO_2 and oxygen exchange. *Kumbhaka* is thus an important technique for increasing our organism's capability to absorb *prana*.

CONTRAINDICATIONS
Please note the contraindications listed under *Ujjayi* with *kumbhaka*.

METHOD
Apart from the *Yoga Upanishads*, which are of unknown age, the first text that describes this method in detail is probably the *Goraksha Shataka*. Goraksha advised inhaling through the left nostril, then performing *kumbhaka* and exhaling through the right.[466] After inhaling through the right nostril, practise *kumbhaka* again and then exhale to the left. This constitutes 1 round. The difference to Vasishta's method here is

466. *Goraksha Shataka* stanzas 43–46

the inclusion of internal (*antara*) *kumbhaka*. Like Vasishta, Goraksha Natha suggests meditating on the moon at the roof of the palate during the inhalation through the left nostril. Notice that moon (*chandra*) is a Sanskrit term, which often doubles up as a name for Ida, the left nostril. Yoga *shastras* often say, 'inhale through the moon' when wanting to suggest breathing in through the left nostril. However, this meditating on the moon is to be continued during the entire Ida cycle, which constitutes inhaling through the left, *kumbhaka* and exhaling through the right. I will explain later what this mysterious moon stands for. With the inhalation through the right nostril, the *Surya* cycle commences. During this cycle Goraksha recommends meditating on the sun in the navel, i.e. the fire *chakra*, *Manipura*. Note that again the term *Surya* here is used for both the right nostril and the fire *chakra*, *Manipura*.

Goraksha is a bit more positive with his remarks on success, and assures us that after performing this technique for three months the *nadis* will be clean, one of the parameters by which this is measured being the fact that one becomes disease free. The *siddha* places particular emphasis on the fact that when one meditates on the ocean of nectar in the 'moon' or the flames of fire in the 'sun', one needs to be happy. This is particularly helpful during the practice.

VISUALIZATION

The *Hatha Yoga Pradipika* also proclaims that during the lunar cycle (inhale left, *kumbhaka*, exhale right) the yogi should meditate on the moon.[467] Jayatarama, in his *Jogapradipyaka*, elaborates – after inhaling on the left side one should contemplate on the moon in the *Ajna Chakra*.[468] Bhavadeva Mishra supports this, saying that *nadi* purification needs to be accompanied by meditation on the moon and sun during inhalation and exhalation respectively.[469]

In my chapter 'Svara and Nadi Balance' I have already explained that the right nostril carries the solar force, which is catabolic (breaking

467. *Hathapradipika* (10 chapters) IV.12
468. *Jogapradipyaka of Jayatarama* stanzas 391–418
469. *Yuktabhavadeva of Bhavadeva Mishra* lxi

254

down tissue), sympathetic (fight or flight response/stress), left-brained (analytical, dissecting mind), fundamentalist ('there is only one truth'), efferent (outgoing nerve currents/action and extrovert psyche) and male. On a *chakra* level the solar force is situated at the navel in *Manipura*, the fire *chakra*. To enhance the effect of the solar breathing cycle, the yogi meditates on the fire *chakra* while performing it.

The left nostril, on the other hand, carries the lunar force, which is anabolic (nurturing/building tissue), parasympathetic (relaxation and recuperation), right-brained (integrating and synthesizing mind), relativistic ('there are many truths'), afferent (incoming nerve currents / contemplative, reflective, introverted psyche) and female. On a *chakra* level the lunar force is situated at the *Ajna Chakra* (third eye). Although we call the *Ajna* the third eye, it is not located on the surface of the forehead. Similarly, we call the *Vishuddha* the throat *chakra* and the *Manipura* the navel *chakra*, but these names refer only to the reference point on the anterior surface of the body. In reality these *chakra*s are far back in the body along the line of the *sushumna*. Shankara, in his *Yoga Taravali*, refers to the *sushumna* as *Pashchima Marga*, i.e. posterior path, for the obvious reason that it is close to the posterior surface of the body, in the vicinity of the spinal cord. The *Ajna Chakra* is in the centre of the brain, specifically the area of its third ventricle, a hollow in the skull filled with cerebrospinal fluid. This ventricle is surrounded by the most important junction of the nervous and endocrine systems, which are the thalamus, hypothalamus, pituitary gland and pineal gland. In this area we need to visualize the disc of the moon, shining like an ocean of silver nectar. If you find it difficult to visualize the moon, then venture out into nature on a clear full-moon night and have a good look at it. It is helpful.

KUMBHAKA WITH JALANDHARA BANDHA

Please study the notes regarding internal *kumbhaka* with *Jalandhara Bandha* under 'Ujjayi with Kumbhakas' and also those in the chapter on *bandha*s.

MANTRA AND BREATH WAVE

The default *mantra* used to count *Nadi Shodhana* is OM. Otherwise it is your *ishtamantra*. Vasishta recommends breaking down the sound OM into its 3 constituents, chanting A on the inhalation, U during *kumbhaka* and M during exhalation.[470] This is the Vedic form of *pranayama*.

The breath wave associated with *Nadi Shodhana* is the three-stage double-up wave. You will be well established in this wave from practising *Nadi Shuddhi*. Place this breath wave inside the technique as described so far and you will find it easier to maintain the visualization, *mantra* and concentration. Without this breath wave, the mind tends to get tamasic, especially during long exhalations.

COUNT AND RATIOS

When adding *kumbhaka* I suggest that you reduce to half the count you used last during Vasishta's *Nadi Shuddhi*. Say you used a 20:40 count; reducing it to half would mean 10:20. We now add an internal *kumbhaka* according to a 1:1:2 ratio, which would let you arrive for your first day at an easy 10:10:20 count, with a total of 40 seconds.

Some teachers insist on again transiting through a *sama vrtti* stage (all components equal length). In this case you would translate your 20:40 count into a *sama vrtti* count of 30:30. Cutting the inhalation into half would be 15 seconds. Applying then the new *sama vrtti* ratio of 1:1:1, you would arrive at a count of 15:15:15, a total of 45 seconds. Seeing that our previous ratios of 20:40 or 30:30 both totalled a minute, neither of these two new counts would pose a problem for you. I repeat that neither of these counts was actually recorded in yogic texts. It was left to the teacher to find out the appropriate ratio, and several possible avenues led to the goal. It is a question of what is common sense, what works and what supports the student, not what is right or wrong.

Choosing in this case the 15:15:15 ratio, inhale through the left nostril for 15 seconds (i.e. fifteen counts of OM) and lift your chest at the end of the inhalation. Swallow, lock the throat, place your chin

470. *Vasishta Samhita* III.1–4

down and retain your breath inside. Count 15 more *OMs* on your
fingers to the ticking of your clock or metronome. Lift your head,
release your throat and exhale slowly for 15 counts. For this entire
45-second cycle meditate on the moon in the centre of the head.

Now commence meditation on the sun in the navel *chakra*. Immediately inhale through the right nostril, counting 15 seconds. Lift your
chest, swallow, lock your throat and place your chin down. Retain
the breath inside for 15 seconds. Lift your head, relax your throat and
exhale through the left nostril for 15 seconds. This constitutes 1 round.

Immediately start the second round and practise in this way for
around 20 minutes per day. You will of course go deeper if you practise
for 30 minutes, but the practice has to fit into your life. Otherwise you
will stop doing it altogether. As your count gets longer you will have
to reduce the number of rounds; otherwise your practice will become
longer and longer. Unless that's what you want.

If you do find the 15:15:15 count easy, then on the next day go to
16:16:16. Remember to practise *Kapalabhati* right before your *Nadi Shodhana*
practice, and ideally your *asana* practice right before *Kapalabhati*. *Kapalabhati*
will enable you to extend your count without strain. Whenever you find
that a particular count becomes too easy – and it can often be discerned
by the fact that the practice is not fully engaging you any more – then
on the next day go one notch up. But do not be ambitious.

Once the length of your breathing cycle has again gone to or above
1 minute, you can graduate to the next higher ratio. For example,
let's say your count was 20:20:20, this would mean that now you
can upgrade to the next *vishama vrtti* ratio (uneven components)
of 1:1:2. Reducing your 20:20:20 to half lets you arrive at 10:10:10.
Increasing now your exhalation according to 1:1:2 will bring you to
a count of 10:10:20. Again you would find this very easy and could
increase on the next day, keeping with the 1:1:2 ratio, to 11:11:22.
Over weeks and if necessary months keep adding on until you have
reached a count of at least 16:16:32.

When you are comfortable with this count, reduce it to half (8:8:16)
and then elongate the *kumbhaka* to make it a 1:2:2 ratio. Your count

257

now would be 8:16:16. Again, you would find this very easy and could increase it on the next day, keeping with the 1:2:2 ratio, to 9:18:18. Keep adding on, if necessary over a period of months, until you have reached a count of 12:24:24.

Realize that your progress depends on many factors such as your nutrition, whether you get enough sleep, your work/rest balance, the quality of your *asana* and *kriya* practice, your family and social life and the amount of stress you are under, but the biggest factor is the quality of your devotion to the Divine. Keep your image of the Divine in front of you during *pranayama* and contemplate it during *kumbhaka*. Remember that *prana* is the perceptible Brahman (*pratyaksha brahman*). *Prana* is nothing but God immanent. To practise *pranayama* is a form of prayer and must be done with devotion. It is a form of harnessing the divine force within us and, if you do remember the Divine while doing so, the work becomes more efficient and will lead to success faster.

Once you have reached a count of 12:24:24, again reduce it by half, arriving at 6:12:12. Now increase the internal *kumbhaka* to the master ratio 1:4:2.[471] The *Yoga Rahasya* says about this ratio that it is the most important.[472] You would now start with a count of 6:24:12. You are likely to find this very easy, and if so increase the next day to 7:28:14. Continue to increase until you meet resistance. Many students who have a good balance in all the factors that I described in the last paragraph can progress relatively smoothly to a ratio of 10:40:20, but do take your time by all means and don't hurry. A lot of *pranayama*'s magic, like burning *karma*, purging the subconscious and fixating *prana* to cure diseases, takes place above those levels. If necessary, read again the section on *kumbhaka* length in the *kumbhaka* chapter and it will now make a whole lot more sense. Ratios of 11:44:22 or 12:48:24 are already very powerful practices, with a lot happening beneath the surface. If you are stuck, don't worry and just continue your daily practice. Analyse, however, which one of

471. Some teachers recommend interpolating a 1:3:2 ratio.
472. *Yoga Rahasya* II.59

the above lifestyle factors could be the problem. If you encounter lots of stress in your profession, eat a lot of fried food, have problems at home or don't sleep enough you are likely to go no further before you have addressed those issues. It is actually better then to stay where you are in your practice, as increasing it would add another layer of stress to your life.

Once you get to this point, do 10 rounds per session. You will find that often the beginning of a session is easy, the middle difficult and the last few rounds easy again because you have settled into it. You will not have this experience if you do 5 or 6 rounds only.

Either way, even if you stay here at this level, a daily 30-minute practice of 12:48:24 will change your entire life and change you as a person. It will be amazingly beneficial. For many students the key to going further is to increase the practice of *Kapalabhati* and add *Bhastrika*, which is the next technique to be described.

Before moving on to *Bhastrika*, however, let's have a look at further extension of the count. Sage Vasishta recommends going to a 16:64:32 count and practising 16 rounds a day, totalling more than 32 minutes in *kumbhaka*,[473] then continuing this practice until perfection is achieved. Do not be disheartened by the call of the *rishi*. Vasishta was one of the most powerful human beings who ever lived, and he had mastered almost all of the ancient arts and sciences. The *Hatha Yoga Pradipika* confirms that the ratio aimed at should be 16:64:32.[474]

Swami Niranjanananda and others teach that the 1:4:2 ratio needs to be expanded until a count of 20:80:40 is reached before any external *kumbhaka*s are added.[475] The Swami suggests that *Nadi Shodhana* should be practised exclusively with internal *kumbhaka* until this count is reached before any other *pranayama*s and/or external *kumbhaka* are tackled.[476] Some teachers do not share this view.

473. *Vasishta Samhita* III.10–12
474. *Hathapradipika* (10 chapters) IV.16
475. Swami Niranjanananda, *Yoga Darshan,* Sri Panchadashnam Paramahamsa Alakh Bara, Deoghar, 1993, p. 328
476. Swami Niranjanananda, *Prana and Pranayama,* Yoga Publications Trust, Munger, 2009, p. 224

External kumbhaka

The opinions on external *kumbhaka* deviate. For example, while the *Hatha Yoga Pradipika* does not mention external *kumbhaka* in the context of *Nadi Shodhana*, some other texts and teachers do. The *Yoga Rahasya* says that *Nadi Shodhana* should be combined with both types of *kumbhaka*,[477] and T. Krishnamacharya practised it in this way.

His student A.G. Mohan teaches external *kumbhaka* before internal *kumbhaka*.[478] External (*bahya*) *kumbhaka* is the form of *kumbhaka* that is explicitly mentioned by Patanjali.[479] Similarly to A.G. Mohan, Swami Ramdev suggests an easy form of external *kumbhaka* outside *Nadi Shodhana* before it is integrated here.[480] External *kumbhaka* is a very important form of practice that clarifies the mind and cleanses and activates the *Svadhishthana* and *Manipura chakras*. If we all waited until we have mastered the 20:80:40 count in *Nadi Shodhana*, few of us would harvest its manifold benefits. An easy approach to external *kumbhaka* is to first learn its application during *Nauli*. After that, external *kumbhaka*s may be integrated into various *mudra*s, such as *Tadaga Mudra* and *Yoga Mudra*, at the end of one's practice. These two postures become truly *mudra* only through the integration of external *kumbhaka* with full *Bahya* (external) *Uddiyana*. The advantage of starting the application of external *kumbhaka* here is that one does not have to count the retentions and only needs to hold them to capacity.

Once proficiency is gained in these *mudra*s and in *Nauli*, external *kumbhaka*s should next be integrated into *Bhastrika*. *Bhastrika* provides vast amounts of excess oxygen, which are well utililized by learning to perform external *kumbhaka*s according to breath count. Once external *kumbhaka*s are mastered in the context of *Bhastrika*, they can be integrated first into *Ujjayi* and then here into *Nadi Shodhana*.

477. *Yoga Rahasya* I.103
478. A.G. Mohan, *Yoga for Body, Breath, and Mind*, Shambala, Boston & London, 2002, p. 166
479. *Yoga Sutra* I.34
480. Swami Ramdev, *Pranayama Rahasya*, Divya Yog Mandir Trust, Hardwar, 2009, p. 93

In any case, if external *kumbhaka* is integrated into *Nadi Shodhana* it is good practice to start again with a *sama vrtti* ratio of via 1:1:1:1. Seeing that you would have practised a 1:4:2 ratio lately in *Nadi*

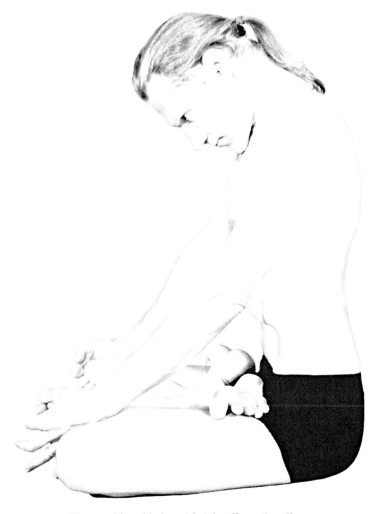

External kumbhaka with Jalandhara Bandha

Shodhana, I suggest the following transition formula. Keep the length of your inhalation and give each of the four components of the new ratio that length. This way you have kept the length of the inhalation, and reduced the total length spent in *kumbhaka* and exhalation by half.

261

This will give you ample leeway to integrate the more demanding external *kumbhaka* with *Bahya Uddiyana*.

Example: Suppose you recently practised a count of 12:48:24, with 48 seconds being the length of you internal *kumbhaka*. The new count would now be 12:12:12:12. Both *kumbhaka*s together would be 24 seconds long, that is half of what your previous internal *kumbhaka* was, and additionally the exhalation would be reduced to half.

You would then inhale through the left nostril to the count of 12, initiate *Jalandhara Bandha* and hold internal *kumbhaka* for a count of 12, then exhale through the right nostril for 12 seconds. At the end of the exhalation, apply *Bahya Uddiyana* and, if you have mastered it, *Jalandhara Bandha* too, but be aware of the additional stretch due to the dropped chest. This constitutes the entire lunar cycle, during which we meditate on the moon in the centre of the cranium. At the end of external *kumbhaka*, inhale through the right nostril with all elements of the solar cycle (during which we meditate on the sun in the navel) having the same length. Together this constitutes 1 round. Practise this for 20 to 30 minutes daily. Again add on the ratio slowly and eventually split to a 1:1:2:1 ratio. After adding on, apply a 1:2:2:1 then 1:2:2:2, and finally a 1:4:2:2 ratio, with the last digit always referring to external *kumbhaka*. Some teachers allow a more straightforward approach, teaching that one may go from a 1:4:2 ratio straight to 1:4:2:2 – which is, however, not as easy as it sounds. I found it much easier to slowly integrate external *kumbhaka* through the above steps.

The royal ratio for this most important of all *pranayama* techniques, *Nadi Shodhana*, is 1:4:2:2. It should form the foundation of every *pranayama* practice and be practised daily. Only after a certain proficiency in *Nadi Shodhana* has been achieved should one move on to practise other *pranayama*s. The reason for achieving proficiency in *Nadi Shodhana* first is the injunction of the *shastras* that higher yoga can only succeed if the *nadis* are purified beforehand. *Nadi Shodhana* is the main method for achieving this aim.

BHASTRIKA

Bhastrika, a rapid-breathing technique, has the largest breath volume and is the most powerful *pranayama* method. It is used to supercharge the entire organism with *prana*. It simultaneously reduces and ejects all three *dosha*s (humours), *vata*, *pitta* and *kapha*. Thus it can be practised, similarly to *Nadi Shodhana*, without creating an imbalance in the humours.

DISAMBIGUATION OF THE VARIOUS FORM OF BHASTRIKA
I have learned in India, from various teachers and institutions, forms of *Bhastrika* that are so different in regard to the technique and its effects that they can hardly go under the same name. Rather than 'believing' that one of them taught correctly, I have practised the various techniques, studied their effects and compared them to the effects as outlined in yoga *shastra*. Additionally, I have analysed most accounts of *Bhastrika* as published in current printed media.

I have found four schools of thought in regard to *Bhastrika*. Of those four, three claim that *Bhastrika* is a form of abdominal bellowing, in other words nothing but a modified *Kapalabhati*. The fourth school claims that *Bhastrika* is thoracic bellowing and thus completely independent of and different from *Kapalabhati*.

Schools of thought on Bhastrika
• Those who hold that *Bhastrika* constitutes *Kapalabhati* with throat constriction. This would make *Bhastrika* a combination of *Kapalabhati* and *Ujjayi*.
• Those who simply see *Bhastrika* as *Kapalabhati* with an added *kumbhaka*.
• Those who teach that *Bhastrika* is abdominal bellowing like *Kapalabhati* but with an added active inhalation, whereas in *Kapalabhati* only the exhalation is active.
• The fourth school considers *Bhastrika* a completely different technique and, although its approach somehow constitutes an outlier

from the three other schools, numerically this school has the greatest number of proponents. Swami Ramdev, for example, says that abdominal breathing is useless during *Bhastrika*,[481] and the chest has to get utilized instead.[482] Andre Van Lysebeth teaches that *Bhastrika* is a complete yogic breathing cycle, but done much faster than normally.[483] Shyam Sunder Goswami is probably the clearest when calling *Bhastrika* thoracic short-quick breathing,[484] as opposed to *Kapalabhati*, which he calls abdominal short-quick breathing.[485] The *Hatha Yoga Pradipika* clearly takes sides in this discussion, stating that in *Bhastrika* the air should be filled up to the lotus of the heart,[486] which clearly indicates the thorax. The *Yoga Kundalini Upanishad* also proclaims that during *Bhastrika* the breath should be inhaled up to the heart.[487] Other teachers who taught or teach *Bhastrika* as thoracic bellowing include K. Pattabhi Jois, B.N.S. Iyengar and Swami Maheshvarananda.

DIFFERENCE BETWEEN BHASTRIKA AND KAPALABHATI

The confusion becomes apparent when even students of the same master offer different opinions on the technique. For example some of T. Krishnamacharya's students tend to the abdominal camp whereas others teach *Bhastrika* as a thoracic technique. To find a solution to this problem I analysed the statements of the *shastras* in regard to both methods and compared them with the effects that I achieved with both abdominal and thoracic bellowing. The *Yoga Kundalini Upanishad* declares that *Bhastrika* pierces the three *granthis*[488] and reduces *kapha* and *pitta*.[489] The *Hatha Tatva Kaumudi* explains that *Bhastrika* reduces all three humours, a claim that is confirmed by the *Hatha Ratnavali of*

481. Swami Ramdev, *Pranayama Rahasya*, Divya Yog Mandir Trust, Hardwar, 2009, p. 38
482. Swami Ramdev, *Pranayama*, Divya Yog Mandir Trust, Hardwar, 2007, p. 26
483. Andre van Lysebeth, *Die Grosse Kraft des Atems*, O.W. Barth, Bern, 1972, p. 192
484. Shyam Sunder Goswami, *Laya Yoga*, Inner Traditions, Rochester, 1999, p. 307
485. Shyam Sunder Goswami, *Laya Yoga*, Inner Traditions, Rochester, 1999, p. 323
486. *Hatha Yoga Pradipika* II.61
487. *Yoga Kundalini Upanishad* I.33
488. *Yoga Kundalini Upanishad* I.39
489. *Yoga Kundalini Upanishad* I.37–38

Shrinivasayogi.[490] The *Hatha Yoga Manjari* enthusiastically proclaims that *Bhastrika* removes the *doshas*, awakens Kundalini and the 6 *chakras*, and pierces the 3 *granthis*.[491] *Kapalabhati*, however, has completely different effects. The *Hatha Yoga Pradipika* states that *Kapalabhati* reduces *kapha*, but not the other two *doshas* (*pitta* and *vata*).[492] Most authorities agree that *Kapalabhati* either cannot be increased or should be reduced during the hot season.

This is corroborated by experience: If you practise 10 or 15 minutes of *Kapalabhati* in summer during heat, you will quickly notice how the rising *pitta* (the humour that produces heat) will deprive you of sleep or manifest other detrimental effects. This is due to the fact that *Kapalabhati* is nothing but *Nauli* stage 1 / *agnisara* without the added *kumbhaka*. *Agnisara* means fire fanning. The digestive fire is fanned through the flapping of the abdominal wall. You can literally visualize the abdominal wall functioning like a fan, which, when moved, awakens the gastric fire. This movement of the abdominal wall in *Kapalabhati* is very similar to *Nauli* stage 1 / *Agnisara*. In both methods the movement raises *agni* / *pitta* and at the same time reduces *kapha*. A technique that includes flapping of the abdominal wall and increasing *pitta* cannot simultaneously decrease all three humours, *vata*, *pitta* and *kapha*. Therefore *Bhastrika* cannot be a technique based on abdominal bellowing.

Kapalabhati is an abdominal form of bellowing or, as S.S. Goswami put it, 'abdominal short-quick breathing', which increases *pitta* and reduces *kapha*. It is plain therefore that a bellowing technique that reduces all humours and not just *pitta* cannot be abdominal but must engage the whole torso. *Bhastrika* therefore must include thoracic bellowing but is not restricted to it. It could even be called 'whole torso bellowing'. As *Bhastrika* is an accelerated complete yogic breathing cycle with high breath volume, each breath initiates and terminates in the abdomen. However, at high speeds (up to 120

490. *Hatha Ratnavali of Shrinivasayogi* II.25
491. *Hatha Yoga Manjari of Sahajananda* III.14–17
492. *Hatha Yoga Pradipika* II.35–36

strokes per minute) it appears that only the thorax moves. For this reason the term thoracic bellowing is acceptable to distinguish it from *Kapalabhati*, which is exclusively abdominal bellowing. Realistically speaking, in *Bhastrika*, depending on the speed, 75–95% of bellowing will take place in the thorax.

The *Yoga Kundalini Upanishad* explains that, during *Bhastrika*, exhalation and inhalation are done in the same way.[493] This means that *Bhastrika* cannot be *Kapalabhati* with an added *kumbhaka*, because in *Kapalabhati* the exhalation is short and active and the inhalation is long and passive.

Whereas *Bhastrika* is enthusiastically lauded as breaking through the three energetic knots (*granthi*s),[494] there are no such claims about *Kapalabhati*. Let's have a look where these knots are located. Yoga proposes that along the spine there are three energetic blockages that block the ascent of spiritual energy and thus one's spiritual evolution. These knots are confusingly named after the three main representations of the Divine, Brahma, Vishnu and Shiva (Rudra is the Vedic name of Shiva), which represent the creating, maintaining and destroying functions of one and the same Godhead. The knots are so called because they deal with areas of human life that the three deities represent. The *Brahma granthi* deals with blockages in the area of creation of human life, that is blockages of sexual and survival functions. These blockages are thought to be located in the pelvic and lower abdominal region. In terms of *chakra*s they are *Muladhara* (root or earth *chakra*) and *Svadhishthana* (water *chakra*). The *Vishnu granthi* is symbolic of blockages relating to the maintenance of human life. These include assimilation (of food and wealth), claiming one's space within society (symbolized by the expansion of the chest during inhalation) and expressing oneself as a complete, integrated human being (related to the heart *chakra*). The *Vishnu granthi* includes the upper abdominal area (*Manipura* or fire *chakra*) and predominantly the thorax (heart *chakra*). Finally, the *Rudra* (Shiva) *granthi* deals with areas of life that

493. *Yoga Kundalini Upanishad* I.34–35
494. *Hatha Yoga Pradipika* II.67

266

we can access only when we go beyond and leave behind our individuality. Shiva is therefore called the destroyer or dissolver of the ego. The *Rudra granthi* represents realizing universal and divine law (related to the throat *chakra*, the *Vishuddha*) and recognizing the Divine with form (related to the third-eye *chakra*, *Ajna*, in the cranium). The *Rudra granthi* blocks rising Kundalini from reaching those two *chakras*.

While all of this at first hand may sound abstract it really is very down to earth and experiential. One category of disorders, for example, includes individuals who cannot sufficiently take care of themselves (survival issues) or have either a complete blockage of their sexual function or an obsession with it. These obstacles come under the heading of *Brahma granthi* and need to be overcome before major spiritual states can be experienced. A blockage in the area of the *Manipura Chakra* can mean that either the person does not have enough monetary success in their life or is so obsessed with material gain that they cannot progress any further. Moving on to the next *chakra*, if a person cannot take their place in society as a fully integrated, responsible and caring individual then, in yogic parlance, the heart *chakra* is blocked. Both the *Manipura* and *Anahata chakras* are part of the *Vishnu granthi* and it also needs to be pierced before a major spiritual state can ensue. Once these *chakras* are opened, the two highest *chakras*, which are located in the throat and head and related to the *Rudra granthi*, may be opened. Even a person who is procreative, proactive, successful in society and caring towards others doesn't automatically experience the transcendental states.

The interesting thing about the yogic *granthi* model is that yoga does not see these blockages as just psychological but as actual energetic blockages located in the pranic body. These are located along the entire length of the spine. It is apparent that a breathing method that only includes the lower abdomen cannot break through the blockages located in the chest. For this reason the abdominal bellowing was never used for this purpose. A technique that does break through the energetic blockages sitting along the entire spine must therefore include the entire torso and particularly the thorax. Hence *Bhastrika* must include thoracic bellowing, which means that Goswami's term 'thoracic short-quick breathing' and van Lysebeth's 'accelerated complete yogic breathing cycle' represent the correct view of *Bhastrika*.

Please don't get me wrong. I am not against *Kapalabhati*. In fact I practise it daily and like to do so extensively. What I'm saying is that *Kapalabhati* and *Bhastrika* are two completely different techniques. To get maximum benefits, the skilled yogi should practise daily both *Kapalabhati* and *Bhastrika*, which are separate techniques providing different benefits.

A WORD OF CAUTION

If practised as thoracic bellowing, *Bhastrika* is the most powerful breathing technique ever conceived. Properly introduced into the practice of a well-prepared yogi, it will accelerate spiritual growth faster than almost anything else. If it is mishandled, however, it can comprehensively backfire. Listen to my account:

During the 1960s, in what was then Czechoslovakia, the psychiatrist Stanislav Grof researched the potential therapeutic application of the hallucinogen LSD. While it was still legal at the time, it was soon declared illegal and Grof's supply dried up. He looked for ways to simulate the effect of LSD and realized that one of its effects was that it strongly enriched the brain with oxygen. Based on his research, Grof developed a breathing method that he called holotropic breathing, which is quite similar to *Bhastrika*. Another breathing technique developed by Leonard Orr, called rebirthing, also had surprising similarities to *Bhastrika*. During the late 1970s a mix of both breathing methods had trickled out from their use by psychologists into the mainstream of the Human Potential movement in the form of group therapies. Such breath therapy was thought to release the birth trauma, which impinged on our vital expression.

I attended such a group therapy workshop during the early 1980s. We were instructed to lie down and breathe very deeply up into the chest, a process that was to be continued for over an hour. Soon after I began, some very powerful sensations took over and I began screaming, convulsing, beating and kicking. This process was called catharsis, a cleansing and releasing breakdown of one's defences. I don't know what exactly got stirred up that day and whether it was the birth trauma or not. One of the problems was probably the fact that there were about 30 people on the floor with only one therapist and one assistant, so that not too much attention could be given to individual problems. Whatever got stirred up did not get released, and on that afternoon I entered a depression that was to last for 18 months. Within a day I turned from a jolly young fellow into a dark, brooding, pessimistic character.

Looking back, what I did was practise *Bhastrika* for about 90 minutes without any preparation. I do recommend *Bhastrika*, but I suggest doing it for about 90 seconds to start with, not 90 minutes. In other words I received 60 times the dosage that I would give to a beginner. Ninety or even 105 minutes of *Bhastrika* is a form of practice that is used by very advanced yogis,[495] who will combine it with 90 minutes of *Nauli*, 90 minutes of *Surya Bhedana* and 90 minutes of head and shoulder stands to raise Kundalini. You would need to have mastered *asana*, *kriya* and *Nadi Shodhana* through long years of practice to attempt 90 minutes of *Bhastrika*, and even then you would introduce it very slowly.

What happened to me on that day in terms of yoga would be interpreted as, without any adequate preparation, forcing up Kundalini, which then burned its path through existing blockages and closed *chakras*. The *Hatha Tatva Kaumudi* says that, when being excessively electrified by *Bhastrika*, the great serpent (i.e. the Kundalini) hisses and, spreading her hood, rises up.[496] Without first slowly perfecting the various yogic limbs, this may open Pandora's box. I'm not per se against rebirthing or holotropic breathing. I do

495. *Hatha Yoga Manjari of Sahajananda* IX.7
496. *Hatha Tatva Kaumudi of Sundaradeva* XLIV.12

respect Stanislav Grof's work and I'm sure that there are well-qualified therapists out there achieving good results in appropriate settings. Possibly in my case the therapist was not adequately trained or the group was just too large. However, *Bhastrika* is the most powerful breathing method on earth and its surging waves of *prana* must be slowly and effectively harnessed. It needs to be introduced very slowly and responsibly and only into soil that is adequately prepared. If it is introduced properly, however, then it is absolutely safe and very effective.

PREREQUISITES

Bhastrika is the most athletic *pranayama*. For *Bhastrika* practice you need to be proficient in *Kapalabhati* and *Nadi Shodhana*. You also need to be proficient in a high-quality meditation posture, ideally *Padmasana*. The better your general *asana* practice the further you will be able to go in *Bhastrika*. It is also advisable to be proficient in long inversions.

If the practice is limited to around 3 minutes, or as described and supervised by a yoga therapist, then the above prerequisites may be partially waived.

CONTRAINDICATIONS

Bhastrika is contraindicated during pregnancy and menstruation, and in cases of high blood pressure, epilepsy, stroke, heart disease and deep-vein thrombosis. A mild form of *Bhastrika* can be advantageous with ailments such as hypertension, heart disease or clogged blood vessels if those ailments have not progressed too far and *Bhastrika* is phased in slowly enough. Practice in these cases needs to be supervised by an experienced yoga therapist.

Do not practise *Bhastrika* when your nostrils are blocked or almost blocked. The strain placed on the tender alveoli could in the long run lead to emphysema.

BENEFITS

Through its forceful vibrations, *Bhastrika* can be utilized to clear obstructed blood vessels.[497] Obviously a yoga therapist must be consulted in this case also, and the exercise phased in slowly. *Bhastrika* increases oxygen saturation in the brain and it also speeds up the pulsating rhythm of the brain that is linked to the breath. *Bhastrika* speeds up the blood circulation throughout the entire body. Extended practice of *Bhastrika* lets every cell in the body vibrate, supplying it with oxygen and *prana*. The great Swami Kuvalayananda called *Bhastrika* the best exercise ever invented for the body.[498] *Bhastrika* also makes the body alkaline, improves resistance to cold, purifies the blood, increases lung capacity and makes the lungs more vital, increases *prana* uptake, helps with many diseases, increases and purifies *agni* and makes purified *agni* eject and reduce the *dosha*s (humours and impediments of the body, i.e. *vata*, *pitta* and *kapha*), breaks through the *granthi*s (energetic blockages), activates the *chakra*s and raises Kundalini. The list could be continued at nauseam.

SEQUENCE OF PRANAYAMA TECHNIQUES

Kapalabhati and *Nadi Shodhana* must be mastered before *Bhastrika*. However, once *Bhastrika* is introduced, it is good to practise it before *Kapalabhati* and *Nadi Shodhana*. After a successful *Nadi Shodhana* practice, breath ratio and heart rate have slowed down to such an extent that practising *Bhastrika* now appears counterintuitive. A useful sequence is:

1. *Asana* practice including shoulder stand and headstand
2. *Bhastrika* with subsequent *kumbhaka*s
3. *Kapalabhati*
4. *Nadi Shodhana*
5. Meditation
6. Relaxation

497. Swami Ramdev, *Pranayama Rahasya*, Divya Yog Mandir Trust, Hardwar, 2009, p. 49
498. *Yoga Mimamsa* III.1

TECHNIQUE

In the *shastras* you will find different techniques referred to with the name *Bhastrika*. You may find thoracic bellowing on its own or combined with internal or external *kumbhaka*. Additionally the texts describe *Bhastrika* as bellowing through both nostrils at the same time or through alternate nostrils.

All of these methods are extremely powerful, and an advanced yogi will find it beneficial to use them all. However, the fundamental technique that should be mastered first is *Bhastrika* as thoracic bellowing through both nostrils and without *kumbhaka*. The actual thoracic bellowing mechanism lies at the heart of all *Bhastrika* variations, and you need to master it before taking on any additional layers of difficulty.

To perform *Bhastrika* you need to sit in a proper meditation/ *pranayama* posture with your knees on the floor, palms and soles of the feet facing up and spine, neck and head in a straight line. Many teachers insist that *Bhastrika* should be performed in *Padmasana*, which is the only posture that, due to its foot lock, provides the necessary stability. This is certainly the case if you go even near to the maximum of 120 breaths per minute. During *Bhastrika* keep the whole body absolutely still. Don't lift your shoulders when inhaling and also keep your head steady. Do not rock your torso back and forth or from side to side.

BHASTRIKA WITHOUT KUMBHAKA AND WITHOUT ALTERING NOSTRILS

Advanced *Bhastrika* consists of a complete yogic breathing cycle with increased volume and accelerated speed. However, to come to terms with the increased volume, we will not initially increase the speed. Take a few breaths to establish the complete yogic breathing cycle. Exhale all air available and exhale it from all areas of the torso. When inhaling, fill all available areas of the torso and inhale close to the maximum volume (without brimming or straining). Be especially particular about the upper lobes of the lungs.

The next step is to add *Bhastrika*'s native breath wave, which is the two-stage up-and-down wave. All rapid breathing methods need to be exercised using a two-stage wave, since when you breathe fast you will not be able to isolate the three levels of the torso. We will start *Bhastrika* very slowly and it will seem to you as if you could use a three-stage wave. That this is impossible will become apparent once you use higher respiratory rates. In distinction from *Kapalabhati*, we will here use the thorax for bellowing. This means we will actively expand the thorax to breathe in and actively compress it to pump air out. That's why, instead of a double-up wave as in *Kapalabhati*, we use here an up-and-down down wave, which makes the thorax the active part in inhalation and exhalation. Once a high respiratory rate is achieved, it appears as if only the thorax is used and the abdomen remains static.

Using the two-stage up-and-down wave, fill up the torso from the pubic bone to the collarbones and then eject the air starting from the uppermost part. In order to learn this movement without tensing up it is necessary to slow it right down. Most students start *Bhastrika* much too fast and therefore never learn it properly. If the average person breathes about 16 times per minute, each breathing cycle takes on average 3.75 seconds.

I suggest starting with *Bhastrika* below that, taking about 6 seconds per breath (i.e. 3 seconds for inhalation and 3 seconds for exhalation) so that you will only take 10 breaths per minute. If you combine that with the fact that you will use close to your maximum breath volume, after 90 seconds or 15 breaths you will already feel a clear effect.

In the beginning even just 15 breaths with such a huge volume may make you light-headed, a sign that *prana* is entering your head. There are two ways to prevent that. One is not to breathe all the way up to the collarbones. Instead of that you may breathe up to about the third or fourth rib. Do so until the light-headedness abates. The other method is to slightly contract your throat, as you would do in *Ujjayi* but to a lesser extent. This method, suggested by Swami Sivananda, will limit the volume of air breathed and thus prevent

273

light-headedness.[499] Its disadvantage is that it puts strain on the alveoli. I found this method helpful for *Bhastrika* in the beginning, but it is important that the throat be constricted only very mildly, with the breath barely discernible audibly. Also, to prevent putting strain on the alveoli, it is preferable that this method be faded out once your organism has adjusted to the increased amount of oxygen and decreased amount of carbon dioxide in your blood.

If each breathing cycle is to be 6 seconds, each inhalation and each exhalation will be 3 seconds long. While under normal circumstances it may not be that difficult to time a breathing cycle to exactly 6 seconds, you will find it a different story altogether when experiencing the onslaught of huge amounts of oxygen. I found the use of a metronome made *Bhastrika* much more accessible, and it enables you to replicate a certain exercise every day under similar conditions without a lot of fluctuations. If you set your metronome to 20 ticks per minute there will be one tick per 3-second inhalation and one tick per 3-second exhalation. I found this to be a good initial setting, which allows you to distribute your breath volume evenly over the 3 seconds.

For some students it will be enough to take 10 full high-volume breaths in this fashion to reach their capacity. If so, stay at this level but make sure you perform the exercise daily. Other students will be comfortable with 15 breaths. Do not go beyond the 2-minute mark in the first few days. Initially your intercostal muscles may get sore and you need to prepare them slowly for this vigorous exercise. In the second week you may go to 2.5 minutes of practice, in the third week to 3 minutes, but you may also progress much more slowly if you prefer. At this early point 3 minutes should be the limit for an uninterrupted session of *Bhastrika*.

Once you are able to practise 3 minutes of *Bhastrika* with a breathing cycle length of 6 seconds there are several ways to intensify your practice. The first and most obvious is to expand your breath

499. Swami Sivananda, *The Science of Pranayama*, BN Publishing, 2008, p. 79

volume by breathing further up into the chest and making sure that all air is exhaled subsequently. The second step is to increase your breath ratio. At a breath ratio of 10 breaths per minute we are looking at a very introductory practice of *Bhastrika*. I suggest increasing that slowly and step by step. You should have a teacher to check your progress and determine whether you are ready to increase speed. The next step in making your practice more effective is to add internal and then external *kumbhakas*. Like no other breathing method, *Bhastrika* supplies you with huge quantities of oxygen. Rather than just sitting and watching the oxygen dissipate, it should be used for *kumbhaka*.

BHASTRIKA WITH INTERNAL (ANTARA) KUMBHAKA

I am assuming that you are comfortable with the steps described above and capable of practising thoracic bellowing (*Bhastrika*) at 10 breaths per minute with maximum volume uninterrupted for 3 minutes. Immediately after you have concluded your bellowing, using *Shanka Mudra* close your left nostril and inhale only through the right nostril. Then, employing *Jalandhara Bandha*, practise *kumbhaka*. Finally lift your head, close the right nostril and exhale through the left nostril. Once you have completely exhaled, immediately inhale again through the left nostril, perform *kumbhaka* with *Jalandhara Bandha* and then exhale through the right nostril. If performed by itself, this breathing technique is called *Agnisoma Pranayama*, with *agni* (fire) standing for the right nostril and *soma* (nectar) for the left. Here, however, it simply forms part of *Bhastrika*. The general rule that we commence each *pranayama* with the left nostril is waived here, because *pitta* is suspended trough the thoracic bellowing. Note that this is not possible after abdominal bellowing (*Kapalabhati*).

Since we are here switching from rapid bellowing to slow breathing, we will now use the three-stage double-up wave, which we know already from *Nadi Shodhana*. Together with the thoracic bellowing, these two breath cycles constitute 1 round of *Bhastrika* with internal *kumbhaka*. Initially use the same count that you are currently using in *Nadi Shodhana*. You will find that this count is very easy to perform after thoracic bellowing, and that usually it is not necessary to re-start here with a *sama vrtti* ratio. I repeat here that you must be proficient in *Kapalabhati* and *Nadi Shodhana* before working with this most powerful breathing technique, *Bhastrika*.

INCREASING THE BREATH COUNT

You will quickly notice that with those massive amounts of oxygen available you can comfortably extend your count. Do so responsibly. Say, for example, you have been bellowing for 3 minutes and find that your *Nadi Shodhana* count of 11:44:22 still leaves you with large amounts of oxygen. You can now extend your count to 12:48:24, but be sure to stay here until this count is fully integrated before you again extend it. *Bhastrika* confers great powers but they must be used responsibly.

After you have established yourself here for a number of days, concluding your exhalation through the right nostril, you could now include a second round of *Bhastrika*, consisting again of bellowing with two subsequent *kumbhaka*s, one initiated through the right, the second initiated through the left nostril. If you do practise a second round, I suggest you limit your bellowing to 2 minutes per round, making 4 minutes in total. After you have established yourself at this level of practice you can slowly extend each round again to 2.5 or 3 minutes, totalling then 6 minutes of bellowing. This is enough for now, as you still need afterwards to practise 5 minutes of *Kapalabhati* and 10 rounds of *Nadi Shodhana*, which still should be your main form of *pranayama* practice. Note that if you wish to add more rounds of *Bhastrika*, considering that your *kumbhaka*s can be made very long you could quickly come to a 1-hour-long *pranayama* practice. This is too long during the early stages. I suggest therefore limiting yourself at this stage to no more than 2 rounds of *Bhastrika*.

ACCELERATING THE BREATH RATIO

The next step now is to increase your breath ratio during the bellowing. So far we have worked with a breathing-cycle length of 6 seconds, leaving 3 seconds for each inhalation and exhalation respectively. This equates to 20 ticks on the metronome per minute. Now change your metronome to 21 ticks. This reduces the breathing cycle from 6 to approximately 5.7 seconds, and it means that you will, for example, fit 10.5 breathing cycles instead of only 10 into 1 minute. This is only a slight increase, but if you proceed at this level your increases will eventually compound to an incredible practice, whereas otherwise you will possibly discontinue your practice for one reason or another. What is important is that you do not sacrifice breath volume for speed; otherwise there is no point in increasing the breath ratio. Maintain your volume and increase speed in small increments.

Once you have practised for a while an accelerated breath ratio of 21 full-volume breaths per 2 minutes, you may find that you are able to increase *kumbhaka* again. If so, then, following our example above, go to 13:52:26. If you are not yet ready to increase your count, stay here and wait until you can again accelerate the breath ratio. Setting your metronome to 22 ticks per minute, each inhalation or exhalation will now be 2.73 seconds long and a full breathing cycle 5.45 seconds. You will now fit 22 full-volume breaths into 2 minutes or 11 into 1 minute. This is still very slow for *Bhastrika*, but you need to get used to this powerful practice before accelerating too fast.

From here on, alternately increase the breath ratio (breaths per minute) and the breath count, which determines the total length of each breathing cycle and thus the time spent in *kumbhaka*. In *kumbhaka* do not be idle but spend the time pronouncing your chosen *mantra* or otherwise *OM*, and meditate on your chosen form of the Divine. If you do not tell your mind what to do, it will pick its own tasks/entertainment at random or as determined by your past conditioning. The outcome of your *sadhana* (spiritual practice) then becomes random.

Slowly, slowly, over months of practice, increase your breath ratio until you hit 60 strokes/breaths per minute and at the same time increase your breath count accordingly. At this level you will easily reach a count of 16:64:32. This is a powerful form of practice, and you will certainly need guidance from an experienced teacher. The maximum for *Bhastrika* is 120 strokes per minute, at which level *kumbhakas* of several minutes are accessible.

BHASTRIKA WITH EXTERNAL KUMBHAKA

Due to the large amount of oxygen available, *Bhastrika* is the ideal practice to be combined with external *kumbhakas*. These are extremely powerful and need to be integrated slowly. They are the prime means of purifying the *Svadhishthana* (2nd) and *Manipura* (3rd) *chakras*, with some teachers opining that they are the only means. Some teachers hold that the *sutra* in which Patanjali suggests clearing the mind by retaining the breath outside to refer to *Bhastrika* with external *kumbhakas*.[500] This is quite possibly the case. The practice is said to activate the brain, to improve concentration, to increase vitality, to decrease stress and anxiety, to burn through the *granthis* (energetic blockages), to destroy *karma* and to induce *prana* into *sushumna*.

Do not practise external *kumbhakas* during the first three days of menstruation, as *Bahya Uddiyana* (sucking the abdominal contents into the thoracic cavity), which is required during external *kumbhaka*, will stop the menstrual flow.

If you have followed the instructions in regard to external *Uddiyana* (*Bahya Uddiyana*) and *Nauli*, you will already have a firm footing in external *kumbhaka*. Other good places to integrate them into your practice are *Tadaga Mudra* after back-bending and before inversions and in *Yoga Mudra* at the end of your *asana* practice The difference between applying external retention during *Nauli* or *mudra* and practising them as formal external *kumbhaka pranayama* is that during *Nauli* and *mudra* you do not need to observe count. The instruction will always be to 'practise to capacity'. However, here in your *pranayama* practice you will need to observe count, which adds another layer of complexity. Hence it is good to become familiar with external *kumbhaka* in the above-mentioned places.

500. *Yoga Sutra* I.34

278

COUNT

If you do have a strong *Nadi Shodhana* practice with internal *kumbhaka*s, your teacher may determine at this point that you should devote your *Bhastrika* practice to external *kumbhaka*s.

Because external *kumbhaka*s are more demanding, they are often practised with a count of 1:2:2, with 1 referring to inhalation, 2 to external *kumbhaka* and 2 to exhalation. *Bhastrika* can be an exception in the regard that a 1:2:4 ratio could be applied. If you did have a committed internal *kumbhaka* practice in *Bhastrika*, you could for example switch to external *kumbhaka* merely by cutting the internal *kumbhaka* ratio count into half. For example, if your internal *kumbhaka* ratio in *Bhastrika* was 16 (inhalation) : 64 (internal kumbhaka) : 32 (exhalation), a realistic initial external *kumbhaka* ratio would be 8 (inhalation) : 16 (exhalation) : 32 (external *kumbhaka*). Since external *kumbhaka* is more *agni*-increasing than internal *kumbhaka*, the question whether you need to start with the left or right nostril needs to be determined by your teacher, depending on your current state and the season and temperature of the place of practice.

In this example I am assuming that you complete your bellowing with an exhalation through both nostrils and start your *kumbhaka* ratio with an inhalation through the left nostril to counteract the additional *agni*. Inhale through the left nostril to a count of 8 seconds, using digital counting and your *mantra*. Then exhale through the right nostril to a count of 16. At the end of the exhalation, contract your throat, perform a faked inhalation and suck your abdominal contents up into the thoracic cavity, thus performing *Bahya* (external) *Uddiyana*. If in doubt, read again all the instruction in the chapter on *bandha*s. Hold external *kumbhaka* with *Bahya Uddiyana* for 32 seconds. Then inhale through the right nostril to a count of 8, followed by an exhalation through the left nostril for 16 seconds. Again apply *Bahya Uddiyana* and hold *kumbhaka* for 32 seconds.

If your previous internal *kumbhaka* count was 16:64:32, this new external *kumbhaka* count should pose no problem for you. In all likelihood you will be able to increase it soon, in line with the new ratio

8:16:32. After that you may enter into a second round of *Bhastrika* followed by 2 external *kumbhaka*s, or go on to *Kapalabhati* followed by *Nadi Shodhana*.

Once you have familiarized yourself with external *kumbhaka*s with count, you may also integrate *Jalandhara Bandha*. This is helpful especially if you practise lengthy external *kumbhaka*s. Adequately prepare yourself by increasing the time you spend in *Sarvangasana* and *Halasana*, which are the postures that induce the correct *Jalandhara Bandha* position. Only then will your neck be sufficiently prepared for the additional workload. Additionally, practise your external *kumbhaka*s right after your *asana* practice. This intense practice is not to be toyed around with, and your body must be fully baked in the fire of *asana* practice to withhold its pranic intensity. When practising *Jalandhara Bandha* during external *kumbhaka*, lift your chest as high as you can and additionally draw your shoulders forward so that the sternum and clavicles move forward and upwards to meet the chin.

Once you have mastered external *kumbhaka*s here, you may integrate them first into *Ujjayi* together with internal *kumbhaka*s into one single count. Once you have adapted to this, take them across into *Nadi Shodhana* with the aim of the final ratio of 1:4:2:2.

ALTERNATE NOSTRIL BHASTRIKA

An even more powerful form of *Bhastrika* is alternate nostril *Bhastrika*. You need to be proficient in *Kapalabhati*, *Nadi Shodhana* and *Bhastrika* through both nostrils to attempt this intense practice. You also need to have reasonably open nostrils, as bellowing through a half-closed nostril could lead in the long term to emphysema. Be sure to practise *Jala Neti* (*Neti* with water) daily, and if this does not give the desired results *Sutra Neti* (*Neti* with a thread) is applicable.

Benefits

Alternate Nostril Bhastrika induces *prana* into *sushumna* and raises Kundalini. It has many therapeutic applications too.

Method

Using the powerful thoracic bellowing, close your right nostril and inhale through the left, then close the left nostril and blow the air out through the right. Immediately suck the air back in through the right nostril and exhale through the left. In principle, alternate nostril bellowing is a rapid version of *Nadi Shodhana* with a huge breath volume.

Since the method is more strenuous, start it with the same speed initially used for *Bhastrika*, that is 3 seconds per inhalation and 3 seconds per exhalation. You will notice that it is harder to bellow through one nostril only, and the friction is higher. Increase the speed slowly and initially limit the technique to 3 minutes. As it is an exceedingly powerful technique, you need to be under the supervision of an experienced teacher. Also this method can be combined with internal and external *kumbhaka*s, applying the same considerations as when bellowing through both nostrils.

A course in *Kapalabhati, Nadi Shodhana* and *Bhastrika* is suitable for all. In the case of *Bhastrika* this is limited to those who are of average health and already sufficiently established in *asana, pranayama* and *kriya*. In contrast to that, the *pranayama*s described from here on are not suitable for all. They influence the *dosha* make-up of the individual, and hence must be tailored by an expert to the individual.

DOSHA-CHANGING PRANAYAMAS

The *pranayama*s and *kumbhaka*s in this section have a distinct medical function and can therefore be prescribed by a yoga therapist, a person who applies yogic techniques in a therapeutic context rather than a primarily spiritual one. They can also be used as spiritual *sadhana*sif the doshic make-up of the student is taken into consideration. Before venturing into these techniques it is important to understand their effects, as none of them is a stand-alone balanced form of practice. Because they are imbalanced they can be used to address and correct an assisting imbalance of the *dosha*s. In a therapeutic setting, *Surya Bhedana* is used to lower *vata* and *kapha*; *Ujjayi Kumbhaka* is used to reduce *kapha*; *Chandra Bhedana*, *Shitali* and *Sitkari* are utilized to lower *pitta*.

If applied in a therapeutic setting, a rather short, non-intense practice is prescribed. This is entirely different from their use for spiritual purposes. Once *Nadi Shodhana* is mastered here, the spiritual practitioner uses these methods to raise Kundalini. For this purpose they are practised for a very long time with very long *kumbhaka*s; hence their effect is entirely different. For example a 10- to 15-minute practice per day of one of these *pranayama*s could be used to restore balance of the *dosha*s. The same method for Kundalini-raising would demand a practice of 1 to 1.5 hours a day combined with other practices of the same magnitude. Such a Kundalini practice needs to be preceded by mastery of *asana*, *kriya* and *Nadi Shodhana*; otherwise the delicate *nadi* system will not withstand the onslaught of the ascending serpent power (Shakti).

Keep in mind, therefore, when reading and dealing with these techniques, that the same ones are applied by two completely different groups of people in two completely different settings. Be clear what the use is, as there are no shades of grey. For example, suppose you are a yoga therapy patient with relatively minor exposure to yoga but with an aggravated *vata* disorder. You may then use *Surya Bhedana* daily for 10 minutes to reduce your *vata* and become more balanced. Once you have achieved that, you cannot decide to change the purpose of the method and crank up your *Surya Bhedana* to 1 hour per day with long *kumbhaka*s. If you wish to do that you first need to achieve a certain level of mastery over *asana*, *kriya* and *Nadi Shodhana*. This needs to be understood clearly because, due to the dual purpose of these methods, there is a lot of confusion about their responsible use.

The two following techniques, *Surya* and *Chandra bhedana*, are mirror images of each other and combine to form *Nadi Shodhana*. While *Nadi Shodhana* corrects *nadi* imbalances slowly, if the imbalance is properly diagnosed *Surya* or *Chandra bhedana* can be used to correct it quickly, after which *Nadi Shodhana* practice is resumed.

Surya Bhedana

Surya Bhedana means 'sun piercing' referring to the fact that all inhalations are processed through the right, solar nostril.

The Yoga Kundalini Upanishad,[501] *Hatha Yoga Pradipika*[502] and *Yoga Rahasya*[503] all list *Surya Bhedana* among the most important *kumbhaka*s that are thought to alleviate diseases. Apart from its capacity to remove diseases caused by aggravation of *vata*,[504] *Surya Bhedana* finds its main application in raising Kundalini.[505] It is then often combined with *Bhastrika*, *Nauli* and other techniques. If used in yoga therapy to reduce *vata*, *Surya Bhedana* needs to be handled with care, as it also increases *pitta*. In fact *Surya Bhedana* also reduces *kapha*, although for this purpose generally *Ujjayi Kumbhaka* is used, which is not quite as heating.

To neutralize *Surya Bhedana*'s *pitta*-increasing effect, it is often combined with *Shitali*, which reduces *pitta*. In yoga therapy *Surya Bhedana* is generally limited to about 10 minutes and usually without – or with only very short – *kumbhaka*s. When *Surya Bhedana* is used as a spiritual

501. *Yoga Kundalini Upanishad* I.21
502. *Hatha Yoga Pradipika* II.11–12
503. *Yoga Rahasya* II.61
504. *Kumbhaka Paddhati of Raghuvira* stanzas 129–130
505. *Hatha Yoga Manjari of Sahajananda* IX.8

283

sadhana it is practised for 45 to 90 minutes a day and combined with other practices. It is then a powerful practice for increasing *agni* (inner fire) with the purpose of raising Kundalini. Needless to say, such a use should only be pursued under the guidance of a teacher experienced in the subject.

One of the problems that we face with *Surya Bhedana* is that it is not in itself a balanced practice like *Nadi Shodhana* or *Bhastrika*. In the process of igniting *agni*, *Surya Bhedana* activates all parameters associated with the right nostril, i.e. the sympathetic chain (fight/ flight response), efferent nerve currents (outgoing signals and outgoing personality), left brain hemisphere, catabolism (breaking down tissue) and analytical fundamentalist mind (there is only one truth), whereas it suppresses or weakens tendencies towards those connected to the left nostril, viz. the parasympathetic chain (rest and relaxation response), afferent nerve currents (incoming signals, introspective personality), right brain hemisphere, anabolism (nurturing and building up tissue) and intuitive/relativistic mind (there are many truths).

Upon re-reading that list slowly you will find word by word the drama of Western versus ancient Indian culture. Western culture is hopelessly *Surya* or solar predominant, whereas traditional Indian culture was predominantly lunar. If you study the views of 19th- and early-20th-century western indologists about Indian culture and religion, you will usually find the typical lack of understanding that people raised in a solar culture will have towards a lunar culture. In days of yore *Surya Bhedana* was a panacea for all imbalances faced by a typical medieval or ancient Indian yogi, who centuries ago would have needed a good dose of *Surya Bhedana* to create the necessary fervour and thrust to burn through lunar obstacles. On the other hand, the average contemporary Western yogi, at least at the time of writing this text, already has far too much solar, sympathetic, left-brained, efferent, fundamentalist, catabolic, analytical and extrovert tendencies. Examples are not only the testosterone-driven bulldozing of the rainforests but also the testosterone-driven bulldozing of the

284

safe deposits of almost the entire planetary population into the fire of the global financial crisis.

While strongly represented in modern white males, this tendency also increasingly grips women and members of Oriental cultures. Greatly simplified, the constant call for increase of Gross Domestic Product and its main motor, domestic consumption, increase the solar attitude of the population and thus make it more catabolic (breaking down and burning resources), extrovert (working longer hours and performing more difficult work-related tasks), sympathetic (more stressed through more work and ever higher education requirements) etc. While all of this was for a long time considered a white male domain, economists have long found out that global economic output can only continue its rise if the entire female population and the populations of formerly undeveloped countries are recruited as well. Solar, male culture has overrun lunar, female culture and, if this tendency continues, the global organism will burn out in a similar way to the highly stressed and highly strung ambitious individual, a tendency that is usually associated with breathing predominantly through the right nostril. The *shastras* state that if you breathe through the *Surya* (right nostril) consecutively for three days you will live for only one more year.[506]

Simplified *Surya Bhedana* will make you less mental, less self-reflective and more physical, less easy-going and more in-your-face, less intuitive and more analytical, more outgoing and less introspective, more interested in breaking down existing structures (even if they are useful) than in nurturing them, and more interested in the one truth (often yours) than in others that also may have a point. *Surya Bhedana* is a powerful technique for those who have too much of the opposite, lunar tendencies. While it may have been possible to prescribe this *pranayama* technique unanimously to most/all yogis in India, say 1000 or 2000 years ago, one needs to ask whether many modern yogis have not already imbibed too much of this medicine. This technique should be practised only when prescribed and tailored

506. *Hatha Tatva Kaumudi* LVI.8

by a knowledgeable teacher to the needs of an individual student. Swami Niranjanananda says that *Surya Bhedana* should be used only by those who have a preponderence of the lunar *nadi* (Ida), as *Surya Bhedana* activates the sympathetic nervous system, creates heat and produces extroversion.[507] Only if you are lacking these qualities should you practise it. Do not self-medicate with *Surya Bhedana*. An experienced teacher has to determine whether this practice or *Chandra Bhedana* is appropriate for you, and the selection might even change according to season and place of practice. If in doubt, simply continue the practice of *Nadi Shodhana*.

CONTRAINDICATIONS

Do not practise *Surya Bhedana* during a summer heatwave or when pregnant (because it's catabolic). Do not practise it when your *pitta* is already aggravated, as *Surya Bhedana* increases *pitta*. Do not practise it with high blood pressure, hyperthyroidism or when suffering from acidity and related *pitta* diseases such as ulcers and gastritis. Do not practise it with heart problems such as angina pectoris.

Do not practise this technique if you are very analytical/ logical and not intuitive enough. Do not practise it when the female, compassionate, caring aspects of your personality are already under-developed. Do not practise it when you are very physical, ambitious and materialistic, and cannot relate at all to lofty concepts and idealism. Do not practise it when you tend to stress easily, are tense, are a type A personality, have heart problems or stomach ulcers, cannot relax, suffer from interrupted sleep, overheat easily or suffer from excess *pitta*. In other words do not practise it if you are a solar personality and body type.

If you are practising *Surya Bhedana* and notice that you are starting to project internal conflicts into the outer world (i.e. living out in your surroundings and relationships conflicts that would be resolved better through a mental understanding and recognition process)

507. Swami Niranjanananda, *Prana and Pranayama*, Yoga Publications Trust, Munger, 2009, p. 280

then this may be an indication to stop the technique and replace it with *Nadi Shodhana*.

BENEFITS

The *Hatha Tatva Kaumudi* recommends *Surya Bhedana* in winter (to warm up) or to cure diseases cause by aggravated *vata* and *kapha*.[508] It is excellent to practise up in the mountains or during the cold season and is good for purifying and stoking *agni* (inner fire). *Surya Bhedana* can be used to cure pulmonary disorders, such as colds, sinusitis, bronchitis and other *vata* and *kapha* disorders. It is also good in cases of depression or when feeling weak and helpless, as this technique gives energy. It is an excellent way to alleviate excess lunar symptoms such as lethargy and being dull and unspirited. *Surya Bhedana* increases vitality and strengthens the body. It makes you dynamic, successful and outgoing. It is applicable when incredible physical feats or those of willpower are required, such as during warfare.

Since it increases catabolism it can be used to decrease weight, i.e. the breaking down and disposal of adipose tissue. Swami Ramdev recommends that for this purpose 27 rounds should be done twice a day.[509] Internal *kumbhaka*s are not added in this case, but external *kumbhaka*s would increase the catabolic effect if the student were capable of practising them without strain.

TECHNIQUE WITHOUT KUMBHAKA

This is a slow-breathing method and its native breath wave is the three-stage double-up wave. Sitting in a meditation *asana*, form *Shanka Mudra* with your right hand. Close your left nostril with your ring and little finger and inhale through the right nostril. Then, closing your right nostril with your thumb, exhale through the left nostril. This constitutes one round. Immediately close the left nostril again, and inhale through the right nostril. Again close the

508. *Hatha Tatva Kaumudi Kaumudi of Sundaradeva* X.1
509. Swami Ramdev, *Pranayama*, Divya Yog Mandir Trust, Hardwar, 2007, p. 35

right nostril and exhale through the left. In *Surya Bhedana* all inhalations are taken through the right nostril and all exhalations are taken through the left.

Start with a 1:1 ratio and do 10 rounds or as many as your teacher recommends. If using *Surya Bhedana* in a yoga therapy setting, practise it only to the extent necessary to reduce lunar symptoms. Slowly, without ever straining or forcing yourself, extend your count until you have reached 30:30, that is 30 seconds inhalation and 30 seconds exhalation. Then reduce the inhalation to half and go to a 1:2 breath ratio. From here extend the breath count again until one breathing cycle exceeds 1 minute. During the entire breathing cycle, meditate on the sun in the navel as during the solar cycle of *Nadi Shodhana*. Unless your teacher gives you another *mantra*, use the *mantra* of catabolism, *Ram*. When using *Surya Bhedana* for an extended period, even without *kumbhaka*, you need the advice of a knowledgeable teacher, who must scout for signs of aggravating the solar *nadi*.

TECHNIQUE WITH KUMBHAKA

If you are using the technique as a spiritual *sadhana* to purify and ignite *agni*, thus rousing Kundalini, you must add *kumbhaka*. The *kumbhaka*s themselves and the length of the entire practice session must become quite long. In this case supervision is even more important. Once a count of 20:40 is achieved, reduce the inhalation to half and add internal *kumbhaka* according to a 1:1:2 ratio.[510] The new count would then be 10:10:20, that is 10 seconds for the inhalation, 10 seconds for internal *kumbhaka* and 20 seconds for the exhalation. Extend the count until each breathing cycle again exceeds 1 minute and then switch to a 1:2:2 ratio. From here, following the same method, go to a 1:3:2 ratio and finally the 1:4:2 ratio.

510. Unless your teacher insists that you again transit through a *sama vrtti* ratio of 1:1:1. If you are firmly established in *Nadi Shodhana*, an alternative possibility is to bring your *Nadi Shodhana* ratio across and just reduce it by about 10%. The reduction pays tribute to the fact that *Surya Bhedana* is simply a *Nadi Shodhana* without its (cooling) lunar cycle. This means that initially you will have to reduce slightly the heating *kumbhaka*s.

In order to raise Kundalini, the method must be combined with other techniques, such as *Nauli* and *Bhastrika*, but Kundalini-rousing is not the subject of this book. If you create too much heat and suffer from its symptoms, increase *Shitali* or *Sitkari*. If you aggravate the solar *nadi*, i.e. increase the preponderance of solar symptoms, counteract this through *Chandra Bhedana*, which is described later. In the case of acute aggravation, immerse yourself in water and drink large or, if you can, extremely large quantities of milk. An Indian teacher told me that if practising the technique backfired I should drink 300 glasses of milk and the symptoms would subside!

If we think of an average glass containing 0.2 litres, 300 glasses would make 60 litres of milk. That would be more than you would expect the average corner shop to stock. This is obviously why many traditional Indian yogis never ventured too far from the next cow. In any case this drives home the necessity of getting the advice of a teacher if advanced breath ratios are practised.

Chandra Bhedana

Chandra Bhedana (moon piercing) is so called because all inhalations are taken through the left nostril and all exhalations through the right. The technique is a mirror image of *Surya Bhedana*.

While not popular in the golden days of ancient India, *Chandra Bhedana* has become more important today for the following reasons:
• Since air pollution in modern cities often rules out *Shitali* and *Sitkari* (which take the inhalation through the mouth), *Chandra Bhedana* is now the *pitta*-reducing, cooling *pranayama* of choice for modern urban yogis.
• Due to the solar predominance of modern societies, many contemporary yogis suffer from an aggravated solar *nadi*. This can easily be counteracted through this lunar *nadi*-empowering *pranayama*.

Chandra Bhedana is less lauded in *shastra* than *Surya Bhedana*, but as described earlier *Surya Bhedana* was much more applicable in ancient India, which was then a very lunar culture. In days of yore the average Indian yogi was brought to balance through *Surya Bhedana.*

Chandra Bhedana is, however, described in the *Yoga Chudamani Upanishad.*[511] It is also recommended in Raghuvira's *Kumbhaka Paddhati,* where it is said to bring nourishment.[512] In the field of therapy, *Chandra Bhedana* can be used to lower *pitta* and raise *kapha,* but it can also be used to raise Kundalini.

The greatest advertisement for *Chandra Bhedana* is found in Sundaradeva's *Hatha Tatva Kaumudi,* where he explains that poison flows through *Surya;*[513] therefore the yogi should not practise *pranayama* when Pingala flows. On the other hand, the nectar of immortality flows through Ida, and the yogi should practise inhalation and *kumbhaka* through that nostril only, whereas the right nostril is useless. Sundaradeva calls this the great secret taught by Lord Shiva. The fact that poison flows through *Surya* and nectar (*amrita*) through Ida is repeated twice in the *Hatha Tatva Kaumudi*[514] and confirmed in the *Kumbhaka Paddhati.*[515]

Opposed to that, *Chandra Bhedana* is considered off limits by Swami Satyananda and his disciples. Swami Niranjanananda says that in Satyananda's tradition *Chandra Bhedana* is almost never taught but considered a restricted technique, since it creates extreme introversion that can turn into depression.[516] Opposed to *Surya Bhedana,* which awakens *prana Shakti,* i.e. physical power, *Chandra Bhedana* awakens *manas Shakti,* that is mental power. Swami Satyananda feared that practitioners could turn lunatic when practising this technique. In fact the very term lunatic indicates that a person has an aggravated lunar *nadi.*

511. *Yoga Chudamani Upanishad* stanza 95
512. *Kumbhaka Paddhati of Raghuvira* stanza 130
513. *Hatha Tatva Kaumudi of Sundaradeva* XXX.8
514. *Hatha Tatva Kaumudi of Sundaradeva* XLIV.47–48
515. *Kumbhaka Paddhati* stanza 14
516. Swami Niranjanananda, *Prana and Pranayama,* Yoga Publications Trust, Munger, 2009, p. 261

I have not, however, come across any other Indian yogic school of thought that places these restrictions on *Chandra Bhedana*. Yogeshwaranand Paramahamsa taught *Chandra Bhedana* with both *antara* and *bahya kumbhaka*s without giving any restrictions.[517] Similarly, in the tradition of Swami Kuvalayananda it was handed down in the same way as other *pranayama*s. His student and collaborator M.L. Gharote describes *Chandra Bhedana* without giving any restrictions.[518]

The practitioner using *Chandra Bhedana* needs, however, to understand that she will activate all functions associated with the left nostril at the same time. It is not possible to activate some and leave out the others. *Chandra Bhedana* activates the parasympathetic chain (rest and relaxation), afferent nerve currents (incoming signals and introvert personality – in extreme cases leading to a brooding disposition), right intuitive brain hemisphere, anabolism (building up tissue, nurturing) and synthesizing/holistic/relativistic mind (developing a predisposition to embrace the many truths and being incapable of seeing the one truth). On the other hand it suppresses or weakens tendencies towards the right nostril connection, viz. the sympathetic chain (fight/flight response), efferent nerve currents (outgoing signals and outgoing personality), left brain hemisphere, catabolism (breaking down tissue) and analytical/fundamentalist mind (developing a preponderant inclination to the one truth and being incapable of seeing the many truths).

Chandra Bhedana is a very powerful tool, useful to those who have an outgoing, analytical, sympathetic, stressed or Type A personality that needs to be balanced with properties associated with the lunar culture of ancient India, such as psychic abilities, deep spirituality, ability to meditate deeply, appreciation of the Divine in all beings, consideration towards others, humility to the extent of self-denial etc.

Do not self-medicate with *Chandra Bhedana*. An experienced teacher has to determine whether this practice or *Surya Bhedana* is

517. Yogeshwaranand Paramahamsa, *First Steps to Higher Yoga*, Yoga Niketan Trust, New Delhi, 2001, p. 346
518. Dr M.L. Gharote, *Pranayama: The Science of Breath*, Lonavla Yoga Institute, Lonavla, 2003, p. 75

appropriate for you, and the selection may even change according to season and place of practice.

BENEFITS

Chandra Bhedana is a good *pranayama* during pregnancy, due to its nurturing, anabolic and feminine quality. It reduces *pitta* and alleviates its associated disorders such as acidity, ulcers and inflammation. Due to its cooling quality, it is a good practice in summer or in hot places. It also relieves fatigue and calms the mind. Since it is not as dependent on premium air quality as *Shitali* and *Sitkari*, it is an important tool in reducing *pitta*.

It stimulates the right brain hemisphere and awakens psychic abilities. It increases empathy and compassion for others. It makes you intuitive, develops holistic and integrative tendencies in your mind and enables you to appreciate complex artworks and mysticism. It is helpful in cases of extreme extraversion – that is, if you have no awareness of your own feelings and are dependent on ongoing external stimulation. It is helpful for meditation.

Chandra Bhedana activates Ida *nadi*, the *nadi* that circulates *soma*, the nectar of immortality. It activates the parasympathetic nervous system, meaning it is relaxing. It can therefore be used to relieve hypertension. It can also be used to raise Kundalini, and in this case it can be combined with *Bhastrika*, *Ujjayi* and *Kapalabhati*, which are all heating. S.S. Goswami also recommends combining *Chandra Bhedana* with *Nauli* to raise Kundalini.[519]

CONTRAINDICATIONS

Chandra Bhedana should not be used if suffering from depression, lethargy, dullness or low motivation. Do not practise it in winter and cold countries or high up in the mountains. Do not practise it when suffering from aggravated *kapha* and its related diseases such as colds, flue, bronchitis, pneumonia and asthma. Only those who lean towards Pingala and all its associated tendencies should use

519. Shyam Sunder Goswami, *Laya Yoga*, Inner Traditions, Rochester, 1999, p. 91

Chandra Bhedana. It should not be used when incredible physical feats or those of great willpower are required. For example it is unsuitable for military personnel during conflict. Since it is anabolic, do not use it if you have a tendency to adiposity and want to lose weight. Do not practise *Chandra Bhedana* if you are too introverted already and want to become more expressive. Do not practise it if you have too much self-doubt and do not feel in control of your life.

If you are practising *Chandra Bhedana* and notice that you are starting to somatosize internal conflicts (i.e. living out in your body conflicts that would better be resolved through a mental understanding and recognition process) then this may be an indication that you should stop using the technique and replace it with *Nadi Shodhana*.

TECHNIQUE WITHOUT KUMBHAKA

It being a slow-breathing method, *Chandra Bhedana* has the three-stage double-up wave as its native breath wave. Sit in a meditation *asana* and form *Shanka Mudra* with your right hand. Close your right nostril with your thumb and inhale through the left nostril. Then, closing your left nostril with your ring and little finger, exhale through the right. This constitutes one round. Immediately close again the right nostril and inhale through the left. Close the left nostril once more and exhale through the right. In *Chandra Bhedana* all inhalations are taken through the left nostril and all exhalations through the right.

Start with a 1:1 ratio and perform 10 rounds or as many as your teacher recommends. If using *Chandra Bhedana* in a yoga therapy setting, practise it only to the extent necessary to reduce solar symptoms. Slowly, without ever straining or forcing yourself, extend your count until you have reached 30:30, that is 30-second inhalations and 30-second exhalations. Then reduce the inhalation to half and go to a 1:2 breath ratio. From here, extend the breath count again until 1 breathing cycle exceeds 1 minute. During the entire breathing cycle, meditate on the moon in the centre of the head in the area of the third ventricle of the brain, as you did during the lunar cycle of *Nadi*

Shodhana. This method of concentration is suggested in the *Yoga Chudamani Upanishad.*[520]

Unless your teacher gives you another *mantra,* use *OM. OM* is a safer bet than using the water *bija, Vam. Vam* is a safe *mantra* when using it in conjunction with the fire *bija, Ram,* during *Nadi Shodhana.* During *Chandra Bhedana* the probability of *Vam* bringing you into contact with the lower emotional mind is too high: it would tend to make you a slave to your emotional urges. Using *OM* instead will bring you in contact with the higher spiritual mind. Alternatively, you may use the *ishtamantra* associated with your preferred form of the Divine.

If using *Chandra Bhedana* for an extended period, even without *kumbhaka,* you need the advice of a knowledgeable teacher, who must scout for signs of aggravation of the lunar *nadi.*

TECHNIQUE WITH KUMBHAKA

The *Yoga Chudamani Upanishad* states that, during *Chandra Bhedana, kumbhaka* must be held for as long as possible. In this case supervision is even more important. Once a count of 20:40 is achieved, reduce the inhalation to half and add internal *kumbhaka* according to a 1:1:2 ratio. The new count would then be 10:10:20, that is 10 seconds for the inhalation, 10 seconds for internal *kumbhaka* and 20 seconds for the exhalation. Extend the count until it again exceeds 1 minute and then switch to 1:2:2. From here, following the same method go to a 1:3:2 ratio and finally the 1:4:2 ratio. Experienced practitioners may be able to import the count they used during *Nadi Shodhana,* but it is suggested you consult with an experienced teacher.

In order to raise Kundalini, the method must be combined with other techniques such as *Nauli* and *Bhastrika,* but this is not the subject of this book. Be on your guard for any symptoms of an aggravated lunar *nadi* developing, such as feeling cold or experiencing kapha-related disorders, self-doubt, depression, lethargy, dullness, low motivation, extreme introversion or any type of lunacy. Like *Surya*

520. *Yoga Chudamani Upanishad* stanza 96

Bhedana, this method is extremely powerful but calls for supervision by an experienced teacher.

THE TRIAD NADI SHODHANA, SURYA AND CHANDRA BHEDANA AND THEIR CULTURAL CONSIDERATIONS

Nadi Shodhana consists of one round of *Chandra Bhedana* combined with one round of *Surya Bhedana*. *Chandra* and *Surya bhedana* constitute the isolated lunar and solar cycles of *Nadi Shodhana* respectively. *Nadi Shodhana* is the default *pranayama* technique that should be practised by all in most cases. In the long term, *Nadi Shodhana* will achieve most or all of the benefits that the other two *pranayama*s can supply. However, the time taken can be significantly shortened if a skilled teacher recognizes the imbalances of the individual student and is capable of interpreting them in conjunction with other factors such as season, climate and location. So a student with an aggravated solar *nadi* may return to balance faster if her *Nadi Shodhana* practice is replaced with *Chandra Bhedana* during the hot season or summer weeks/months. The same student living in the Rocky Mountains, Siberia or Nepal would require less *Chandra Bhedana* to return to balance. On the other hand, if she lived in Mexico or the Sahara belt, she would require more time practising *Chandra Bhedana* than in the previous case.

Cultural influences

The *shastras* state that if one wants to perform heroic actions in warfare one needs to make the solar *nadi* flow. It is astonishing how much nostril and *nadi* predominance seems to be linked to cultural background. There is a strong aggravation of the solar nadi in people who come from a country that either was a colonial power during the last few centuries or stood out through prowess in the military arena. Hence I have found that there is a significant occurrence of solar aggravation in students of Anglo-Saxon (USA, UK and Australia), Germanic or Japanese origin, many of whom will benefit from practising some *Chandra Bhedana* during the hot season (supervised only). Since the end of the great wars, many of the descendants of these cultures have shifted the playground of their solar aggravation to academic and economic prowess. Hence we now find in these countries many individuals with high stress levels, interrupted and insufficient sleep, overlong work hours and other solar symptoms such as peptic ulcers and heart disease. Again, a responsible use of *Chandra Bhedana* can go a long way here to restoring balance.

On the other hand, descendants of cultures and nations that were dominated by solar nations and became colonies are inclined to have an aggravated lunar *nadi*. They may benefit (only after taking into consideration individual circumstances) from practising *Surya Bhedana*, particularly during the cold months of the year and even more if living in cold countries or at high altitudes.

Generally speaking women used to be more lunar and males more solar. However, in the wake of globalisation and consumerism, many women today also suffer from an aggravated solar *nadi*. Similarly, cultures that used to be lunar are becoming solar in the wake of the triumph of the solar cultures. A typical case is India. It used to be the spiritual, lunar powerhouse of the planet, but of course on the battle-field was no match for the solar Great Britain. After being subjected for centuries to British education and economy, India has learned its solar lessons so well that it may soon outdo its erstwhile master in solar qualities and become one of the rulers of the world. Thus it is likely the day will come when Indians will be able to benefit from *Chandra Bhedana* practice to cure their solar aggravation.

If you have reached your goal and come to a state of balance of nostril dominance and brain hemisphericity, then cease practising *Surya / Chandra Bhedana* and return to *Nadi Shodhana*. The state of balance can be recognized from the fact that no symptoms of solar or lunar aggravation are present, or both of them to the same extent. It is then time to replace either of the two techniques through *Nadi Shodhana*, which combines them both.

If you have overshot your mark and started to manifest symptoms of aggravation of the opposite *nadi*, you may switch to the opposite technique before returning to *Nadi Shodhana*. Example: You suffered initially from excess solar symptoms such as being aggressive, tending to get involved in conflict, having high stress levels and being talkative, outgoing, physical and go-getting. Your teacher advises you to practise a course of *Chandra Bhedana* to return to balance. After several weeks you find yourself too introspective or melancholic; you can't find the motivation to get out of bed; you are putting on weight; you entertain excess internal dialogue. You wonder what others are thinking about you and are slow to make decisions that previously seemed obvious. This would constitute a typical case of an aggravated lunar *nadi*. In this case practise *Surya Bhedana* for about 50% of the time that you practised *Chandra Bhedana* and then return to *Nadi Shodhana*.

Discussed next are *Shitali* and *Sitkari*. Both are excellent cooling *pranayama*s but, since the inhalations are taken through the mouth, they require superior air quality, nowadays difficult to obtain in cities. Hence these *pranayama*s point towards an increased importance for *Chandra Bhedana*.

Shitali

Shita (with a long *i*) means cool. This is a cooling *pranayama*. The *Hatha Yoga Pradipika* lists it among the essential *pranayama*s.[521] The *Yoga Rahasya* also gives it a prime spot in stating that *Ujjayi*, *Nadi Shodhana*, *Surya Bhedana* and *Shitali* together remove all diseases.[522]

Shitali forms a triad with *Surya Bhedana* and *Ujjayi*. Yoga therapy uses the triad to address any imbalance between the three *dosha*s, with *Ujjayi* reducing *kapha*, *Surya Bhedana* reducing *vata* and *Shitali* reducing *pitta*. A combination of the three can be used to restore balance. *Shitali* also is an excellent method for balancing the heating properties of *Kapalabhati* and *Bhastrika*. *Kapalabhati* is certainly heating and *Bhastrika* can be, depending on your condition. You may

521. *Hatha Yoga Pradipika* II.11–12
522. *Yoga Rahasya* II.61

find that over the long term your body heats up through the practice of *Kapalabhati* and *Bhastrika*, especially if you practise in a hot climate. The easiest way to cope with this is to reduce the time spent on these exercises, which may be necessary during a heatwave. However, then you would not derive the benefit either. Other means include practising in a tub of cool water or placing a wet sheet on your body. Both should be used only when the environmental temperature is very high. Another method is to go up into the mountains, where it is cooler. This is one of the main reasons why yogis disappeared into the Himalayas. T. Krishnamacharya, for example, learned in the Himalayas that he could melt ice around him through *kumbhaka*. Not wanting to go to any such extremes, apart from *Chandra Bhedana*, *Shitali* is the most straightforward method for cooling down.

Shitali and its cousin *Sitkari* have, however, a major disadvantage. Both involve inhaling through the mouth – through the rolled tongue in the case of *Shitali* and through the crevices of the teeth and the tongue in the case of *Sitkari*. The cooling effect in both *pranayama*s is created by enriching the air with evaporating saliva, in much the same way that an evaporative air-conditioning system functions.

We do not usually inhale through the mouth because the nose is purpose-built to filter out of the air foreign particles, toxins and pollutants. This does not take place when inhaling through the mouth. If practised in polluted cities, *Shitali* and *Sitkari* may be harmful and contribute to bronchitis, pneumonia and other pulmonary diseases. They have to be used with caution. If living in an inner-city apartment, the use of an air filter may make *Shitali* more beneficial. Often location within a city plays a role. At the time of writing this text I live in the Australian city of Perth. My residence is in an outer suburb close to the ocean. The air here is good enough for me to practise *Shitali* daily without demerit. My yoga studio, however, is closer to the city – conveniently located for most of my students. When I practise *Shitali* there for a few days in a row I get a sore throat, since the air is more polluted.

You do not necessarily have to practise *Shitali* or *Sitkari* right after

298

your *asana* and *pranayama* practice. For many people a solution would be to combine a sunset outing to the beach with *Shitali* practice on the waterfront, if the the wind blows from the ocean at that time of day.

CONTRAINDICATIONS
Do not practise in polluted air. Use only sparsely in winter. Do not use if suffering from low blood pressure or colds, coughs, bronchitis, pneumonia or tonsillitis.

BENEFITS
Shitali is good during pregnancy, as it dissipates excess heat. In a yoga therapy setting it can be used to reduce excess *pitta*. It is also effective in reducing excess *pitta* created through the practice of other yogic techniques such as *Surya Bhedana* and *Kapalabhati*. *Shitali*, if done without *kumbhaka*, can be used to reduce high blood pressure. The *Yoga Yajnavalkya* recommends *Shitali* for asthma and diabetes.[523] The *Hatha Yoga Pradipika* also suggests its use to reduce hunger and thirst, and as an antidote to poisons,[524] a claim also made by the *Yoga Kundalini Upanishad*.[525] It is good practice to stay cool in summer[526] and also helpful in reducing inflammations and ulcers. It is good *pranayama* to practise before bedtime for letting go of the heat of the day, particularly if you are a *pitta* type. It is also helpful in reducing acidity and is reputed to prevent the onset of old age. Some yogic texts claim that it will even turn grey hair black.[527]

   Shitali also has a strong spiritual effect. Since we are inhaling through the rolled tongue, there is stimulation of the central energy channel (*sushumna*), a branch of which goes through the tongue.[528] To increase this effect it is necessary to place the tongue into *Jihva*

523. *Yoga Yajnavalkya* VI.39–49
524. *Hatha Yoga Pradipika* II.58
525. *Yoga Kundalini Upanishad* I.31
526. *Hatha Tatva Kaumudi of Sundaradeva* X.1
527. *Hatha Tatva Kaumudi of Sundaradeva* X.15–17
528. M.M. Gharote et al. (eds), *Therapeutic References in Traditional Yoga Texts*, Lonavla Yoga Institute, Lonavla, 2010, p. 215

Bandha upon exhalation. Here it comes into contact with the uvula, which is also connected to *Sushumna*.

TECHNIQUE WITHOUT KUMBHAKA

Since this is a slow-breathing *pranayama*, the three-stage double-up wave is utilized.

Stick your tongue out slightly and roll it so that it forms a tube. Then inhale through the rolled tongue, which moistens the incoming air far more than the mucous membranes of the nose would do. You will find that after a long inhalation the tongue becomes quite dry, so make sure you supply it with enough saliva to sustain the cooling effect throughout the length of the inhalation. During the exhalation place the tongue into *Jihva Bandha* and bring it into contact with the uvula. A ratio of 1:1 is preferable to a 1:2 ratio in most cases, as it extends the length of the cooling inhalation. In the beginning do only a few rounds and repeat this daily. If you do not have a reaction after a few days, you can presume that the air quality in your location is good enough. You can now increase to 10 rounds, but many more can be done if one suffers from excess *pitta*.

Notice whether the effect is sufficient to give you the required cooling, otherwise increase your rounds to up to 20. More rounds are possible, but the situation should be assessed by a qualified teacher or yoga therapist. If you develop a sore throat, cough, angina or bronchitis, discontinue the technique, as it indicates the presence of copious air pollutants.

TECHNIQUE WITH KUMBHAKA

The *Yoga Kundalini Upanishad* describes the technique as drawing up the breath through the tongue while producing the sibilant *sa*, performing *kumbhaka* and then exhaling slowly through both nostrils.[529] *Kumbhaka* should be performed with *Jalandhara Bandha* and simultaneous *Jihva Bandha*. Unlike the technique without *kumbaka*, *Shitali* with *kumbhaka* is not suitable for lowering blood pressure as *kumbhaka* itself has, at least

529. *Yoga Kundalini Upanishad* I.30

in its initial stages, the effect of raising blood pressure. Also, the cooling effect of the technique is somewhat reduced by performing *kumbhaka*, which is in itself heating. If you do combine the *Shitali* with other *pranayama* methods containing *kumbhaka*s, practise *Shitali* without *kumbhaka* to enhance its cooling effect.

Some students are not capable of rolling their tongue, an ability that is apparently genetically determined. If you cannot roll your tongue you may resort to *Sitkari*, which is described next.

Sitkari

Sitkari (with a long *i*) means 'hissing-sound maker'. The hissing sound is not produced by the teeth but by the tongue.

The *Hatha Yoga Pradipika* counts this *pranayama*, together with *Surya Bhedana*, *Ujjayi*, *Shitali* and *Bhastrika*, among the important *kumbhaka*s,[530] but other *shastra*s see it as secondary to *Shitali*. The *Pradipika* also says that it makes one near immortal.[531] The *Hatha Ratnavali of Shrinivasayogi* proclaims, somewhat excitedly, that through *Sitkari* one becomes like a god of love and free from suffering.[532] The *Jogapradipyaka of Jayatarama* recommends practising *Sitkari* only in summer, not in winter.[533]

BENEFITS

Sitkari is an excellent replacement for *Shitali* for those who cannot roll their tongue. It reduces *pitta* and its related diseases such as inflammation, ulcers, acidity and fever. It also cures insomnia related to excess *pitta*. Additionally, it is believed to develop the intellect. *Sitkari* can be used to increase *kapha* when needed, and in this case it needs to be done without *kumbhaka*. It also removes lethargy, hunger and thirst. If the tongue is held in the right way, air is diverted to cool the upper palate, which leads to secretion of *amrita* (nectar).

530. *Hatha Yoga Pradipika* II.11–12
531. *Hathapradipika* (10 chapters) IV.47
532. *Hatha Ratnavali of Shrinivasayogi* II.16–17
533. *Jogapradipyaka of Jayatarama* stanzas 481–485

The enthusiastic promises in *shastras* related to longevity stem from this effect.

CONTRAINDICATIONS

Do not practise *Sitkari* when *kapha* is already aggravated. Do not practise it in winter, when feeling cold or when high up in the mountains. Do not practise it when air pollution is present. In this regard it is similar to *Shitali*. Since we evade the filtering mechanism of the nose, we achieve greater cooling qualities but are more likely to get a sore throat or throat infection if air quality is poor.

TECHNIQUE WITHOUT KUMBHAKA

The native breath wave for this *pranayama* is the three-stage double-up wave. Open your lips wide as if striking a Hollywood grin (maybe that's where the claim about the god of love comes from) but keep your teeth together. Now press your tongue against the hard palate and expand it laterally so that it almost touches your molars in most places. Now inhale, creating a hissing sound. The hissing sound is created by the air getting past your tongue, which almost blocks its path. Create enough friction to allow you to significantly extend the inhalation. Shape the tongue in such a way that the air strikes the upper soft palate. When the inhalation is complete, close your lips, place the tongue into *Jihva Bandha* and slowly exhale through the nose. This constitutes one round. In the beginning do only a few rounds and repeat this daily. If you do not have a reaction after a few days you can presume that the air quality in your location is good enough. You can now increase to 10 rounds, but many more can be done if you are suffering from excess *pitta*. A ratio of 1:1 is preferable to a 1:2 ratio, as it extends the length of the cooling inhalation.

TECHNIQUE WITH KUMBHAKA

As *kumbhaka* is heating and mitigates to a certain extent the cooling effect of this *pranayama* to counteract the heating *pranayama*s, *Sitkari* is often practised without *kumbhaka*. If *Sitkari* with *kumbhaka* is desired, draw the breath in through the crevices of your teeth and your tongue positioned as described above. At the end of your inhalation place the tongue into *Jihva Bandha*, swallow, contract the throat and place the chin against the sternum (*Jalandhara Bandha*). At the end of *kumbhaka*, lift the head, release the contraction of the throat and exhale through the nose, while keeping the tongue in *Jihva Bandha*. This constitutes one round. Repeat as often as desired.

Ujjayi Kumbhaka

I have described Ujjayi twice already. First it was used as an introductory technique to extend and slow down the breath with the purpose of leading you to alternate nostril breathing. After describing the basic alternative nostril breathing technique, *Ujjayi* was again used to introduce internal and external breath retentions (*kumbhaka*s).

The *Ujjayi* mentioned here is a therapeutic *kumbhaka* used for the purpose of reducing *kapha*. The standard *Ujjayi* breathing, which combines a sibilant inhalation with an aspirate exhalation, is not as effective in destroying *kapha* but is more suitable as a general tonic; hence it can be used during the vinyasa practice. Different from the multi-purpose *Ujjayi* breathing, the *Ujjayi Kumbhaka* described here uses a silent exhalation through the left nostril.

Ujjayi Kumbhaka is the last of the important *kumbhaka*s[534] and the last of the three techniques that are used to readjust the balance of the three humours (*vata*, *pitta* and *kapha*). Ujjayi Kumbhaka reduces *kapha*. The *Yoga Rahasya* declares that it is capable of curing all diseases when combined with *Nadi Shodhana*, *Surya Bhedana* and *Shitali*.[535]

The Hatha Yoga Pradipika states that *Ujjayi* consists of a sonorous inhalation through both nostrils, a breath retention and a concluding exhalation through the left nostril.[536] The fact that the exhalation is to be made through the left nostril is also proclaimed by the *Yoga*

534. *Hatha Yoga Pradipika* II.11–12
535. *Yoga Rahasya* II.61
536. *Hatha Yoga Pradipika* II.51–52

Kundalini Upanishad,[537] which adds that the method produces the rare feat of cooling the head and reducing *kapha* (phlegm) elsewhere by increasing *agni.*[538] The *shastra*s agree that *Ujjayi* (meaning here the sibilant inhalation and aspirate exhalation through both nostrils) can be practised anywhere and any time (even when walking), which makes it suitable for practising it during *asana*. If so, there is no breath retention and exhalation takes place through both nostrils with a sonorous sound. This is the difference between the formal sitting practice of *Ujjayi Kumbhaka* described here and the less potent, multi-purpose, informal *Ujjayi* breathing that was described earlier. The tail end of this present *Ujjayi Kumbhaka* is identical with that of *Surya Bhedana*, where an inhalation through the right nostril is combined with an exhalation through the left. Together they constitute one solar cycle. Exhaling through the left nostril, the second half of the solar cycle of *Surya Bhedana* enhances the *kapha*-destroying/reducing function of *Ujjayi* more than an *Ujjayi* exhalation does.

BENEFITS

Reduces *kapha*-related disorders, especially respiratory ones such as asthma, colds, coughs, bronchitis and pneumonia. Without *kumbhaka* it can be practised during pregnancy, especially when suffering from excess *kapha*. *Ujjayi Kumbhaka* is also beneficial in cases of thyroid disorders, hypertension, rheumatism, ear infections and tonsillitis. *Ujjayi* is also an ancillary technique for rasing Kundalini, although considered somewhat less potent than *Surya Bhedana* and *Bhastrika*.

CONTRAINDICATIONS

Practitioners with a vigorous Ashtanga Vinyasa practice are generally advised not to practise this method too extensively, as quite likely they will have already reduced their *kapha* sufficiently. Additionally, many *vinyasa* practitioners have permanently linked *Ujjayi* with strenuous activity (by always combining the two). This usually triggers a

537. *Yoga Kundalini Upanishad* I.26–27
538. *Yoga Kundalini Upanishad* I.28

response or activation of the sympathetic nervous system as soon as one starts one's *vinyasa* practice. This is counterproductive to a sitting *kumbhaka* practice, in which you need to activate the parasympathetic nervous system to increase *kumbhaka* length. Due to the activation of the sympathetic nervous system, *Ujjayi* might also keep you awake if practised too late and right before going to bed. On the other hand the new link between *Ujjayi* and the sympathetic reflex may be utilized to keep you alert during extensive meditation sessions. Practise *Ujjayi Kumbhaka* only if you have additional excess *kapha* that needs to be reduced.

TECHNIQUE WITHOUT KUMBHAKA

This method would be used in a yoga therapy setting. When *Ujjayi* is practised as a formal sitting *pranayama*, *Jihva Bandha* should accompany it. This is not recommended during the Ashtanga Vinyasa or any other vigorous *asana* practice, as it may lead to excess tension in the head and the palate. Placing the tongue into *Jihva Bandha*, inhale through both nostrils producing a sonorous *Ujjayi* sound. The sound is produced by half-closing the epiglottis much as one does when whispering. Then form *Shanka Mudra* and, closing your right nostril, exhale through the left nostril only. *Ujjayi Kumbhaka* being a slow-breathing *pranayama*, the native breath wave is the three-stage double-up wave. Perform 10 rounds utilizing a 1:1 ratio or as your teacher recommends. Slowly over time extend your breath count until you reach an inhalation and exhalation in excess of 30 seconds. Then reduce the inhalation to half and change the ratio to 1:2, starting with a count of 15:30 or otherwise as your teacher recommends.

TECHNIQUE WITH KUMBHAKA

This method is used as an ancillary technique for raising Kundalini but, due to the additional heat generated in *kumbhaka*, it is also effective in reducing *kapha*. With your tongue in *Jihva Bandha*, inhale through both nostrils, making a sonorous sound. At the end of the inhalation lift your chest and swallow, lock the contraction of the throat and place your chin down on the sternum (breastbone) while keeping *Jihva Bandha*. At the end of *kumbhaka* lift your head, release your throat and, utilizing *Shanka Mudra*, close the right nostril and exhale through the left. Utilize the three-stage double-up wave, meaning the exhalation starts just above the pubic bone and extends upwards from there. Start with a 1:1:2 ratio and extend as previously explained until you reach the 1:4:2 ratio. During *kumbhaka* remember to put emphasis on *Jalandhara Bandha* first, then on *Mula Bandha*. Only when you have mastered both add *Uddiyana Bandha* during internal *kumbhaka*. In any case use exhalation-*Uddiyana Bandha* to drive the air out, starting from the lowest point of the abdominal wall.

KUNDALINI AND MEDITATION PRANAYAMAS

The techniques covered in this section are advanced *pranayamas*. They are utilized once the *nadis* are purified, the *doshas* (humours) are balanced and ejected, and internal and external *kumbhakas* are perfected. At this point the *kumbhakas* are becoming quite long and are then utilized to apply complex yogic meditation techniques involving *chakra* visualization and *mantra*.

An exhaustive description of these advanced *pranayamas* is beyond the scope of this book, but a brief description will give an idea of the direction in which *pranayama* will develop if practice is continued for a long time.

Shakti Chalana Pranayama

Shakti Chalana Pranayama is not the name of a particular *pranayama* technique but a blanket term applied to all yogic techniques that involve *pranayama* and are primarily aimed at raising Kundalini. The terms Shakti, *prana* and Kundalini are often used synonymously. Sometimes the term *prana* is used when the life force circulates, Shakti is used when, through an act of divine grace, life force descends, and it is called Kundalini when, through the effort of the individual, it is made to rise to meet our divine destiny.

The purpose of *asana* is to make the body healthy and steady for *pranayama*. Through *pranayama* the *nadis* are purified and *karma* is deleted.

Then a variety of techniques such as *mantra, pranayama, kriya,* visualization, *bandha* and *mudra* are combined to drive *prana* into the central energy channel (*sushumna*), pierce the energy blockages (*granthis*) and raise *prana* to the *Ajna* (third eye) *Chakra*. Once it is there, *dharana, dhyana* and *samadhi* are experienced almost spontaneously and effortlessly, whereas without this technology the task is tedious. The *Hatha Tatva Kaumudi* states that the vision of the

Divine can be obtained only after *Shakti Chalana* has taken place; hence its importance.[539]

Whereas many yogic schools hold dearly to their own individual recipe of *Shakti Chalana*, Sundaradeva's *Kaumudi* is a veritable encyclopaedia of its many varieties. *Shakti Chalana* can for example take place through:

- Practising *Utkarsha Pranayama* combined with all five *bandha*s (*Mula, Uddiyana, Jalandhara, Jihva* and *Maha bandha*) and *Maha Mudra*.[540]
- Practising *Surya Bhedana* for 90 minutes in both the morning and the evening[541] and then turning *apana* up, i.e. the path of fire and air.
- Sitting in *Siddhasana* blocking the *Muladhara Chakra* with the left heel and then practising *Bhastrika*.[542]
- Closing the nine gates (i.e. *Siddhasana* + *Yoni Mudra*) combined with external *kumbhaka*[543] and additionally *bandha, mudra* and *Utkarsha Pranayama*.
- Contracting *Surya* (right nostril) and engaging *Mula Bandha*; subsequently *Uddiyana Bandha* drives Kundalini up through *kumbhaka*.[544]
- Sitting in *Siddhasana*, closing the nine gates (*Siddhasana* + *Yoni Mudra*) and inhaling through the crow beak *mudra*, then performing *kumbhaka* and, listening to the inner sound, raising fire and *apana*.[545]

This is only a small selection of a large catalogue of techniques. The point is that they generally involve *kumbhaka, bandha*s, *mudra*s and *chakra*s, and manipulations of *prana*, or any combination thereof.

---

539. *Hatha Tatva Kaumudi of Sundaradeva* XLIV.39
540. *Hatha Tatva Kaumudi of Sundaradeva* XLIII.20
541. *Hatha Tatva Kaumudi of Sundaradeva* XLIV.5
542. *Hatha Tatva Kaumudi of Sundaradeva* XLIV.16
543. *Hatha Tatva Kaumudi of Sundaradeva* XLIV.36
544. *Hatha Tatva Kaumudi of Sundaradeva* XLIV.41–44
545. *Hatha Tatva Kaumudi of Sundaradeva* LIII.26–27

Bhutashuddhi Kumbhaka

The *Hatha Tatva Kaumudi of Sundaradeva* defines *Bhutashuddhi Kumbhaka* as contemplation of the six *chakras* in sequence in the very same retention (*kumbhaka*). This is a very extensive and minutely detailed technique.

Bhutashuddhi kumbhaka can be practised as a meditation or as a *pranayama*. The meditation technique can also be used as a preparation for the more ambitious task of performing it during *kumbhaka*. *Bhutashuddhi Kumbhaka* is mentioned in *Yoga Rahasya*, handed down through T. Krishnamacharya, and it was from this teacher's student B.N.S. Iyengar that I received this technique. The latter listed it, however, under the blanket name *Shakti Chalana Pranayama* (Kundalini-rousing *pranayama*). Essentially *Bhutashuddhi Kumbhaka* is a specialized method of *Shakti Chalana*.

Bhutashuddhi Kumbhaka was also taught by *Yogeshwaranand Parama-hamsa*, who called it *Chakra Bhedana*, the piercing of the *chakras*.[546] A useful description of *Bhutashuddhi* is also contained in Sir John Woodroffe's *The Serpent Power*.[547] The effects of performing *kumbhakas* in various *chakras* are listed in Raghuvira's *Kumbhaka Paddhati*[548] and Sundaradeva's *Hatha Tatva Kaumudi*.[549]

A modified version of *Bhutashuddhi* that does not contain *kumbhaka*, and is therefore only called *Bhutashuddhi Pranayama*, was taught by S.S. Goswami.[550] This technique contains all the basic ingredients of yogic meditation.

TECHNIQUE (SIMPLIFIED)

During *kumbhaka*, one visualizes the *Muladhara Chakra* in its (coccygeal) location with its four petals, dark red in colour, associated earth element, *yantra*, sense of smell and *bija mantra Lam*.

546. Yogeshwaranand Paramahamsa, *First Steps to Higher Yoga*, Yoga Niketan Trust, New Delhi, 2001, p. 352
547. Sir John Woodroffe, *The Serpent Power*, Ganesh & Co., Madras, 1995, p. 236
548. *Kumbhaka Paddhati of Raghuvira* stanzas 155–158
549. *Hatha Tatva Kaumudi of Sundaradeva* XXXVIII.121–122
550. Shyam Sunder Goswami, *Laya Yoga*, Inner Traditions, Rochester, 1999, p. 133

One absorbs all qualities into the *bija Lam* and raises the *prana* (through concentration and visualization) to the location of the *Svadhishthana Chakra*. Here one visualizes the *Svadhishthana Chakra* with its its six petals, orange red in colour, with its associated water element, sense of taste and *bija mantra Vam*.

One absorbs all qualities of the *chakra* into the *mantra* and raises the *prana* (through concentration and visualization) to the (lumbar) location of the *Manipura Chakra*. Here one visualizes the *chakra* with its ten petals and blackish blue colour of the storm cloud, associated fire element, sense of form (i.e. visual) and *bija mantra Ram*.

One absorbs all qualities of the *chakra* into the *mantra* and raises the *prana* (through concentration and visualization) to the (thoracic) location of the *Anahata Chakra*. Here one visualizes the *chakra* with its twelve petals, bright red colour of the *Manduka* flower, associated air element, tactile sense and *bija mantra yam*.

One absorbs all qualities of the *chakra* into the *mantra* and raises the *prana* (through concentration and visualization) to the (cervical) location of the *Vishuddha Chakra*.Here one visualizes the *chakra* with its sixteen petals, smoky-purplish colour, associated ether element, sense of sound and *bija mantra Ham*.

One absorbs all qualities of the *chakra* into the *mantra* and raises the *prana* (through concentration and visualization) to the (cranial) location of the *Ajna Chakra*. Here one visualizes the *Ajna Chakra* with its two petals, bright white in colour, associated void element and *bija mantra OM*.

From here the *prana* can be raised to the *Sahasrara Chakra* at the crown of the head with its thousand petals of all colours. This *chakra* is beyond element, beyond sense and beyond *mantra*.

The various layers described in this technique are superimposed onto each other one by one. Each time the yogi adds another layer, *kumbhaka* needs to be extended to accommodate the increasing complexity of the technique. As *kumbhaka* becomes increasingly long, the mind becomes clearer and more luminous. As the mind becomes clearer and more luminous, *prana* becomes steadier and

KUNDALINI AND MEDITATION PRANAYAMAS

kumbhaka can be extended. As *kumbhaka* can again be extended, the power to concentrate and to move *prana* increases. Hence eventually the mind becomes capable of lifting the *prana* to the crown of the head in long *kumbhakas*, a process known as Kundalini-raising (*Shakti Chalana*). This same process has been alluded to by Theos Bernard,[551] known for his incredible physical feats like holding head-stands for three hours and *kumbhakas* for over an hour. He described how during each breath retention he conducted Kundalini through the various *chakras* by means of concentration until it became absorbed into consciousness. This is confirmed by the *Hatha Tatva Kaumudi*,[552] which states that during *kumbhaka* the yogi needs to meditate on Kundalini and move her up through the *chakras* one by one.

Kevala Kumbhaka

The term *Kevala* is related to *Kaivalya*, Patanjali's term for liberation. *Kevala* means free, independent. It is a stand-alone *kumbhaka* that is independent of inhalation and exhalation on the one hand and free of volution and structure on the other.

The general understanding is that *Kevala Kumbhaka* comes about when all other *pranayama* techniques are mastered. Patanjali calls it *chaturtah* – the fourth *pranayama*.[553] According to him it takes place after internal, external and midway suspension are mastered. But the title *chaturtah* that Patanjali chooses also links the *kumbhaka* to *turiya* – the fourth state, described in the *Mandukya Upanishad*. The states are waking state, dream state, deep sleep state and consciousness. This fourth state is the only one that is permanent. It is the state that occurs in all the others. According to some schools of yoga, the pure state of consciousness occurs only when *Kevala Kumbhaka* is present and, according to another view, this *kumbhaka* occurs only when pure consciousness is attained. In any case the two are linked.

Kevala Kumbhaka has also been called the spontaneous *kumbhaka* or

551. Theos Bernard, *Hatha Yoga*, Rider, London, 1950, p. 95
552. *Hatha Tatva Kaumudi* LIII.11–15
553. *Yoga Sutra* II.51

the true *kumbhaka*. It can spontaneously occur when the practitioner enters *samadhi*, and this is true in the regard that no wilful effort is required to achieve it. It is merely entered into when the yogi is ready. *Kevala Kumbhaka* means that he or she is going beyond breath, beyond breathing. It does not mean that the yogi stops the breath wilfully but that the breath stops by itself.

The *Gheranda Samhita* defines *Kevala Kumbhaka* as the confinement of *prana* to the body, meaning it is arrested, fixated. For this reason it cannot leave the body, which would cause death.[554] The *Hatha Tatva Kaumudi* interprets *Kevala Kumbhaka* as the state in which *prana* is evenly distributed all over the body.

The great Shankaracharya, in his *Yoga Taravali*, links *Kevala Kumbhaka* to mastery of the three *bandha*s combined with concentration on the *Anahata* (heart) *Chakra*.[555] He adds that this breathless state, empty of the need to inhale or exhale, is the most important of the *pranayamas*[556] and that, by means of *Kevala Kumbhaka*, *prana* is drawn from Ida and Pingala into the central *nadi* (*sushumna*).[557] Thus this *kumbhaka* awakens the sleeping serpent Kundalini,[558] leading to effortless success in *dharana* and *dhyana*.[559] This last stanza is particularly important, as here the great master confirms that the raising of Kundalini is not something foreign to Patanjali yoga, but it is essential and central to succeeding in and mastering the Ashtanga (eight-limbed) Yoga of Patanjali.

The *Kumbhaka Paddhati* of Raghuvira uses the name *Meru Kumbhaka* instead of *Kevala Kumbhaka*.[560] In teaching that it is attained in 47 stages, Raghuvira seems to be the only authority to define *Kevala Kumbhaka* in a quantitative way, i.e. he judges its attainment by its length. This is very different to Patanjali and Shankara, who give only qualitative definitions for limbs of yoga.

554. *Gheranda Samhita* V.84
555. *Yoga Taravali of Shankaracharya* stanza 9
556. *Yoga Taravali of Shankaracharya* stanza 10
557. *Yoga Taravali of Shankaracharya* stanza 11
558. *Yoga Taravali of Shankaracharya* stanza 12
559. *Yoga Taravali of Shankaracharya* stanza 14
560. *Kumbhaka Paddhati of Raghuvira* stanzas 285–286

TECHNIQUE

There is not one but several ways to access *Kevala Kumbhaka*. As a by-product of *samadhi* it is accessible through the following means:

In Jnana Yoga,[561] one accesses it by rejecting all identification with body, mind, ego and the world and by completely identifying with the formless Absolute (*nirguna brahman*). This is considered the most difficult path. The *Bhakta* achieves it through complete devotion to the *ishtadevata* (personal deity) as a manifestation of the Absolute with form (*saguna brahman*). Chief among the means employed by Laya Yoga[562] is raising the Kundalini through concentration as described under *Bhutashuddhi Pranayama* and *Nadanusandhana* (listening to inner sound). Methods used in Hatha Yoga include the *Bhramari, Shambhavi, Khechari* and *Yoni mudra*s.[563]

Within the system of *pranayama*, there are two primary avenues towards *Kevala Kumbhaka*. The first is to extend the breath count in slow-breathing *pranayama*s such as *Nadi Shodhana* and *Surya* and *Chandra bhedana* more and more. Through long practice, aided by mastery of the *bandha*s, the practitioner slows down the vital functions to such an extent that the breath eventually seems to stop.

The second avenue utilizes the rapid-breathing methods of *Kapalabhati* and *Bhastrika*. If exercised long enough, they enrich the brain with oxygen and deplete carbon dioxide to such an extent that the respiratory centre switches off and does not demand the next breath. Ideally all of the above methods are combined with *bandha*s and internal and external *kumbhaka*s. Such a practice must be tailored by an experienced teacher to the needs of the individual and must take many factors into account, including, for example, season.

---

561. Jnana Yoga is the yoga of knowledge of the Supreme Reality encrypted in the *Brahma Sutra*. It is usually practised after Raja Yoga is mastered.
562. Laya Yoga is the yoga of concentration. It is an alternative term to Kundalini Yoga. Laya Yoga uses aids such as visualization of *chakra*s, pronouncing *mantra*s and listening to inner sounds. Generally it is practised after proficiency in Hatha Yoga has been gained and before Raja Yoga is tackled. Another way of looking at it is to see Laya Yoga as the top tier of Hatha Yoga and the bottom tier of Raja Yoga. The boundaries are rather fluid.
563. *Gheranda Samhita* VII.5

Appendix

PRANAYAMA AS REMOVER OF OBSTACLES

In sutra I.30 of Patanjali's *Yoga Sutra* the sage lists the obstacles to yoga as sickness, rigidity, doubt, laziness, sense indulgence, false views, failure to attain a state and failure to retain it. These obstacles are directly related to the pranic make-up of body and mind. The first obstacle, sickness, is caused by an imbalance of the three *doshas*, *vata*, *pitta* and *kapha*. *Pranayama* is the prime method for bringing the *doshas* back into balance. *Surya Bhedana pranayama* is used to reduce an aggravated *vata*, and *Ujjayi Kumbhaka* is used to alleviate aggravated *kapha*, while *Shitali*, *Sitkari* and *Chandra bhedana* are employed to decrease excess *pitta*. Of all the yogic techniques, *pranayama* is thus the one that, courtesy of its direct influence on the *doshas*, is directly used to cure diseases.

The second obstacle, rigidity, is related to too much *prana* flowing through the solar energy channel, relating to the right nostril (Pingala). Rigidity means to see only your truth and being unable to accept other truths outside of your understanding, which is a solar attitude. Generally speaking *Nadi Shodhana* is the *pranayama* to correct this state, but if solar predominance is strong and persistent it needs to be tackled with *Chandra Bhedana kumbhaka*, i.e. taking all inhalations through the left nostril and exhaling through the right. This diminishes fundamentalism and increases relativism, i.e. being ready to accept the views of others.

The third obstacle, doubt, is the mirror image of the previous one, rigidity. It means that too much *prana* is flowing through Ida, the left nostril. This causes a lunar attitude, which means that one sees truth in everything, starts to believe that truth is a relative thing and in the end becomes so paralysed that one cannot make a decision what to do any more. This obstacle is removed through *Surya Bhedana pranayama*, in which course every inhalation is taken through the right nostril and all exhalation is done through the left. This hightens fundamentalism, i.e. being sure about one's own choices, and decreases relativism.

The fourth obstacle, laziness, indicates an excess of *tamas* in the mind and excess *kapha* in the body. *Kapha* in the body is reduced by *Ujjayi kumbhaka*, whereas *Kapalabhati* and *Bhastrika* reduce *tamas* in the mind. The latter two techniques are used to purify and stoke *agni*, which is the destroyer of *tamas*. Another technique to reduce *tamas* in the mind comprises external *kumbhaka*s, which trigger the sympathetic nervous system. Additionally the length of the inhalation can be increased, which promotes *rajas* and reduces *tamas*.

The fifth obstacle, sense indulgence, can be caused by the aggravation of either *tamas* or *rajas*. The expression 'like a pig in mud', for example, indicates sense indulgence aggravated by *tamas*. The same applies in cases of excess eating caused by depression or 'retail therapy', i.e. combating depression through shopping. On the other hand the demon king Ravana in the *Ramayana* shows us a great example of sense indulgence through aggravated *rajas*. To reduce *tamas*, use the combination of *kumbhaka*s described under the fourth obstacle above, which will all increase the luminosity of the intellect. Extending the exhalations combats sense indulgence brought about through *rajas*. Additionally, *Chandra Bhedana pranayama* is practised, in which all inhalations are taken through the left nostril. This *pranayama* makes one docile and introverted. *Kumbhaka*s can also be employed, but whether they should be external or internal needs to be assessed on a case-by-case basis. It is also beneficial to add meditation.

An obstacle called 'False views' results from an imbalance of Ida and Pingala. In this case, practise *Nadi Shodhana pranayama* to bring about balance and, in extreme cases, use either *Chandra Bhedana* or *Surya Bhedana* to alleviate your particular imbalance.

Patanjali's last two obstacles are 'Failure to attain and failure to sustain a state'. 'Failure to attain' implies a lack of conquering solar attitude. Add *Surya Bhedana* and *Ujjayi*. It is also helpful to increase *agni* through *Kapalabhati* and *Bhastrika*. 'Failure to sustain a state' implies a lack of sustenance. Sustenance is a nurturing, anabolic, lunar quality. Once you have attained a state, use *Chandra Bhedana* to sustain it. The failure to sustain can also be caused by excess *pitta* and lack of *kapha*, in which case *Shitali* and *Sitkari* are employed. Sustaining a state is also related to 'staying power'. Increasing *kumbhaka* length strengthens staying power.

POSSIBLE ORDER OF PRANAYAMA TECHNIQUES
All of these steps must be learned from a qualified teacher.

Step 1
Learn *Nauli, Kapalabhati* and *Neti* and practise them daily.

Step 2
Learn the various breath waves.

Step 3
Practise the complete yogic breathing cycle.

Step 4
Learn to slow down the breath to one breathing cycle per minute using *Ujjayi*.

Step 5
Learn *Nadi Shuddhi*, alternate nostril breathing without *kumbhaka*, and slow down the breath to one cycle per minute.

Step 6
Learn internal and external *kumbhaka*s with all *bandha*s integrated into *Ujjayi*. Keep extending the length of your breathing cycle.

Step 7
Integrate internal and then external *kumbhaka*s into *Nadi Shodhana* (alternate nostril breathing).

Step 8
Learn *Bhastrika* and integrate firstly internal and then external *kumbhaka*s.

Step 9
Learn to replace *Nadi Shodhana* with *Surya* and *Chandra Bhedana*, depending on your tendencies and the season, climate and location. A teacher will need to diagnose you.

Step 10

Learn the application of *Ujjayi Kumbhaka*, *Shitali* and *Sitkari*, depending on whether you need to reduce *kapha* or *pitta*. Use *Surya Bhedana* to reduce *vata* and add a cooling *pranayama* to counteract the heating effect.

SEQUENCE OF YOGIC PRACTICES

Start with *Nauli*, then perform your general *asana* practice and follow it with *asana mudra*s such as *Tadaga Mudra*, *Viparita Karani Mudra* (inversions) and *Yoga Mudra*. Then practise *Kapalabhati* and *Nadi Shodhana*. If you have already graduated to *Bhastrika*, practise it before *Kapalabhati* and eventually add external *kumbhaka*s. After that, practise Kundalini *mudra*s such as *Maha Mudra* and *Maha Vedha Mudra*. Conclude with yogic meditation involving *bandha*, *mudra*, *mantra* and *chakra*.

An alternative order places meditation at the beginning. The rationale here is that one may be too tired to practise meditation at the end of such a long practice session. Also the first part of the early morning – *brahmi muhurta*, the divine time – lends itself readily to meditation.

PRANAYAMA PRACTICE AND STAGE OF LIFE (ASHRAMA)

T. Krishnamacharya said that in ancient society all members were adept in yogic practices.[564] Although, considering the speed with which modern life unfolds, it appears difficult to get back to this state, the following paragraphs look at ways of integrating yoga into one's life, looking at the Vedic categories of *ashrama* (stage of life). The purpose of this information is to give modern yogis the ability to fade in the complete practices of yoga over their entire lifetime.

The most important quantitative consideration for *pranayama* is how to integrate it slowly into our lives. The *Yoga Rahasya* talks about limbs of yoga as applicable to *ashrama*. According to the Vedas, life unfolds in four stages. The first stage, *brahmacharya*, takes up approximately the first 25 years of life. During this time (*brahmacharya ashrama*) we learn and study everything that we need for the rest of our lives. The *Yoga Rahasya* recommends that one focus during this stage on *asana* practice interspersed with certain *mudra*s such as *Maha Mudra* and *Tadaga Mudra*.

The next phase of life, according to the Vedas, is the householder *ashrama* (*Grihastha ashrama*). During this phase we generally marry, start a family and enter professional life or run a business. As a rough guide, *Grihastha ashrama* lasts from age 25 to 50. The *Yoga Rahasya* suggests *pranayama* as one's main form of practice during this phase, while maintaining the level of *asana* practice one had when entering the *ashrama*. If during the householder stage you added 30 minutes of *pranayama* per day to your *asana* practice, you would find yourself well prepared to enter the next phase of your life. The Vedas consider it imprudent, during the householder stage, to reduce the attention dedicated to your family and professional, mercantile or administrative services rendered to society. Please note that the Vedas did not advise dropping out of society to find spiritual freedom. Instead, they accepted that there were four human goals (*purushartha*s): *artha* (acquisition of wealth), *kama* (sexual pleasure), *dharma* (right action) and *moksha* (spiritual liberation). Fulfilment of all four goals makes for a fulfilled life. Generally speaking, as one progresses through the *ashrama*s there is a progression of focus from goal 1 to goal 4, whereas *dharma* (right action) applies at all times, particularly when pursuing *artha* (wealth) and *kama* (sexual pleasure).

The situation changes somewhat when entering the *Vanaprastha ashrama*, which lasts from age 50 to 75 approximately. *Vanaprastha* means forest dweller, referring to the fact that in the ancient days one would move with one's partner into the forest and build a cabin. Today we would call this a sea or tree change; the term *empty nester* refers to the same stage in life. The *Vanaprastha* is still available to family and society in a counselling role, but one's yoga practice time is now significantly increased due to reduced professional duties and the fact that one's children are taking care of themselves. The emphasis on *asana* may become less, while time spent practising *pranayama* may double or triple. A significant meditation and devotional practice is also introduced here. The main focus of the *Vanaprastha* stage of life is spirituality and preparation for *samadhi*.

The final *ashrama*, *Sannyasa* (renunciate), lasts from approximately 75 to 100 years of age. At this point one surrenders all material attachment and focuses solely on one's practice and service to the Divine. When we read of extreme forms of *pranayama* practice, this usually takes place during this stage of life.

The Vedic idea of yoga is that, rather than plunging head-on into extreme forms of practice when young, one should develop one's practice slowly while transiting through the various stages of life fulfilling one's duties to family and society. This view is taken not only in the *Yoga Rahasya* but also, for example, in yogic treatises such as the *Yoga Yajnavalkya* and *Vasishta Samhita*.

Bibliography

Adams, G.C., Jr (transl. & comm.), *Badarayana's Brahma Sutras*, Motilal Banarsidass, Delhi, 1993.

Aranya, H., Sw., *Yoga Philosophy of Patanjali with Bhasvati*, 4th enlarged edn, University of Calcutta, Kolkata, 2000.

Bernard, T., *Hatha Yoga*, Rider, London, 1950.

Bernard, T., *Heaven Lies Within Us*, Charles Scribner's Sons, New York, 1939.

Bhagwan Dev, A., *Pranayama, Kundalini & Hatha Yoga*, Diamond Books, New Delhi, 2008.

Briggs, G.W., *Goraknath and the Kanphata Yogis*, 1st Indian edn, Motilal Banarsidass, Delhi, 1938.

Carroll, J., *The Essential Jesus*, Scribe, Melbourne, 2007.

Chandra Vasu, R.B.S. (transl.), *The Gheranda Samhita*, Sri Satguru Publications, Delhi, 1986.

Chandra Vasu, R.B.S. (transl.), *The Siva Samhita*, Sri Satguru Publications, Delhi, 1984.

Desikachar, T.K.V., *Health, Healing & Beyond*, Aperture, New York, 1998.

Desikachar, T.K.V. (transl.), *Nathamuni's Yoga Rahasya*, Krishnamacharya Yoga Mandiram, Chennai, 1998.

Desikachar, T.K.V. (transl.), *Yoga Taravali*, Krishnamacharya Yoga Mandiram, Chennai, 2003.

Deussen, P. (ed.), *Sixty Upanisads of the Veda*, transl. V.M. Bedekar & G.B. Palsule, 2 vols, Motilal Banarsidass, Delhi, 1997.

Digambarji, Sw. (ed. & comm.), *Vasishta Samhita*, Kaivalyadhama, Lonavla, 1984.

Evans-Wentz, W.Y. (ed.), *The Tibetan Book of the Dead*, Oxford University Press, London, 1960.

Gambhirananda, Sw., *Bhagavad Gita with Commentary of Sankaracarya*, Advaita Ashrama, Kolkata, 1997.

Gambhirananda, Sw. (transl.), *Brahma Sutra Bhasya of Sri Sankaracarya*, Advaita Ashrama, Kolkata, 1965.

Ganguli, K.M. (transl.), *The Mahabharata*, 12 vols, Munshiram Manoharlal, New Delhi, 1998.

Gharote, Dr M.L., *Pranayama: The Science of Breath*, Lonavla Yoga Institute, Lonavla, 2003.

Gharote, Dr M.L., *Yogic Techniques*, Lonavla Yoga Institute, Lonavla, 2006.

Gharote, Dr M.L. (ed. & transl.), *Hathapradipika of Svatmarama* (10 chapters), Lonavla Yoga Institute, Lonavla, 2006.

Gharote, Dr M.L. et al. (eds & transl.), *Hatharatnavali of Srinivasayogi*, Lonavla Yoga Institute, Lonavla, 2009.

Gharote, Dr M.L. et al. (eds & transl.), *Hathatatvakaumudi of Sundaradeva*, Lonavla Yoga Institute, Lonavla, 2007.

Gharote, Dr M.L. et al. (eds & transl.), *Kumbhaka Paddhati of Raghuvira*, Lonavla Yoga Institute, Lonavla, 2010.

Gharote, Dr M.L. and Jha, V.K. (eds & transl.), *Yuktabhavadeva of Bhavadeva Mishra*, Lonavla Yoga Institute, Lonavla, 2002.

Gharote, Dr M.M. et al. (eds), *Therapeutic References in Traditional Yoga Texts*, Lonavla Yoga Institute, Lonavla, 2010.

Gharote, M.L. (transl.), *Brhadyajnavalkyasmrti*, Kaivalyadhama, Lonavla, 1982.

Goldman, R.P. (transl., ed. & comm.), *The Ramayana of Valmiki*, 7 vols, Motilal Banarsidass, Delhi, 2007.

Gosh, S. (transl., ed. & comm.), *The Original Yoga*, 2nd rev. edn, Munshiram Manoharlal, New Delhi, 1999.

Goswami, S.S., *Laya Yoga*, Inner Traditions, Rochester, 1999.

Gupta, R.S., *Pranayama: A Conscious Way of Breathing*, New Age Books, Delhi, 2000.

Hatha Yoga Manjari of Sahajananda, Kaivalyadhama, Lonavla, 2006.

Holy Bible, New King James Version, Thomas Nelson Publishers, London, 1982.

Iyengar, B.K.S., *Pranayama*, HarperCollins Publishers India, New Delhi, 1993.

Jois, K.P., *Yoga Mala*, Astanga Yoga Nilayama, Mysore, 1999.

Joshi, Dr K.S., *Yogic Pranayama*, Orient Paperbacks, Delhi, 1982.

Kaivalyadhama Yoga Institute, *Yoga Mimamsa* (research journal), Lonavla, 1924–2004.

Krishnamacharya, T., *Yoga Makaranda*, rev. English edn, Media Garuda, 2011. (The authenticity of the currently available editions of the Yoga Makaranda is disputed. There could well be interpolations by a later commentator.)

Kunjunni Raja, K., editor, *Hathayogapradipika of Swatmarama*, The Adyar Library and Research Centre, Madras, 1972.

Kaivalyadhama, Lonavla, 2006.

Kuvalayananda, Sw., *Pranayama*, 7th edn, Kaivlayadhama, Lonavla, 1983.

Kuvalayananda, Sw. & Shukla, Dr S.A. (eds and transl.), *Goraksasatakam*,

Madhavananda, Sw. (transl.), *The Brhadaranyaka Upanisad*, Advaita Ashrama, Kolkata, 1997.

Maehle, G., *Ashtanga Yoga: Practice and Philosophy*, New World Library, Novato, 2007.

Maehle, G., *Ashtanga Yoga: The Intermediate Series*, New World Library, Novato, 2009.

Maheshananda, Sw. et al. (eds & transl.), *Jogapradipyaka of Jayatarama*, Kaivalyadhama, Lonavla, 2006.

Mallinson, J., *The Gheranda Samhita*, Yoga Vidya, Woodstock, 2004.

Mohan, A.G., *Krishnamacharya: His Life and Teachings*, Shambala, Boston & London, 2010.

Mohan, A.G. (transl.), *Yoga-Yajnavalkya*, Ganesh & Co, Madras.

Mohan, A.G., *Yoga for Body, Breath, and Mind*, Shambala, Boston & London, 2002.

Muktibodhananda, Sw., *Swara Yoga*, Yoga Publication Trust, Munger, 1984.

Muktibodhananda, Sw. (transl. & comm.), *Hatha Yoga Pradipika*, 2nd edn, Yoga Publications Trust, Munger, 1993.

Muller, M. (ed.), *The Sacred Books of the East*, 50 vols, Motilal Banarsidass, Delhi, 1965.

Nikhilananda, Sw. (transl.), *The Gospel of Ramakrishna*, Ramakrishna Math, Madras, 1942.

Niranjanananda, Sw., *Prana and Pranayama*, Yoga Publications Trust, Munger, 2009.

Niranjanananda, Sw., *Yoga Darshan*, Sri Panchadashnam Paramahamsa Alakh Bara, Deoghar, 1993.

Radhakrishnan, S. (ed.), *The Principal Upanisads*, HarperCollins Publishers India, New Delhi, 1994.

Radhakrishnan, S. (transl. & comm.), *The Bhagavad Gita*, HarperCollins Publishers India, New Delhi, 2002.

Rama, Sw., *Path of Fire and Light*, vol. 1, Himalayan Institute Press, Honesdale, 1988.

Ramaswami, S., *Yoga for the Three Stages of Life*, Inner Traditions, Rochester, 2000.

Ramdev, Sw., *Pranayama*, Divya Yog Mandir Trust, Hardwar, 2007.

Ramdev, Sw., *Pranayama Rahasya*, Divya Yog Mandir Trust, Hardwar, 2009.

Rosen, R., *The Yoga of Breath*, Shambala Publications, Boston, 2002.

Rosen, R., *Pranayama: Beyond the Fundamentals*, Shambala Publications, Boston, 2006.

Satyadharma, Sw., *Yoga Chudamani Upanishad*, Yoga Publications Trust, Munger, 2003.

Satyananda Saraswati, Sw., *Moola Bandha*, 2nd edn, Bihar School of Yoga, Munger, 1996.

Satyananda, Sw., *A Systematic Course in the Ancient Tantric Techniques of Yoga and Kriya*, Yoga Publications Trust, Munger, 1981.

Satyananda, Sw., *Asana, Pranayama, Mudra and Bandha*, Yoga Publications Trust, Munger, 1969.

Shrikrishna, *Essence of Pranayama*, 2nd edn, Kaivalyadhama, Lonavla, 1996.

Sinh, P. (transl.), *The Hatha Yoga Pradipika*, Sri Satguru Publications, Delhi, 1915.

Sivananda, Sw., *The Science of Pranayama*, BN Publishing, 2008.

Tiwari, O.P., *Concept of Kundalini*, DVD, Kaivalyadhama, Lonavla.

Tiwari, O.P., *Kriyas and Pranayama*, DVD, Kaivalyadhama, Lonavla.

Van Lysebeth, A., *Die Grosse Kraft des Atems*, O.W. Barth, Bern, 1972.

Woodroffe, J., *The Serpent Power*, Ganesh & Co., Madras, 1995.

Yogeshwaranand, P., *First Steps to Higher Yoga*, Yoga Niketan Trust, New Delhi, 2001.

Index

Author information

Gregor Maehle started his yogic practices 30 years ago. In the mid-1980s he commenced yearly travels to India, where he studied with various yogic and tantric masters and traditional Indian *sadhus*. Among other associations, he studied for 14 months with K. Pattabhi Jois in Mysore, and in 1997 was authorized by him to teach. Since then he has gone on to research the anatomical alignment of postures and the higher limbs of yoga. In India he also received eight months of mostly one-on-one instruction in scripture and the higher limbs of yoga from B.N.S. Iyengar, a student of T. Krishnamacharya. Additionally, he studied Sanskrit under Professor Narayanachar and Dr Chandrasekhar. He lived for several years as a recluse, spending his days studying Sanskrit and yogic scripture, and practising yogic techniques. In 1996, together with his wife, Monica, he founded 8 Limbs in Perth. Today, along with maintaining a daily practice of the Primary, Intermediate and Advanced series of Ashtanga Yoga postures, he engages in yoga research, his main focus being on *pranayama*, Kundalini and meditation.

Gregor has already published *Ashtanga Yoga: Practice and Philosophy* and *Ashtanga Yoga: The Intermediate Series,* which have been translated into several foreign languages. He has been invited to many countries to teach and has contributed to and been interviewed by many yoga magazines.

Today Gregor teaches an anatomically sophisticated interpretation of classical vinyasa yoga, integrated into the practice of the higher limbs in the spirit of Patanjali and T. Krishnamacharya. His zany sense of humour, his manifold personal experiences, his vast and in-depth knowledge of scripture, Indian philosophies and yogic techniques combine to make his teachings applicable, relevant and easily accessible to all his students.

He teaches speciality workshops, retreats and part-time and full-time teacher-training courses. He also offers a 4-week teacher-training intensive in Bali, Indonesia, for international students. For those who do not have a senior teacher available locally, Gregor offers consultation services through the medium of the internet.

For more information, sign up for his newsletter at www.8limbs.com or visit www.facebook.com/gregor.maehle

Lightning Source UK Ltd.
Milton Keynes UK
UKOW04f1501011015

259654UK00002B/55/P